The Impact of Beverages on Ingestive Behavior

The Impact of Beverages on Ingestive Behavior

Special Issue Editor

Shanon L. Casperson

MDPI • Basel • Beijing • Wuhan • Barcelona • Belgrade

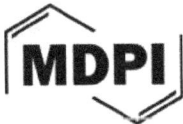

MDPI

Special Issue Editor
Shanon L. Casperson
USDA-ARS
USA

Editorial Office
MDPI
St. Alban-Anlage 66
4052 Basel, Switzerland

This is a reprint of articles from the Special Issue published online in the open access journal *Nutrients* (ISSN 2072-6643) from 2017 to 2018 (available at: https://www.mdpi.com/journal/nutrients/special_issues/beverage_ingestive)

For citation purposes, cite each article independently as indicated on the article page online and as indicated below:

LastName, A.A.; LastName, B.B.; LastName, C.C. Article Title. *Journal Name* **Year**, *Article Number, Page Range.*

ISBN 978-3-03897-812-1 (Pbk)
ISBN 978-3-03897-813-8 (PDF)

Contents

About the Special Issue Editor

Shanon L. Casperson, Ph.D., is a research biologist currently working at the Grand Forks Human Nutrition Research Center. Dr Casperson's research focuses on the metabolic role of dietary intake patterns in weight control. Most Americans consume a skewed diet in which the majority of their total daily calories and protein intake occurs during the evening meal. In addition, approximately 16% of total calories come from added sugars, with the largest source of added sugar being sugar-sweetened beverages (9%). These dietary intake patterns may be responsible for a disruption in the homeostatic regulation of food intake and body weight. Dr. Casperson's current research examines how dietary intake patterns affect energy metabolism and between-meal snacking and how the inclusion of a sugar-sweetened beverage with meals affects substrate utilization and cravings for high-sugar snack foods.

Preface to "The Impact of Beverages on Ingestive Behavior"

Today, the number of beverage choices in the supermarkets is greater than at any other time in our history. We know from the growing body of literature that beverage choice has a substantial impact on metabolism, food reinforcement, and eating behaviors. Accounting for 17 to 19 percent of total caloric intake, what we drink can be as important to our health as what we eat. This collection showcases original articles from research groups around the world (i.e., United State of America, Australia, China, Spain, France) that provide insight into our perceptions, intake patterns, and post-ingestive consequences related to the beverages we consume. The variety of the topics and the interdisciplinary content will appeal to a large audience. Specifically, clinicians will be able to utilize these findings to better develop nutritional interventions to implement in their daily practice, and researchers will be able to build on the outcomes in future studies.

Shanon L. Casperson
Special Issue Editor

nutrients

MDPI

Article

Beverage Consumption Patterns among Overweight and Obese African American Women

Terryl J. Hartman [1,*], Regine Haardörfer [2], Brenda M. Greene [3], Shruti Parulekar [1] and Michelle C. Kegler [2]

1   Department of Epidemiology and Emory Prevention Research Center, Rollins School of Public Health and Winship Cancer Institute, Emory University, Atlanta, GA 30322, USA; Shrutiparulekar28@yahoo.com
2   Department of Behavioral Sciences and Health Education and Emory Prevention Research Center, Rollins School of Public Health, Emory University, Atlanta, GA 30322, USA; regine.haardoerfer@emory.edu (R.H.); mkegler@emory.edu (M.C.K.)
3   Southwest Health District, 8-2, Division of Public Health, Georgia Department of community Health, Albany, GA 31710, USA; bmgreene@dhr.state.ga.us
*   Correspondence: tjhartm@emory.edu; Tel.: +1-404-727-8713

Received: 3 November 2017; Accepted: 6 December 2017; Published: 11 December 2017

Abstract: The goal of this research was to assess patterns of beverage consumption and the contribution of total beverages and classes of beverages to overall energy intake and weight status. We conducted an analysis in a community-based study of 280 low-income overweight and obese African American women residing in the rural South. Participants provided baseline data including demographic characteristics, weight and two 24-h food and beverage dietary recalls. Mean energy intake from beverages was approximately 273 ± 192 kcal/day or 18.3% of total energy intake. The most commonly reported beverage was plain water, consumed by 88.2% of participants, followed closely by sweetened beverages (soft drinks, fruit drinks, sweetened teas, sweetened coffees and sweetened/flavored waters) consumed by 78.9% of participants. In multiple regression analyses total energy and percent energy from beverages and specific categories of beverages were not significantly associated with current body mass index (BMI). It is widely accepted that negative energy balance may lead to future weight loss. Thus, reducing consumption of beverages that contribute energy but not important nutrients (e.g., sugar sweetened beverages) could be an effective strategy for promoting future weight loss in this population.

Keywords: beverages; sugar sweetened beverages; overweight; obesity

1. Introduction

It is estimated that over one-third of all U.S. adults are obese. However, substantial disparities exist among racial/ethnic minorities [1]. For example, approximately 56.9% of adult African American women are obese compared to 45.7% of Hispanic and 35.5% of Caucasian women [2]. Obesity and weight gain and their accompanying metabolic abnormalities have been linked to several chronic diseases including cardiovascular disease, type 2 diabetes and cancer at several sites [3]. Energy-containing beverages could promote weight gain because they are substantial sources of energy in the U.S. diet [4]. In nationally representative data, Storey and colleagues [5] and more recently, Han and Powell [6] reported that beverage consumption by adults varied by race/ethnicity, socioeconomic status, age and sex. Overall, for women, beverage energy intake peaked at ages 20–39 years contributing approximately 19% of total energy intake, or 380 kcal/day. Han and Powell [6] observed that mean beverage energy intake ranged from 362 kcal/day among Mexican American women and was highest among African American women at 405 kcal/day. Racial minorities were more likely to report consuming more sugar sweetened beverages overall, and among children, adolescents and adults [6]. Added sugar is one factor which could contribute to obesity and related chronic diseases, thus, sugar-sweetened beverages, the largest source of added sugar in the diet of the US population, have been a major focus of obesity prevention efforts [7].

The objective of the present study was to describe the contribution of total beverages and classes of beverages, particularly sugar sweetened beverages, to overall energy intake and to evaluate the associations between beverage consumption and body mass index (BMI) in a population of overweight and obese African American women.

2. Materials and Methods

2.1. Population and Data Collection

The Healthy Homes/Healthy Families (HHHF) study is a randomized controlled intervention trial designed to test the effectiveness of home-based coaching to promote healthier home food and physical activity environments for weight gain prevention. Details of the study and data collection procedures have been reported [8]. The trial, developed by the Emory Prevention Research Center (EPRC) in partnership with the Cancer Coalition of South Georgia and the EPRC Community Advisory Board (CAB) followed a community based participatory research model. The CAB is comprised of residents of southwest Georgia representing local organizations such as churches, businesses, health departments, and civic organizations.

All data collection procedures for HHHF were approved by the Institutional Review Board at Emory University and participant verbal informed consent was obtained by telephone. Overweight and obese (body mass index ≥ 25) female participants ages 35–65 were recruited from February 2011 to December 2012 from nine southern Georgia clinic sites affiliated with three federally qualified health centers. Eligible individuals had to speak English, live with at least one other person, and reside within 30 miles of a participating community health center. We excluded those with contraindications for a medically unsupervised intervention that focused on healthy eating and physical activity to promote weight gain prevention (e.g., pregnant women). Trained interview staff collected data by telephone at baseline, six and 12 months. Participants provided demographic (e.g., age, educational status, income, residence, number of children living in the household–defined as sleeping in that home at least three nights per week) and health-related information including physical activity, anthropometry (height in feet and inches and weight in pounds used to calculate body mass index–BMI kg/m^2), completed a series of home food environment questions, and completed two 24-h dietary recalls (one week and one weekend day) at each time point. The data included in the present report are from baseline, prior to any intervention, and include only overweight and obese African-American participants ($n = 280$).

2.2. Dietary Assessment

Dietary data were collected on one weekday and one weekend day on unannounced, non-consecutive days using the Nutrition Data System for Research (NDSR, Version 2010, Nutrition Coordinating Center, University of Minnesota, Minneapolis, MN, USA). Participants were mailed a printed food booklet to assist them when estimating portion sizes for foods and beverages. Data were cleaned by examining 100% of foods, records, and meal quality assurance reports produced by NDSR. Reports were reviewed for irregular food and beverage weights, total energy and fat amounts; database minimum/maximum amount flags; and food detail notes. Missing foods were resolved by comparing nutrients to product nutrition labels per product websites. Nutrient values were compared to similar NDSR entries and matched by the following set of nutrient tolerances per 100 g of food: 85 kcal; 2.5 g of fat; 100 mg of sodium; 10 g of carbohydrates; 5 g of protein. Results from the two days of intake were averaged. Aggregate beverage groups and nutrients of interest contributed by beverage groups were calculated from the NDSR dietary intake data Food Group Serving Count File and Food File with online guidance from the developers. We grouped beverages into the following categories: 100% fruit/vegetable, milk unsweetened, non-dairy milk, sweetened/flavored milk, sugar sweetened (soft drinks, fruit drinks, sweetened teas, coffees and waters), artificially sweetened, unsweetened (tea, coffee), alcohol, and water (without additions). Non-alcoholic substitutes were rarely consumed and were not included. Meal replacement drinks were considered "food" and were not included. For the aforementioned categories we determined any/no consumption (number, % any) and calculated both volume (mL) and energy (kcal) estimates of absolute intake, percent total beverage volume (%), and percent total energy contribution (%). For analyses, we excluded participants with only one recall or who reported dietary intakes <400 or >5000 kcal total energy/day (adapted from guidelines by Willett [9]).

2.3. Statistical Analyses

Statistical analyses were conducted using SAS 9.4 (SAS Institute Inc., Cary, NC, USA). Analyses included 280 participants with complete data. Initial analyses examined the distribution of the beverage and other variables and evaluated distributions and potential outliers. In univariate analyses we evaluated the association between demographic characteristics with total beverage intake as servings, absolute volume (mL), absolute energy (kcal) and percent energy contributed by beverages (%). The associations between demographic and lifestyle characteristics with beverage groups (Table 1) are reported as a percentage of participants who reported consuming any of the category. In subsequent univariate analyses we evaluated the association between groups of beverages with overweight/obesity reflected by categories of body mass index (BMI-kg/m^2) (Table 2). For these analyses, within each beverage group, we included only those respondents who were consumers. Results are reported as means with standard deviations (SD) (for continuous data) or number and percent (for categorical data) by strata of participant characteristics of interest. Multivariate linear and multinomial regression models were constructed with BMI as the outcome variable coded as continuous and categorically (overweight, obese, morbidly obese), respectively. The results of the multivariate linear and multinomial regression analyses were similar; thus, only the multivariate linear results are presented in results. We evaluated the associations for BMI with total beverage energy variables (continuous total beverage energy (kcal) and % energy from beverages). We also evaluated the associations among BMI with a priori selected grouped beverage variables (continuous 100% fruit/vegetable juices, dairy/non-dairy milks, sugar sweetened beverages, and alcohol) entered into models either as absolute beverage energy (kcal) or percent total energy (%kcal). Results (beta, standard errors (SE) and *p*-values) are reported for all variables under consideration with model fit statistics (total *r*-squared) reported separately. In sensitivity analyses we repeated the above regression analyses for a reduced sample (*n* = 244) which eliminated participants reporting <24 oz. total beverage/day and were considered potential beverage under-reporters. The results for the reduced sample were similar to the overall results; thus, the full sample results are presented throughout. All statistical tests were two-sided and *p*-values < 0.05 were considered statistically significant.

3. Results

Table 1 presents total and grouped beverage consumption by demographic and lifestyle characteristics of the population. Overall, in this population of overweight and obese African American women mean energy intake from beverages was approximately 273 ± 192 kcal/day or 18.3% of total energy intake. The most commonly reported beverage was plain water, consumed by 88.2% of participants, followed closely by sweetened beverages (soft drinks, fruit drinks, sweetened teas, sweetened coffees and sweetened/flavored waters) consumed by 78.9% of participants. Unsweetened beverages (tea, coffee, not including water) and artificially sweetened beverages (diet soft drinks, diet fruit drinks, diet tea and diet coffee beverages) were reported by 46.8% and 29.3% of participants, respectively. Milk consumption (without additions) was reported by 68.2% of participants, overall. Study participants who were younger, lived with children, and had more education tended to report greater energy intakes from beverages either for absolute intake (kcal/day) or relative to total energy intake (i.e., percentage of energy intake). Morbidly obese participants reported more absolute energy contributed by beverages (~300 kcal/day) than either obese or overweight (249 and 278 kcal/day, respectively) participants; however, percentage of energy intake from beverages was similar for overweight (19.9%) and morbidly obese (19.3%) participants. Obese participants reported 17.1% of energy from beverages. There were no significant differences in the percentage of participants reporting any (v. no) consumption of sweetened beverages by strata of demographic characteristics. Table 2 presents mean beverage consumption for categories of beverages among consumers with results stratified by BMI (overweight, obese, morbidly obese). Among participants who reported consuming sugar sweetened beverages, those who were morbidly obese reported the highest daily energy intakes from beverages (187 kcal) compared to overweight (161 kcal) and obese participants (150 kcal). Morbidly obese participants also reported a lower percentage of their total beverage intake as water (48.8% total volume (mL)) compared to either overweight (53.4%) or obese (51.7%) participants. In multiple regression analyses total energy from beverages and percent energy from beverages were not significantly associated with BMI modeled as a continuous outcome (Table 3). Similarly, no clear patterns emerged for energy intake from beverages in multinomial regression models where BMI was considered as a categorical outcome variable [10]. Finally, in multivariate regression models, none of the a priori selected grouped beverage variables were associated with BMI as a continuous outcome (Table 3) or as a categorical outcome [10].

Table 1. Total Beverage Consumption (Mean and Standard Deviation -SD) and Percent Reporting Any Consumption (%) of Selected Subgroups of Beverages, by Participant Characteristics.

Characteristic	n (%)	Total Intake (serv.)	Total Volume (mL)	Total Energy from Beverages (kcal)	% Energy From Beverages (%)	100% Fruit/Vegetable Beverages (% Any)	Milk Beverages (No Additions) (% Any)	Non-Dairy Milk Beverages (% Any)	Sweetened, Flavored Milk Beverages (% Any)	Sweetened Beverages (% Any)	Artificially Sweetened Beverages (% Any)	Unsweetened Beverages (% Any)	Alcohol (% Any)	Water (% Any)
Sample	280 (100.0)	6.0 (2.8)	1355.2 (657.2)	272.9 (192.2)	18.3 (10.6)	112 (40.0)	191 (68.2)	7 (2.5)	10 (3.6)	221 (78.9)	82 (29.3)	131 (46.8)	16 (5.7)	247 (88.2)
Age (years) (missing = 1)														
35–50	131 (47.0)	6.2 (3.0)	1404.5 (704.3)	304.2 (203.1)	19.6 (11.4)	55 (42.0)	83 (63.4)	5 (3.8)	5 (3.8)	106 (80.9)	33 (25.2)	50 (38.2)	13 (9.9)	116 (88.5)
50+	148 (53.1)	5.8 (2.6)	1311.5 (614.0)	244.2 (178.2)	17.2 (9.7)	56 (37.8)	107 (72.3)	2 (1.4)	5 (3.4)	114 (77.0)	49 (33.1)	80 (54.1)	3 (2.0)	130 (87.8)
Education (missing = 1)														
<HS/GED	59 (21.2)	4.8 (2.5)	1088.4 (578.0)	207.9 (152.4)	15.2 (9.0)	19 (32.2)	45 (76.3)	0 (0.0)	1 (1.7)	42 (71.2)	19 (32.2)	32 (54.2)	2 (3.4)	53 (89.8)
≥HS	220 (78.9)	6.3 (2.8)	1427.0 (661.4)	290.2 (198.7)	19.2 (10.8)	92 (41.8)	145 (65.9)	7 (3.2)	9 (4.1)	178 (80.9)	63 (28.6)	98 (44.5)	14 (6.4)	193 (87.7)
Residence														
Urban	153 (54.6)	6.1 (2.8)	1389.0 (663.1)	265.9 (181.2)	17.5 (9.6)	60 (39.2)	98 (64.1)	3 (2.0)	4 (2.6)	118 (77.1)	45 (29.4)	81 (52.9)	11 (7.2)	133 (86.9)
Rural	127 (45.4)	5.8 (2.8)	1314.5 (650.3)	281.3 (205.1)	19.3 (11.6)	52 (40.9)	93 (73.2)	4 (3.1)	6 (4.7)	103 (81.1)	37 (29.1)	50 (39.4)	5 (3.9)	114 (89.8)
Living (missing = 1)														
No children	130 (46.6)	6.0 (2.8)	1358.3 (666.0)	250.8 (186.9)	17.2 (10.1)	50 (38.5)	90 (69.2)	1 (0.7)	5 (3.8)	100 (76.9)	41 (31.5)	71 (54.6)	8 (6.2)	114 (87.7)
Children	149 (53.4)	5.9 (2.8)	1343.4 (644.5)	290.2 (194.8)	19.3 (11.0)	62 (41.6)	101 (67.8)	6 (4.0)	5 (3.4)	120 (80.5)	41 (27.5)	60 (40.3)	8 (5.4)	132 (88.6)
BMI														
Overweight	34 (12.1)	5.3 (2.1)	1211.3 (506.9)	278.0 (176.9)	19.9 (11.4)	14 (41.2)	21 (61.8)	0 (0.0)	0 (0.0)	30 (88.2)	7 (20.6)	17 (50.0)	0 (0.0)	28 (82.4)
30–<40	133 (47.5)	6.0 (3.0)	1349.3 (685.8)	249.3 (192.5)	17.1 (10.1)	56 (42.1)	84 (63.2)	5 (3.8)	6 (4.5)	103 (77.4)	41 (30.8)	70 (52.6)	8 (6.0)	114 (85.7)
>40	113 (40.4)	6.2 (2.8)	1405.5 (661.2)	299.1 (194.3)	19.3 (10.9)	42 (37.2)	86 (76.1)	2 (1.8)	4 (3.5)	88 (77.9)	34 (30.1)	44 (38.9)	8 (7.1)	105 (92.9)
Income (missing = 6)														
$10,000 or under	95 (34.7)	5.0 (2.6)	1146.6 (598.9)	247.4 (177.7)	18.7 (12.1)	34 (35.8)	63 (66.3)	1 (1.1)	2 (2.1)	73 (76.8)	30 (31.6)	42 (44.2)	3 (3.2)	80 (84.2)
$10,001–$25,000	106 (38.7)	6.4 (3.0)	1452.1 (685.5)	272.2 (182.9)	18.2 (9.7)	45 (42.5)	74 (69.8)	4 (3.8)	4 (3.8)	83 (78.3)	28 (26.4)	49 (46.2)	7 (6.6)	95 (89.6)
$25,000 or more	73 (26.6)	6.5 (2.5)	1486.6 (606.4)	303.3 (219.3)	17.9 (10.0)	30 (41.1)	49 (67.1)	2 (2.7)	4 (5.5)	60 (82.2)	22 (30.1)	39 (51.3)	6 (8.2)	66 (90.4)

Note: Standard deviation (SD) or percentage (%) in parentheses. Percentages may not add up to 100 due to rounding.

Table 2. Mean (SD) Beverage Volume (mL), Percent Total Beverage Volume (%) and Mean (SD) Energy Contribution (kcal) from Selected Subgroups of Beverages by BMI.

Beverage	Overweight				BMI 30–<40				BMI ≥ 40			
	% Any Use	Mean (SD) (mL) *	% Total mL	Mean (SD) Energy (kcal) *	% Any Use	Mean (SD) (mL) *	% Total mL	Mean (SD) Energy (kcal) *	% Any Use	Mean (SD) (mL) *	% Total mL	Mean (SD) Energy (kcal) *
Water	82.4%	719.1 (513.6)	53.4 (24.3)	0.0	85.7%	794.9 (623.4)	51.7 (23.0)	0.0	92.9%	755.7 (621.6)	48.8 (25.1)	0.0
100% Fruit/veg	41.2%	101.6 (88.7)	10.8 (12.1)	89.6 (52.1)	42.1%	133.1 (137.4)	11.8 (12.5)	101.6 (81.4)	37.2%	132.3 (94.0)	11.2 (9.3)	94.4 (96.6)
Milk	61.8%	64.7 (98.4)	7.7 (10.9)	155.4 (166.4)	63.2%	75.6 (118.3)	6.3 (7.1)	118.9 (106.0)	76.1%	66.3 (78.2)	5.7 (8.3)	134.9 (96.5)
Non-dairy milk	0.0	0.0	0.0	0.0	3.8%	150.2 (109.2)	11.6 (11.5)	94.2 (68.5)	1.8%	354.9 (167.3)	16.7 (1.1)	209.6 (76.3)
Milk, sweetened, flavored	0.0	0.0	0.0	0.0	4.5%	147.9 (83.1)	7.3 (3.7)	110.8 (87.9)	3.5%	170.0 (69.9)	13.8 (5.8)	123.6 (28.5)

Table 2. Cont.

Beverage	Overweight				BMI 30–<40				BMI ≥ 40			
	% Any Use	Mean (SD) (mL) *	% Total mL	Mean (SD) Energy (kcal) *	% Any Use	Mean (SD) (mL) *	% Total mL	Mean (SD) Energy (kcal) *	% Any Use	Mean (SD) (mL) *	% Total mL	Mean (SD) Energy (kcal) *
Sugar sweetened other than milk	88.2%	418.8 (361.6)	36.1 (24.9)	161.4 (137.5)	77.4%	370.4 (294.3)	31.7 (23.8)	150.1 (123.3)	77.9%	468.9 (341.9)	37.9 (24.5)	187.1 (135.5)
Artificially sweetened	20.6%	268.9 (143.8)	25.2 (13.5)	2.9 (1.8)	30.8%	384.6 (246.5)	30.8 (19.0)	5.1 (6.4)	30.1%	408.0 (377.4)	27.3 (21.9)	5.0 (4.6)
Unsweetened not including water	50.0%	224.6 (103.7)	19.7 (9.9)	4.3 (4.2)	52.6%	268.8 (186.4)	22.0 (16.6)	3.2 (2.8)	38.9%	256.3 (176.5)	18.8 (13.5)	9.6 (38.3)
Alcohol	0.0	0.0	0.0	0.0	6.0%	99.9 (65.8)	8.4 (5.8)	193.0 (146.9)	7.1%	78.2 (74.3)	7.1 (7.8)	110.3 (90.6)

This is among users so zero's will not be averaged in. * Standard deviation (SD) in parentheses.

Table 3. Regression Analyses of the Relationship between BMI (continuous outcome) with Total and Percent Energy from Total Beverages and Classes of Beverages (continuous exposures) Adjusting for Demographic Characteristics *.

Variable	Estimate (SE)	p-Value	Model r^2	Model Pr > F
Total Beverage Energy (kcal)	0.0041 (0.003)	0.15	5.10%	0.05
% Energy Total Beverages (% kcal)	0.0005 (0.0005)	0.30	4.74%	0.07
Energy: 100% Fruit/Vegetable (kcal)	−0.0057 (0.008)	0.47	5.59%	0.13
Unsweetened Milks **	0.0037 (0.005)	0.45		
Sweetened Beverages ***	0.0053 (0.004)	0.19		
Alcohol	0.0103 (0.01)	0.41		
% Energy: 100% Fruit/Vegetable (% kcal)	−0.1088 (0.12)	0.35	5.72%	0.11
Unsweetened Milks **	0.0359 (0.07)	0.62		
Sweetened Beverages ***	0.0958 (0.07)	0.15		
Alcohol	0.1468 (0.24)	0.53		

* All models adjusted for age, education (<HD/GED v. ≥HS), residence (urban vs. rural), living with children (yes vs. no), income (≤$10,000, $10,001–25,000, ≥$25,000) Models use continuous outcome (BMI in kg/m², estimate with standard error (SE) and continuous exposure variables (kcal, % kcal); ** Includes dairy and non-dairy milks, unsweetened; *** Includes all sugar sweetened beverages (e.g., sodas, fruit drinks, sweetened coffee/teas, milk beverages with added sugar and flavor).

4. Discussion

In this population of low-income overweight and obese African American women mean beverage energy intake was 272 (±195) kcal/day or approximately 18% of total daily energy intake. The most commonly consumed beverages were water (88.2%), sugar sweetened beverages (78.9%) and milk without additions (68.2%).

Daily consumption of sugar sweetened beverages was common across all demographic characteristics considered in our analyses. Approximately 79% of our participants reported consuming sugar sweetened beverages, similar to the 82% observed by Bleich [11] among US Non-Hispanic Black adults. Although consumption was more common among overweight than obese participants in our study, among consumers, mean energy intake (kcal/day) from sugar sweetened beverages was highest among the morbidly obese (187 ± 135 kcal/day). This value exceeds the American Heart Association's recommendation for no more than 100–150 kcal/day from all added sugar [12]. For those who were morbidly obese and reported consuming sugar sweetened beverages, 38% of their total fluid intake was from sugar sweetened beverages.

In multivariate regression analyses we did not observe any associations between intakes of energy-contributing beverages (total), sugar sweetened beverages, or other categories of beverages with current weight. However, based on our data, we cannot reject the possibility that energy-containing beverages could be a contributing factor to future weight gain. In a randomized controlled crossover design including 44 women, DellaValle et al. [13] observed that energy-containing beverages consumed with a meal added to energy intake without significantly affecting satiety. Similarly, a recent systematic review concluded that energy consumed in liquid form is more difficult to offset in subsequent meals and could promote positive energy balance [7]. Energy intakes from sugar sweetened beverages of the magnitude reported in this study (e.g., 1000–1300 kcal/week), which appear relatively modest, could lead to weight gain on the order of one or more pounds per month in the context of overall energy intakes above the requirements for weight maintenance. In addition, a growing body of research suggests that regular consumption of sugar sweetened beverages may be associated with incidence of cardiometabolic disease, independent of obesity [14].

Previous research of the relationship between sugar sweetened beverage consumption and weight among adults has been summarized in a number of recent comprehensive reviews. A systematic review of sugar-sweetened soft beverages and obesity by Gibson [15] concluded that the effect of sugar sweetened beverages on obesity among adults was likely small except in susceptible individuals or at very high intakes. Gibson [15] described results from six previous reviews of sugar sweetened beverages and obesity; two citing the evidence as strong, one probable, and three inconclusive or negligible. Notably, in prospective studies the strongest associations between sugar sweetened beverage consumption and increases in weight have been observed among participants who increased their consumption over time compared to those who maintained either a high or a low consumption. Another recent review focusing on the evidence of common beliefs in obesity research stated that although increased consumption of energy-contributing beverages tends to be coupled with increased total energy intake, associations with BMI have rarely been observed [16]. In contrast, Hu [17] concluded that when all the evidence is considered, the relationship between consumption of sugar sweetened beverages and weight is modest but compelling and important from a public health perspective.

Beverage intakes are of interest beyond the contribution to energy intake. Milk is a source of key nutrients, including calcium and vitamin D, and in some emerging research has been linked with cardiovascular health benefits [18,19]. In contrast to our results where more than 2/3 of participant reported consuming milk, in nationally representative data for Non-Hispanic Black adults for 1999–2004, Bleich and colleagues [11] reported that only 31% of those ages 20–44 consumed milk on any given day (data were not stratified by gender). Vitamin C, a water-soluble antioxidant, is an essential nutrient with well-established roles in a number of biological processes including immune function, collagen synthesis, and protein metabolism. There is at least some evidence that citrus juices may have potential benefits for chronic disease prevention [17,18]. 100% fruit and vegetable juices, important contributors to vitamin C and phytochemical intake, were consumed by 40% of respondents in our study. In the study by Bleich et al. [11] 24% of Non-Hispanic Black adults 20–44 years old reported consuming 100% fruit and vegetable juices.

This research had several strengths. We report results for consumption of total beverage and categories of beverages among a unique population of low-income overweight and obese African American women in South Georgia. Demographic data and two days of beverage intake data were collected and processed by trained staff using standardized methods. Despite these strengths, there are several limitations with our study. This population was recruited as part of an intervention study focusing on weight management; therefore, all of the participants were overweight or obese, and the results may not be generalizable to similar adults of healthy weight. This analysis is cross-sectional, and includes self-reported data for both weight and dietary intake data, and thus could be subject to confounding or bias. Although these data were collected at baseline and prior to any intervention, if obese and morbidly obese persons, had already decreased their consumption of energy-containing beverages or replaced consumption of caloric beverages with non-caloric alternatives to facilitate weight loss, then we would underestimate the relationship between beverage energy intake and weight. We are unable to completely explore this possibility with our data. Compared to overweight women (20.6%) more morbidly obese women (30.1%) reported any consumption of artificially sweetened beverage; yet, the percent of total beverage volume contributed by artificially sweetened beverages among the morbidly obese women (27.3%) was not strikingly different than overweight women (25.2%). Under-reporting of energy intake by overweight and obese persons has been consistently reported [20]. If under-reporting of energy-containing beverages was more substantial among women with higher BMIs, as a result, we could underestimate the relationship between energy-containing beverages and BMI. We cannot completely rule out this possibility; however, mean sugar sweetened beverage volume was greatest among morbidly obese participants in this population.

5. Conclusions

To conclude, in this study of overweight and obese African American women, we did not observe a significant association between intakes of overall energy-containing beverages or categories of beverages with current weight status. Due to the cross-sectional nature of this data we cannot estimate the prospective relationship between beverage intake and obesity incidence or weight gain. For example, we cannot rule out the possibility that energy from beverages contributed to positive energy balance and weight gain over time. In a future analysis we may further explore the potential contribution of intervention-related changes in sugar sweetened beverage consumption on weight loss. An important consideration is that our tailored intervention model allowed intervention participants to select healthy actions to focus on and not all intervention participants ($n = 89$) selected decreasing sugar sweetened beverage intake as a behavior they wished to modify. Nonetheless it is widely accepted that negative energy balance leads to weight loss. Thus, reducing consumption of beverages that contribute energy but not important nutrients (e.g., sugar sweetened beverages) could be an effective strategy for promoting future weight loss in this population.

Acknowledgments: This publication was supported by Cooperative Agreement Number # 5U48DP001909 from the Centers for Disease Control and Prevention. The findings and conclusions in this journal article are those of the authors and do not necessarily represent the official position of the Centers for Disease Control and Prevention. The authors wish to thank members of the Emory Prevention Research Center Community Advisory Board for their guidance in the design and implementation of this research. We also wish to thank Iris Alcantara, our interviewers, the Cancer Coalition of South Georgia, and study participants for their valuable contributions to this research.

Author Contributions: Authors M.C.K., R.H. and B.M.G. designed the study. Authors R.H., S.P. and T.H. planned and conducted the statistical analysis. T.H. wrote the first draft of the manuscript and all authors contributed to and have approved the final manuscript.

Conflicts of Interest: The authors declare no conflict of interest.

References

1. Ogden, C.L.; Carroll, M.D.; Kit, B.K.; Flegal, K.M. Prevalence of childhood and adult obesity in the united states, 2011–2012. *JAMA* **2014**, *311*, 806–814. [CrossRef] [PubMed]
2. Ogden, C.L.; Carroll, M.D.; Fryar, C.D.; Flegal, K.M. *Prevalence of Obesity among Adults and Youth: United States, 2011–2014*; National Center for Health Statistics: Hyattsville, MD, USA, 2015.
3. American Institute for Cancer Research. Updated Estimate on Obesity-Related Cancers. Available online: http://www.aicr.org/cance-research-update/2014/march_19/cru-updated-estimate-on-obesity-related-cancers.html (accessed on 1 October 2017).
4. Nielsen, S.J.; Popkin, B.M. Changes in beverage intake between 1977 and 2001. *Am. J. Prev. Med.* **2004**, *27*, 205–210. [CrossRef] [PubMed]
5. Storey, M.L.; Forshee, R.A.; Anderson, P.A. Beverage consumption in the us population. *J. Am. Diet. Assoc.* **2006**, *106*, 1992–2000. [CrossRef] [PubMed]
6. Han, E.; Powell, L.M. Consumption patterns of sugar-sweetened beverages in the united states. *J. Acad. Nutr. Diet.* **2013**, *113*, 43–53. [CrossRef] [PubMed]
7. Malik, V.S.; Schulze, M.B.; Hu, F.B. Intake of sugar-sweetened beverages and weight gain: A systematic review. *Am. J. Clin. Nutr.* **2006**, *84*, 274–288. [PubMed]
8. Kegler, M.C.; Alcantara, I.; Haardorfer, R.; Gazmararian, J.A.; Ballard, D.; Sabbs, D. The influence of home food environments on eating behaviors of overweight and obese women. *J. Nutr. Educ. Behav.* **2014**, *46*, 188–196. [CrossRef] [PubMed]
9. Willett, W.C. *Nutritional Epidemiology*, 3rd ed.; Oxford University Press: New York, NY, USA, 2013.
10. Hartman, J.K. Emory University: Atlanta, GA, USA, Unpublished work. 2017.
11. Bleich, S.N.; Wang, Y.C.; Wang, Y.; Gortmaker, S.L. Increasing consumption of sugar-sweetened beverages among us adults: 1988–1994 to 1999–2004. *Am. J. Clin. Nutr.* **2009**, *89*, 372–381. [CrossRef] [PubMed]
12. Johnson, R.K.; Appel, L.J.; Brands, M.; Howard, B.V.; Lefevre, M.; Lustig, R.H.; Sacks, F.; Steffen, L.M.; Wylie-Rosett, J. The American Heart Association Nutrition Committee of the Council on Nutrition, Physical Activity; Metabolism and the Council on Epidemiology and Prevention. Dietary sugars intake and cardiovascular health: A scientific statement from the american heart association. *Circulation* **2009**, *120*, 1011–1020. [PubMed]
13. DellaValle, D.M.; Roe, L.S.; Rolls, B.J. Does the consumption of caloric and non-caloric beverages with a meal affect energy intake? *Appetite* **2005**, *44*, 187–193. [CrossRef] [PubMed]
14. Imamura, F.; O'Connor, L.; Ye, Z.; Mursu, J.; Hayashino, Y.; Bhupathiraju, S.N.; Forouhi, N.G. Consumption of sugar sweetened beverages, artificially sweetened beverages, and fruit juice and incidence of type 2 diabetes: Systematic review, meta-analysis, and estimation of population attributable fraction. *BMJ* **2015**, *351*, h3576. [CrossRef] [PubMed]
15. Gibson, S. Sugar-sweetened soft drinks and obesity: A systematic review of the evidence from observational studies and interventions. *Nutr. Res. Rev.* **2008**, *21*, 134–147. [CrossRef] [PubMed]
16. Casazza, K.; Brown, A.; Astrup, A.; Bertz, F.; Baum, C.; Brown, M.B.; Dawson, J.; Durant, N.; Dutton, G.; Fields, D.A.; et al. Weighing the evidence of common beliefs in obesity research. *Crit. Rev. Food. Sci. Nutr.* **2015**, *55*, 2014–2053. [CrossRef] [PubMed]
17. Hu, F.B. Resolved: There is sufficient scientific evidence that decreasing sugar-sweetened beverage consumption will reduce the prevalence of obesity and obesity-related diseases. *Obes. Rev.* **2013**, *14*, 606–619. [CrossRef] [PubMed]
18. Helm, L.; Macdonald, I.A. Impact of beverage intake on metabolic and cardiovascular health. *Nutr. Rev.* **2015**, *73* (Suppl. 2), 120–129. [CrossRef] [PubMed]
19. Frei, B.; Birlouez-Aragon, I.; Lykkesfeldt, J. Authors' perspective: What is the optimum intake of vitamin C in humans? *Crit. Rev. Food. Sci. Nutr.* **2012**, *52*, 815–829. [CrossRef] [PubMed]
20. Murakami, K.; Livingstone, M.B. Prevalence and characteristics of misreporting of energy intake in us adults: NHANES 2003–2012. *Br. J. Nutr.* **2015**, *114*, 1294–1303. [CrossRef] [PubMed]

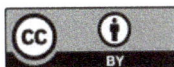

nutrients

MDPI

Article

Plant-Based Beverages as Good Sources of Free and Glycosidic Plant Sterols

Anneleen I Decloedt [1,2,*], Anita Van Landschoot [1,3], Hellen Watson [1], Dana Vanderputten [3] and Lynn Vanhaecke [2]

[1]   Faculty of Bioscience Engineering, Laboratory of Biochemistry and Brewing, Ghent University,
       Valentin Vaerwyckweg 1, B-9000 Ghent, Belgium; Anita.Vanlandschoot@ugent.be (A.V.L.);
       Hellen.Watson@ugent.be (H.W.)
[2]   Faculty of Veterinary Medicine, Department of Veterinary Public Health and Food Safety, Laboratory of
       Chemical Analysis, Ghent University, 133 Salisburylaan, B-9820 Merelbeke, Belgium;
       Lynn.Vanhaecke@ugent.be
[3]   Faculty of Science and Technology, Department of Biosciences and Food Sciences, University College Ghent,
       Valentin Vaerwyckweg 1, B-9000 Ghent, Belgium; Dana.Vanderputten@hogent.be
*   Correspondence: Anneleen.decloedt@ugent.be; Tel.: +32-9-264-7316

Received: 25 October 2017; Accepted: 18 December 2017; Published: 29 December 2017

Abstract: To address the ever-growing group of health-conscious consumers, more and more nutritional and health claims are being used on food products. Nevertheless, only very few food constituents, including plant sterols, have been appointed an approved health claim (European Commission and Food and Drugs Administration). Plant sterols are part of those limited lists of approved compounds for their cholesterol-lowering properties but have been praised for their anti-inflammatory and anti-carcinogenic properties as well. Despite this indisputable reputation, direct quantitative data is still lacking for naturally present (conjugated) plant sterols in beverages. This study aimed to fill this gap by applying a validated extraction and UPLC-MS/MS detection method to a diverse range of everyday plant-based beverages. β-sitosterol-β-D-glucoside (BSSG) showed to be by far the most abundant sterol in all beverages studied, with concentrations up to 60–90 mg per 100 mL in plant-based milk alternatives and fresh fruit juices. Ergosterol (provitamin D_2) could be found in beers (0.8–6.1 µg per 100 mL, from the yeast) and occasionally in juices (17–29 µg per 100 mL). Overall, the results demonstrated that the concentrations of water-soluble sterol conjugates have been underestimated significantly and that specific plant-based beverages can be good, low-fat sources of these plant sterols.

Keywords: (conjugated) plant sterols; beverages; cholesterol-lowering; ergosterol; anti-aging; coronary heart disease; health claims; anti-inflammatory; anti-carcinogenic

1. Introduction

Over the last decade, the beverage industry has taken a serious jump into the future by introducing a broad range of new, convenient, natural, and functional beverages. These beverages, often called health drinks, include (iced) teas and juices but also shakes and "super drinks" such as pomegranate juice or *Aloe vera* extract–based drinks. For most of these products, a range of different nutrition and health claims are being formulated on the label and in advertisements. These claims stimulate the consumer to purchase these particular beverages in order to increase their personal health status. Popular health claims are "free from" claims such as gluten-free or lactose-free but also vegan, organic, "helps to prevent coronary heart disease" and "lowers cholesterol" claims are being used quite often. To streamline these claims, FDA (Food and Drug Administration) and EC (European Commission) rules have been adopted on the use of nutrition and health claims on foods. Up until now, only very few compounds have been appointed an approved health claim by both organizations. Plant sterols are part of that limited list of approved compounds for their cholesterol-lowering properties (FDA Health Claim; Phytosterols and Risk of Coronary Heart Disease) (EFSA, Article 14 (1)(a) "Reduction of disease risk" of the Regulation on nutrition and health claims 1924/2006). Less well-known, but perhaps even more promising, are a range of other suggested health benefits related to the consumption of plant sterols such as anti-carcinogenic, anti-inflammatory, and anti-oxidative effects [1–6]. Despite this general interest, quantitative data on the concentration of these sterols in day-to-day consumption goods and especially beverages are extremely scarce.

Plant sterols, or phytosterols, are one of the main constituents of plant membranes, playing an important role in cell membrane stability and as signal transducers [7]. Ergosterol (provitamin D_2), on the other hand, takes up a similar role in protozoa and fungi (e.g., yeast) and is a provitamin form of vitamin D_2 or ergocalciferol. Exposure of ergosterol to ultraviolet (UV) light causes a photochemical reaction that produces vitamin D_2. This happens naturally to a certain extent, and quite often, mushrooms are irradiated after harvest to increase their Vitamin D_2 content [8]. Fungi are also grown industrially so that ergosterol can be extracted and converted to Vitamin D_2 for sale as a dietary supplement and food additive [9]. Chemically, ergosterol (provitamin D_2) and plant sterols are very alike and similar to their human and animal counterpart, cholesterol (Figure 1). They contain a stereo-specific oriented methyl or ethyl substitution at the C24 position of the sterol side chain and, in the case of stigmasterol, ergosterol, and brassicasterol, an additional double bound between C22 and C23 [4,10] (Table 1). Upon human consumption, these structural and functional resemblances allow plant sterols and ergosterol to interfere with cholesterol absorption in the intestinal tract through displacement of cholesterol from the micelles and/or competition with cholesterol binding proteins. As a result, low-density lipoprotein (LDL) cholesterol levels will decrease, lowering the risk for coronary heart failure [11,12].

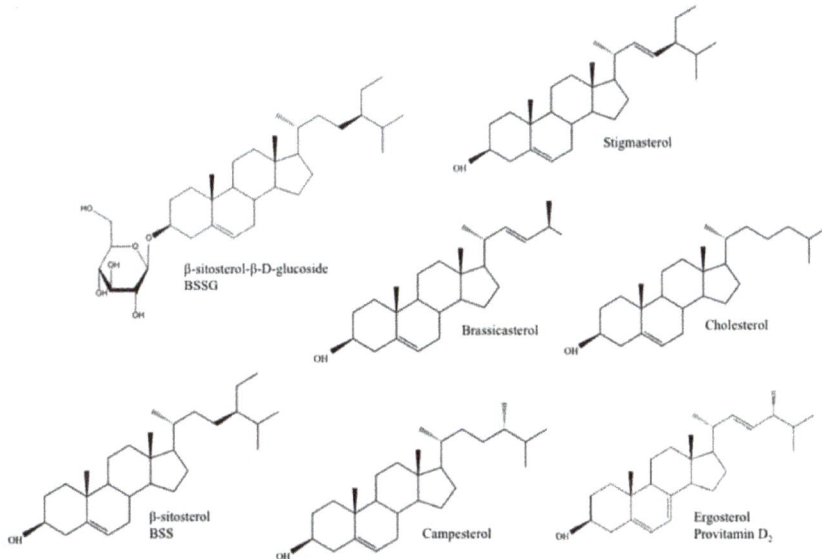

Figure 1. Chemical structure of the main free and conjugated plant sterols (campesterol, stigmasterol, brassicasterol, β-sitosterol (BSS), and β-sitosterol-β-D-glucoside (BSSG)), cholesterol (animal sterol), and ergosterol (fungal/yeast sterol, provitamine D_2).

Table 1. Chemical similarities and structural differences between cholesterol, ergosterol (provitamin D_2) and plant sterols. Listed characteristics include mean mass, molecular formula, number of double bounds, position of double bounds, and alkyl group present at C24 (none, methyl, or ethyl).

Sterol Name	Mean Mass (Da)	Molecular Formula	Structural Characteristics		
			Double Bounds	Position Double Bounds	Alkyl Group at C24
Cholesterol	386.654	$C_{27}H_{46}O$	1	C5–C6	/
Ergosterol (Provitamin D_2)	396.648	$C_{28}H_{44}O$	3	C5–C6 C7–C8 C22–C23	Methyl
β-sitosterol-β-D-glucoside (BSSG)	576.847	$C_{35}H_{60}O_6$	1	C5–C6	Ethyl
β-sitosterol (BSS)	414.707	$C_{29}H_{50}O$	1	C5–C6	Ethyl
Brassicasterol	398.675	$C_{28}H_{46}O$	2	C5–C6 C22–C23	Methyl
Stigmasterol	412.691	$C_{29}H_{48}O$	2	C5–C6 C22–C23	Ethyl
Campesterol	400.691	$C_{28}H_{48}O$	1	C5–C6	Methyl

The European Food Safety Authority (EFSA) and FDA concluded that, relative to a placebo, blood LDL cholesterol levels can be reduced by 7 to 12.5% if a person consumes 1.5 to 3 grams of plant sterols and stanols (expressed as free sterols) a day (EFSA claim, article 14(1)(a)) [13,14]. A recent meta-analysis by Ras et al. (2014) (124 studies, 202 stratas) extended these findings; they found that plant sterol intakes of 0.6 to 3.3 g per day gradually reduce LDL-cholesterol concentrations by, on average, 6 to 12% [15]. The cholesterol-lowering effect is usually established within two to three weeks after diet change and could be sustained for months [16]. No significant alterations in high-density-lipoprotein (HDL)-cholesterol (the "good" cholesterol), or triglycerides in general, were reported. Effectiveness of this approach has been positively tested in hypercholesteraemic patients as well as in individuals with normal cholesterol levels [17].

FDA and EC rules on novel food and novel food ingredients (in force since 1997) require all new ingredients to go through an applicant-specific authorization procedure that involves a rigorous safety assessment before they can be placed on the market (Regulation (EC) No 258/97, concerning novel foods and novel food ingredients). Under these rules, approval has been given for the addition of plant sterols in a range of foods, but these are mostly high-fat products such as yellow fat spreads, dairy products (e.g., yogurt), mayonnaise, and salad dressings. Unsaturated forms of plant sterols, phytostanols, have also been added to food. An example hereof is a non-fatty alternative, chewable plant stanol ester gum, for which efficacy has been confirmed recently [18]. Nevertheless, high concentrations of phytostanols are not natural, as high concentrations of phytostanols are very rare in most plants (with the exemption of a few cereal species and their derived products such as rice oil) [7].

Natural water-soluble (glycosidic) plant sterols could be a good alternative for these (fatty) phytostanol- and phytosterol-enriched products [19], especially if they can be obtained from easy to consume low-fat and low-energy natural food sources such as beverages. Unfortunately, only very limited direct, quantitative data is available on the natural presence of (glycosidic) plant sterols. Racette et al. (2009) already noted that glycosylated plant sterols are often excluded from sterol analysis, mostly due to the lack of standards and analytical difficulties [20]. In their study, total plant sterol content, including glycosides, was computed indirectly as the sum of the individual plant sterols determined by double (acidic and alkalic) hydrolysis. Their indirect analyses showed that glycosylated plant sterols (in general) comprised 20% of total plant sterols, in different diets. They also suggested that nuts, seeds, legumes, wheat germ, whole grains, bran, fruit, and vegetables could be important sources of glycosylated plant sterols. The presence of BSSG in dietary supplements and (fatty) foods such as nuts and wheat has also been touched upon by Phillips et al. (2005). The highest concentrations found back then, using indirect detection, were in flaxseed and soybean (up to 11 mg per 100 g dry weight, DW) [21]. Muller et al. (2007) suggested that BSS(G) and ergosterol from beer can compete with cholesterol during protein binding and as such prevent cholesterol uptake. However, he did not succeed in quantifying the true amounts of BSS(G) present in beers [22].

Therefore, this manuscript aimed to extend an extraction method and UPLC-MS/MS detection method, which was recently optimized and fully validated according to EC 2002/657 guidelines and Association of Analytical Chemists (AOAC) MS criteria, with these two compounds of interest (β-sitosterol-β-D-glucoside and ergosterol) (Multiple Reaction Monitoring, MRM) [23]. Campesterol, stigmasterol, brassicasterol, ergosterol (provitamine D$_2$), BSSG, and BSS concentrations were determined in a broad range of plant-based beverages, including a variety of (concentrate-based) juices, vegetable juices, beers, teas, malt-based (non-alcoholic) drinks, and plant-based milk alternatives (e.g., oat or soy beverages). Particular attention was payed to sample selection to cover a range of drinks that is as broad as possible. Plant extract–containing sodas were also included for comparison. Overall nutritional values and other (non-)beneficial compounds used in the formulation were also summarized (e.g., concentrations of proteins, vitamins, and minerals present).

2. Materials and Methods

Chloroform (analytical grade) and HPLC grade methanol (Methanol Optima®) were purchased from Fisher Scientific (Leicestershire, UK). Methanol (analytical grade) was purchased from VWR (Merck, Darmstadt, Germany). HPLC grade, ultrapure (UP) water was acquired from an in-house water purification system (Arium® 611UV, Sartorius Stedium Biotech, VWR, Haasrode, Belgium). Cholesterol (≥99%, from lanolin), β-sitosterol (BSS) (≥97%, from soy beans), brassicasterol (≥95%, from semisynthetic), provitamin D$_2$ (ergosterol) (≥97%, European Pharmacopoeia Reference Standard), and stigmasterol (≥97%, Supelco, Certified Reference Material) were purchased from Sigma Aldrich (St-Louis, Missouri, USA). Campesterol (≥98%, from seeds of *Brassica campestris*) was obtained from Wuhan ChemFaces Biochemical Co., Ltd. (Wuhan, Hubei, China). β-sitosterol-β-D-glucoside (BSSG) (≥95%, from semisynthetic) was purchased from Neuroquest (Halifax, NS, Canada). Stock solutions of each component (500 or 200 ng/μL) and dilutions up to 1 ng/μL were made in HPLC grade methanol. All solutions were kept at 4 °C and protected from direct light (brown flasks and additional aluminum foil coat).

Beverages were purchased from different suppliers/producers including Oat-ly AB (Mälmo, Sweden), 2Food (Soesterberg, The Netherlands), Paulaner Brauerei GmbH & Co. KG (Münich, Germany), AB Inbev (Leuven, Belgium), Olgerdin Egill Skallagrímsson Brewery (Reykjavik, Iceland), Ghent University College (Ghent, Belgium), The Coca-Cola Company (Ghent, Belgium), Melitta België n.v. (Lokeren, Belgium), Dream™ Hain Celestial Group, Inc. (Aalter, Belgium), Continental Foods Belgium (Puurs, Belgium), Pepsico Belux BVBA/SPRL (Zaventem, Belgium). Delhaize Le Lion/De Leeuw (Brussel, Belgium), Alpro, The WhiteWave Foods Company (Wevelgem, Belgium), Forever Living Products (Scottsdale, AZ, USA), Tao family (Ternat, Belgium), NV Brasseries Alken-Maes SA (Malines/Opwijk, Belgium), Haacht Brewery plc (Boortmoorbeek, Belgium), Carlsberg Breweries A/S (Copenhagen, Denmark), Palm breweries (Steenhuffel, Belgium), Brasserie du Bocq (Purnode, Belgium), Duvel Moortgat NV (Puurs, Belgium), Omer Vander Ghinste Brewery (Bellegem, Belgium), Nestle SA (Vevey, Switzerland), and Unilever (Brussel, Belgium).

Statistical model designs were used to optimize the general analytical extraction procedure. Dependent variables that might significantly affect the extraction efficiency were screened with a fractional factorial D-optimal design. These variables were selected on the basis of a literature survey and further optimization of only the influential variables was performed through response surface modeling (RSM) (Modde Pro 12, Umetrics software, Sartorium Stedim Biotech, Umeå, Sweden). The optimal sample volume for liquid samples (beverages) was determined using an additional small-scale full factorial design, and 5 mL was found to be the optimal sample volume, both in relative response per mL and S/N [23] (Table 2).

Table 2. Summary of the validated extraction protocol to extract plant sterols and ergosterol from a diverse range of beverages [23].

1.	5 mL (diluted) $^\Delta$ beverage in a 50 mL tube
2.	Addition of cholesterol (100 μL, 10 ng or 50 ng per μL)
3.	(Calibration samples: fortified with different plant sterols)
4.	Liquid-liquid extraction with 8 mL chloroform:methanol (2:1)
5.	Vortex (30 s) + ultrasonication * (10 min)
6.	Centrifugation (4400× g, 10 min)
7.	Cottonwool filter
8.	Second liquid-liquid extraction (repeat step 2 to 5)
9.	1 mL fresh chloroform:methanol added to the filter (filter wash out)
10.	Transfer 2 mL extract to new tube
11.	15–20 min drying (under liquid N_2, 46 °C)
12.	180 μL methanol (vortex 30 s, ultrasonication * 10 min)
13.	20 μL ultrapure H_2O (vortex 30 s, ultrasonication * 3 min, vortex 30 s)
14.	Centrifugation (12,300× g, 10 min)
15.	Transfer 150 μL to plastic LC-MS vial with insert for analysis

$^\Delta$ Samples were diluted if the first results showed that endogenous concentrations were too high to be able to include calibration points containing two to ten times the endogenous concentration (mostly for BSSG and BSS); * Ultrasonication: power 100, frequency 80 kHz.

An ultra-high performance liquid chromatography tandem mass spectrometry (UPLC-MS/MS) detection method was used for the quantification of free plant sterols, ergosterol, and BSSG in a single run. Previously, this method was fully validated for quantification of campesterol, BSS, stigmasterol, ergosterol, and brassicasterol [23]. Preliminary experiments showed that this method is also suitable for quantification of BSSG. Separation was carried out using an Accela™ High Speed LC (Thermo Fisher Scientific, San Jose, CA, USA) equipped with a Thermo Fisher Scientific™ Hypersil GOLD™ C18 Column (particle size: 1.9 μm, 50 × 2.1 mm I.D.). The mobile phases used were ultra-pure water (solvent A) and methanol (LC-MS grade, solvent B). All analytes could be accurately separated in a total run time of less than 10 min (Table 3). The gradient started with a linear gradient of 90% solvent B (methanol) for the first 2 min, increasing to 100% at 5.5 min, and then held at 100% for 1.5 min (up to 7 min). Afterward, the column was allowed to equilibrate at the initial conditions of 10% A and 90% B for 2 min. The divert valve was used to load the detector from 1.0 to 4.5 min. Scheduling was used to increase sensitivity, by limiting the detection window for each analyte to 0.6 min before and after the expected retention time. Detection was carried out on a TSQ Vantage triple stage quadrupole mass spectrometer equipped with an atmospheric pressure chemical ionization probe (APCI) (Thermo Fisher Scientific, San Jose, CA, USA). Injection volumes were 10 μL each and the APCI source was operated in the positive ion mode. The discharge current was set at ±4 μA. The sheath, sweep and auxiliary gas pressures were set at 20, 2, and 10 arbitrary units, respectively, the capillary temperature at 300 °C, and the vaporizer temperature at 320 °C. The collision gas pressure was kept at 1.5 mTorr, and the cycle time was 0.8 s. Data were acquired in the selected/multiple reaction-monitoring (SRM/MRM) mode. All specified product ions (Table 3) were used for peak integration, ion ratio determinations, and quantification purposes.

Table 3. Selected/multiple reaction monitoring (SRM/MRM) specifics for all compounds of interest: precursor ions, product ions (as m/z, mass over charge), absolute and relative retention time (RT, in minutes, min), appropriate S-Lens amplitude (volt, V), and the corresponding collision energy (CE, in electron volt, eV).

Analyte	Precursor Ion	Product Ions	Mean Relative Ion Abundancy *	Retention Time (Relative)	S-Lens Voltage	Collision Energy
	(m/z)	(m/z)	(%)	(min)	(V)	(eV)
β-Sitosterol-β-D-glucoside BSSG	397.3	91	70	1.80 (0.77)	88	47
		95	73			35
		105	100			40
		147	93			28
Ergosterol Provitamine D$_2$	379.3	69	78	2.04 (0.87)	120	23
		91	100			53
		105	90			34
		15	82			24
Brassicasterol	381.3	105	100	2.27 (0.97)	82	43
		159	67			23
		297	93			14
		311	40			13
Cholesterol internal standard	369.3	91	83	2.35 (1.00)	84	52
		95	69			34
		105	100			40
Campesterol	383.3	81	67	2.61 (1.11)	86	35
		91	85			49
		95	74			34
		105	100			43
Stigmasterol	395.3	81	64	2.63 (1.12)	59	37
		91	91			52
		105	100			44
		297	90			18
β-sitosterol BSS	397.3	91	70	2.90 (1.23)	88	47
		95	73			35
		105	100			40
		147	93			28

* In solvent, at full width half maximum (FWHM) and relative to the product ion with the highest intensity.

Area ratios were calculated relative to the internal standard (ISTD) cholesterol, which was added to both calibration and unknown samples, to compensate for losses during sample preparation and/or variation of the analytical analysis. Cholesterol was considered a suitable internal standard as no significant endogenous concentrations are present in the samples of interest (plant-based) and cholesterol is very similar to the calibrated analytes (Figure 1; Tables 1 and 3), chemically and in retention time but nevertheless chromatographically distinguishable and less expensive than isotopically labeled standards. Applying this method to other samples that, contrary to the samples analyzed in the current study, do contain significant concentrations of endogenous cholesterol would imply the use of another internal standard (e.g., 5α-cholestan-7β-ol or a deuterated (glycosidic) plant sterol).

Of each beverage, at least three non-fortified samples were extracted together with a nine-point matrix-matched calibration curve ($\geq$12 samples per matrix), constructed based upon nine fortification levels (0, 0.25, 0.5, 1, 2, 4, 6, 8, and 10 times the minimal expected endogenous concentration of each plant sterol individually). The minimal expected endogenous concentration was preliminary determined based upon calculated expected endogenous concentrations and standard addition (analysis of matrix matched samples with known added concentrations of plant sterols). Calculations combined available reference values for solid ingredients with their expected minimal contribution (%) to the different beverages. All samples were run twice, to take into account analytical variance, and mean ($n = 6$) ± standard deviation of these duplicate runs are reported in Tables 4 and 5.

Table 4. UPLC-MS/MS determined concentrations of BSS, BSSG, stigmasterol, campesterol, brassicasterol, and ergosterol (provitamin D$_2$) in a diverse range of beverages (fruit juices, vegetable juices, plant-based milk alternatives, gel, sodas, teas, and (non-alcoholic) malt-based drinks and beers).

Category	Product Name	mg per 100 mL		Brassicasterol	µg per 100 mL			
		BSS	BSSG		Campesterol	Stigmasterol	Ergosterol	
Fruit juices	Apple juice	0.21 ± 0.01	4.1 ± 1.2*	NF (<0.75)	27 ± 3	2.6 ± 0.4	ND	
	Orange juice	0.42 ± 0.09	8.3 ± 2.3*	NF (<1.5)	71 ± 12	23 ± 3	ND	
	Pomegranate juice	2.1 ± 0.3	32 ± 7	NF (<3)	139 ± 18	<30	17 ± 6	
	Multifruit-carrot juice	2.5 ± 0.2	16 ± 3	NF (<3)	607 ± 12	224 ± 10	ND	
	Fresh orange-banana juice	5.3 ± 2.2	>90	NF (<3)	846 ± 93	610 ± 35	NF (<3)	
	Tomato juice	0.36 ± 0.02	4.4 ± 0.5	NF (<2)	155 ± 10	331 ± 27	ND	
Vegetable juices	Mixed vegetable juice (a)	0.74 ± 0.05	6.2 ± 0.5	NF (<3)	242 ± 24	596 ± 64	ND	
	Mixed vegetable juice (b)	0.72 ± 0.10	12 ± 3	NF (<3.75)	177 ± 25	359 ± 72	29 ± 4	
	Beetroot juice	0.42 ± 0.07	7.3 ± 1.2	NF (<3)	47 ± 8	40 ± 3	NF (<3)	
	Carrot juice	2.7 ± 0.4	18 ± 4	NF (<3)	677 ± 68	1270 ± 65	NF (<3)	
	Coconut-rice	0.51 ± 0.07	2.8 ± 0.9	NF (<3)	72 ± 10	76 ± 13	ND	
	Rice	1.4 ± 0.1	2.4 ± 0.6	10 ± 3	260 ± 28	234 ± 23	ND	
	Soy	2.5 ± 0.5	4.9 ± 2.1	4.6 ± 0.4	1290 ± 291	998 ± 111	NF (<3)	
Plant-based milk alternatives	Cashew	2.7 ± 0.4	>60	NF (<3)	279 ± 44	15 ± 1	NF (<3)	
	Almond (a) unroasted	2.6 ± 0.6	78 ± 14	NF (<3)	101 ± 30	<30	ND	
	Almond (b) roasted	2.5 ± 0.1	13 ± 2	NF (<2)	62 ± 4	1915 ± 109	ND	
	Oat (a)	2.1 ± 0.2	26 ± 4	NF (<3)	475 ± 30	182 ± 16	ND	
	Oat (b)	3.9 ± 0.7	33 ± 4	217 ± 12	1098 ± 61	<15	NF (<3)	
Gel	Aloe vera gel beverage	0.22 ± 0.03	17 ± 5	NF (<0.75)	23 ± 5	2.2 ± 0.9	ND	
Sodas	Lemonade (a) (orange)	0.48 ± 0.04	1.5 ± 0.3*	NF (<0.75)	73 ± 3	19 ± 2	NF (<0.75)	
	Biolemonade (a) (elderberry)	0.19 ± 0.02	2.3 ± 0.7	NF (<1.5)	24 ± 2	52 ± 15	NF (<0.75)	
	Biolemonade (b) (ginger-orange)	0.17 ± 0.05	2.5 ± 0.7	NF (<0.75)	24 ± 3	4.3 ± 1.0	NF (<0.75)	
	Soda with plant extract (a)	0.05 ± 0.01	1.1 ± 0.2	NF (<0.75)	8.0 ± 1.7	1.3 ± 0.3	NF (<0.75)	
	Soda with plant extract (b) (stevia)	0.05 ± 0.01	0.60 ± 0.10	NF (<0.75)	7.3 ± 1.1	1.9 ± 0.3	NF (<0.75)	
	Soda with plant extract (c) (peach)	0.06 ± 0.01	1.5 ± 0.5	NF (<0.75)	5.8 ± 1.2	0.80 ± 0.31	NF (<0.75)	
Teas	Tea infusion (a)	0.08 ± 0.01	0.67 ± 0.12	NF (<0.75)	9.2 ± 1.7	1.1 ± 0.3	NF (<0.75)	
	Tea infusion (b)	0.06 ± 0.01	0.65 ± 0.17	NF (<0.75)	9.6 ± 1.3	1.5 ± 0.2	NF (<0.75)	
	Tea infusion (c)	0.06 ± 0.01	0.68 ± 0.12	NF (<0.75)	6.9 ± 0.8	2.3 ± 0.2	NF (<0.75)	
	Iced tea (b)	0.06 ± 0.01	0.93 ± 0.32	NF (<0.75)	8.3 ± 1.6	5.8 ± 0.8	NF (<0.75)	
	Iced tea (c)	0.05 ± 0.01	0.84 ± 0.08	NF (<0.75)	6.7 ± 0.8	9.5 ± 1.4	NF (<0.75)	

* Using a group specific calibration curve from respectively pomegranate juice (fruit juices) or lager (a) (beers); ▉ Indicates a plant-based beverage that can be considered a good source of free and conjugated plant sterols; ☐☐ Indicates a plant-based beverage that contains only moderate (yellow) or low concentrations (orange) of plant sterols. NF, not found; ND, not determined.

Table 5. UPLC-MS/MS determined concentrations of BSS, BSSG, stigmasterol, campesterol, brassicasterol, and ergosterol (provitamin D_2) in a diverse range of beverages (fruit juices, vegetable juices, plant-based milk alternatives, gel, sodas, teas, and (non-alcoholic) malt-based drinks and beers).

Category	Product Name	mg per 100 mL		µg per 100 mL			
		BSS	BSSG	Brassicasterol	Campesterol	Stigmasterol	Ergosterol
Non-alcoholic malt drinks	Chinese malt drink	0.07 ± 0.02	0.95 ± 0.33	NF (<0.75)	6.6 ± 2.1	<LOQ (<2)	ND
	Icelandic malt drink	0.14 ± 0.04	2.74 ± 1.31	NF (<1.5)	19 ± 4	2.4 ± 0.9	ND
	Non-alcoholic lager (a)	0.04 ± 0.01	0.50 ± 0.07	NF (<0.75)	6.8 ± 2.4	1.0 ± 0.4	NF (<0.75)
	Non-alcoholic lager (b)	0.07 ± 0.03	1.6 ± 0.5	NF (<0.75)	11 ± 3	1.9 ± 0.8	ND
	Non-alcoholic wheat beer (a)	0.07 ± 0.02	1.0 ± 0.1	NF (<0.75)	7.7 ± 1.9	0.88 ± 0.35	ND
	Non-alcoholic wheat beer (b)	0.12 ± 0.03	1.4 ± 0.2 *	NF (<0.75)	14 ± 3	2.1 ± 0.4	ND
Beers	Lager (a)	0.20 ± 0.04	2.2 ± 0.3	NF (<0.75)	24 ± 5	3 ± 1	NF (<0.75)
	Lager (b)	0.26 ± 0.02	1.7 ± 0.3 *	NF (<0.75)	31 ± 4	5 ± 1	ND
	Lager (c)	0.25 ± 0.04	1.2 ± 0.3 *	NF (<0.75)	39 ± 5	7 ± 1	ND
	Lager (d)	0.23 ± 0.03	1.7 ± 0.3 *	NF (<0.75)	23 ± 4	5 ± 1	ND
	Wheat beer (a)	0.28 ± 0.04	2.8 ± 0.4 *	NF (<0.75)	52 ± 3	6 ± 1	4.1 ± 0.4
	Wheat beer (b)	0.38 ± 0.09	3.2 ± 0.6 *	NF (<0.75)	53 ± 11	7 ± 2	ND
	Wheat beer (c)	0.26 ± 0.02	1.9 ± 0.3 *	NF (<0.75)	30 ± 2	3 ± 1	ND
	Wheat beer (d)	0.27 ± 0.04	3.4 ± 0.4 *	NF (<0.75)	37 ± 6	5 ± 1	ND
	Ale (bottle fermented) (a)	0.37 ± 0.05	2.0 ± 0.3 *	NF (<0.75)	49 ± 7	9 ± 1	0.80 ± 0.18
	Ale (bottle fermented) (b)	0.23 ± 0.03	4.5 ± 0.5 *	NF (<0.75)	36 ± 4	6 ± 1	6.0 ± 0.3
	Ale (bottle fermented) (c)	0.25 ± 0.03	2.5 ± 0.5 *	NF (<0.75)	36 ± 4	4 ± 1	ND
	Ale (bottle fermented) (d)	0.23 ± 0.03	1.3 ± 0.1 *	NF (<0.75)	7 ± 2	2 ± 1	4.6 ± 0.8
	Ale (bottle fermented) (e)	0.09 ± 0.02	0.9 ± 0.1 *	NF (<0.75)	36 ± 4	6 ± 1	ND

* Using a group specific calibration curve from respectively pomegranate juice (fruit juices) or lager (a) (beers); ☐ Indicates a plant-based beverage that contains only moderate (yellow) or low concentrations (orange) of plant sterols. NF, not found; ND, not determined.

For almost half of the samples (n = 19/49), endogenous concentrations of BSSG and/or BSS turned out to be too high to be able to include fortified samples with two to ten times the endogenous concentrations. For those matrices, additional calibration curves were made in diluted samples and additional diluted non-fortified samples were analyzed (diluted 4- to 30-fold with UP water, depending on the matrix). For all samples, endogenous plant sterol concentrations were determined by fitting the compounds' area ratio of non-fortified samples into the corresponding calibration curve. For diluted samples, the concentrations in undiluted samples were recalculated afterward.

3. Results

3.1. Data Analysis and Quality Assurance of the Analytical Method: Limits of Detection and Quantification

Lower limits of quantification (LLOQs) in solvent (90:10 methanol:H_2O) for the method used were between 0.5 and 1.5 ng per mL. In (diluted) beverages, the LLOQ was 0.5–3.0 µg per 100 mL for liquid samples, depending on the general composition of the sample and the compound of interest. In general, fatty and protein rich beverages (e.g., soy and oat beverage) hampered the detection of very low concentrations of plant sterols. Fortunately, most of these beverages were also relatively high in plant sterols. Previous results showed that the limits of detection (LODs) for solid matrices for the different compounds were between 10 and 30 µg per 100 g and LLOQs were between 20 and 100 µg per 100 g [23].

3.2. Quantification of Cholesterol-Lowering (Conjugated) Plant Sterols and Ergosterol (Provitamin D₂) with UPLC-MS/MS

All UPLC-MS/MS determined concentrations of BSS, BSSG, stigmasterol campesterol, brassicasterol, and ergosterol (provitamin D_2) in a diverse range of beverages (fruit juices, vegetable juices, plant-based milk alternatives, gel, soft drinks, teas, (non-alcoholic) malt-based drinks, and beers) have been summarized in Tables 4 and 5.

4. Discussion

Where possible, obtained plant sterol concentrations were compared to previously obtained thin layer chromatography (TLC), gas- or liquid chromatography—mass spectrometry (LC/GC-MS) and GC-FID (Flame Ionization Detector) results available in literature.

4.1. Fruit Juices

BSSG was present in very high concentrations (up to >90 mg per 100 mL). These concentrations are much higher than the mean concentrations determined in corresponding plants in the past, through indirect analysis. These results showed that in general only 20% of the plant sterols found in edible plants (<10 mg per 100 mL) were conjugated [20]. It is thus very likely that glucose-conjugated plant sterols are currently being underestimated in solid matrices, where they are tightly matrix-bound. However, due to their water-soluble nature, they are enriched throughout the production process of plant-based beverages. In addition, it can't be excluded that the previously used indirect method based upon chemical hydrolysis [20] was not sufficient to release conjugated plant sterols from the matrix and complete hydrolysis of the β-glycosidic bound at the same time.

BSS was the most abundant free plant sterol found, in line with mean free plant concentrations in higher plants, where BSS accounted for 50 to 80% of the total amount of plant sterols [24]. The highest concentration of BSS (5.3 ± 2.2 mg per 100 mL) was measured in the fresh orange-banana juice. As a comparison, this is 2.1 and 2.5 times higher than the concentration of BSS in the pomegranate juice and the multifruit-carrot juice, respectively. The lowest concentration of BSS was found in the concentrated orange and apple juice (13 and 25 time lower, respectively).

Interestingly, the two fruit juices that contained orange juice as a main ingredient (80% in fresh orange-banana juice, 100% in the concentrate-based orange juice; Supplementary Materials Table S1) contained very similar ratios of BSSG:BSS:campesterol, but the fresh orange-banana juice had 12 to 14 times higher concentrations. The concentration difference for stigmasterol was 26-fold, but that can be a direct consequence of the 20% banana content. Bananas are typically very high in stigmasterol; containing up to 200 mg per 100 g dry weight of banana pseudostem (pulp) [25–27].

The large difference between both orange juice based beverages can be explained by looking into detail at the results obtained for the apple and orange concentrate based juices, which happened to be produced by the same producer. Their plant sterol concentrations were found to be in linear correlation with the reported concentrations in the corresponding fruits (orange 23–24 mg and apple 12 mg per 100 g fresh weight with 11 mg BSS, 0.3 mg campesterol and 0.05 mg stigmasterol) [23,28–31]. For both juices (100% fruit), only around 2% of the initial plant sterol content of the fruits seemed to end up in the concentrate-based juices (g to mL), which suggests they used similar production processes for both concentrate-based juices, who were unfortunately equally incapable of containing plant sterols into the final juices. This illustrates the possible loss of beneficial compounds during the concentration process. Previous research has shown that the industrial production process can have a significant influence on the final concentrations (e.g., vitamin C and phenols). Previous research also showed that commercial squeezing of oranges extracted 22% more phenols than hand squeezing, however, the freezing process caused a dramatic decrease in phenols and the concentration process caused a mild precipitation of these compounds to the juice cloud [32]. Similar results have been reported for phenols in apple juices, but this could be prevented by using initial high temperature-short time (HTST) treatment and diffusion extraction instead of pressing [33]. Additional research will be needed to elucidate the exact influence of different fruit juice concentrate production processes on the concentrations of plant sterols in the final juice.

In pomegranate juice another peculiar result was detected in the chromatogram for stigmasterol. Stigmasterol could not be quantified as an intense interfering peak appeared at a retention time very close to the retention time of stigmasterol (with the same precursor and fragment ion masses). Upon addition of stigmasterol (matrix-matched calibration curve), it was confirmed that this peak was not stigmasterol. It seems that pomegranate (juice) contains a specific compound/plant sterol, very similar to stigmasterol, or a specific conjugated form of stigmasterol that deconjugates upon ionization (see also 4.6 Other water-soluble glucose-conjugated plant sterols). This illustrates the difficulties caused by the lack of analytical standards for (conjugated) plant sterols. Over 200 different types of plant sterols have been described [7], but for only a very limited number of those plant sterols analytical grade ($\geq$95% purity) standards are available. As such, it is very likely that analytical results still underestimate the contribution of, mostly exotic, novel fruits and other parts of plants that were previously not used for consumption (novel foods list EU 1997, e.g., pomegranate, chia seeds, Aloe vera). Especially as a revision of the novel foods directive is due to come into force in January 2018; the approval process will be significantly shortened and simplified (and thus less expensive) for new fruits or juices as long as a 25 years history of use can be shown in the country of origin (new Directive for Traditional Foods, EC Regulation No. 2015/2283). The introduction of these new fruits or juices onto the market will hamper the accurate detection of plant sterols even more, as these fruits will be accompanied by less well known plant sterols, wherefore no analytical standards are available. Additional research will also be needed to evaluate if these less well-known plant sterols exhibit the same health benefits.

The tropical multifruit-carrot juice was also concentrate-based (18% orange, 19% pine apple, 5% carrot and 3% other fruits including passion fruit, Supplementary Materials Table S1). Orange, pine apple and carrots are moderately high in plant sterols, containing respectively 23, 17 and 12 mg of plant sterols per 100 g edible fresh weight, while passion fruit is high in plant sterols (44 mg per 100 g) [28,31]. However, as with most exotic beverages, the true amount of passion fruit blended into the drink was too low to contribute its beneficial effects (<1%). Nevertheless, the concentrations of plant sterols in this juice were very high, similar to the concentrations measured in fresh juices. When having a look at the results for the carrot juice (4.2 Vegetable juices) it can be noted that the concentrations measured are very alike. So it seems that despite its low contribution percentage-wise, carrot juice does make a strong contribution to the final plant sterol concentrations in the juice. Upon extraction it was already visible that this juice was visually more turbid and more viscous (thicker) than the 100% orange concentrate-based juice. This observation was supported by the ingredient list. This beverage included both juice and sauce concentrates (45%), and not just juice concentrate. Including fruit sauces implies that the cell material rich solid fraction (pulp) is included into the beverage.

No brassicasterol was found in either of these juices, but that is in line with what could be expected, as their ingredient lists (Supplementary Materials Table S1) did not include plants from the Brassicaceae family or products derived from these plants.

4.2. Vegetable Juices

In line with the concentrations measured in fruit juices, BSSG was detected in the highest concentrations, but the difference with BSS was less profound. Respectively, 1.0 ± 0.1 and approximately 10 mg per 100 mL BSS and BSSG were found in the vegetable drinks analyzed. A possible explanation for this is that fruits are typically a lot higher in carbohydrates, and monosaccharides in particular, than vegetables (e.g., orange and pine apple 9 g, apple 10 g, banana 15 g per 100 g fresh weight (FW) versus tomatoes and lettuce 2 g, carrot 6 g, broccoli and cucumber 1 g per 100 g FW), hence the formation of high concentrations of glucose conjugates seems more likely (FDA nutrition facts raw fruits and raw vegetables poster, 2016). This sugar content difference is still detectable in the corresponding juices with mean sugar concentrations of 10 ± 3 and 5 ± 2 g sugar per 100 mL fruit juices and vegetable juices, respectively (Supplementary Materials Table S1), and thus reflected in the conjugated plant sterol concentrations measured. Mixed vegetable juice (b) is a good example thereof, as it contains almost twice as much sugars (5.7 g per 100 mL) as the other mixed vegetable juice (a) (2.7 g per 100 mL), and as a result contained a 2-fold greater amount of BSSG (12 ± 3 versus 6.2 ± 0.5 mg per 100 mL, respectively). The main difference in the ingredient list of both juices is that juice (b) contains less tomato and celeriac/onion juice (2 g sugar per 100 g FW) and more carrot juice (6 g sugar per 100 g FW).

Interestingly, and as touched upon in 4.1 Fruit juices, carrot juice showed to be particularly high in plant sterols, containing two to three times more plant sterols than the other vegetable juices. However, carrots are not particularly high in plant sterols, suggesting that the juice production technology and the true amount of carrots used per mL play an important role as well. Generally, fresh carrots are peeled with steam or mechanical peelers, chopped and eventually cooked to have a better extraction of the juice. The cooked carrots are mashed in a turbo extractor and then cooled and stored in treatment tanks where enzymes can be added (increasing juice yield yet reducing carotene content) [34]. After the enzyme treatment the obtained carrot juice is pasteurized for enzyme inactivation. After that, the carrot juice passes through the decanter to remove fibers and can be concentrated for transport. The main difference with the production of other juices is that these are typically not cooked before juice extraction, which might influence the plant sterol concentrations in the resulting juice. This effect is reflected in the concentrations of plant sterols found in beetroot juice and carrot juice. One of the main differences between both juices is that fresh beets are used to produce beetroot juice, while carrots are boiled before juice extraction. The plant sterol content of their respective raw materials, beetroot and carrot, are very similar (17.1 and 15.3 mg per 100 g FW) [28], yet carrot juice contained at least six times more plant sterols. Despite this lack of plant sterols, beetroot (juice) is being put forward as a promising therapeutic treatment in a range of clinical pathologies associated with oxidative stress and inflammation, due to the presence of other anti-oxidative constituents [35].

Botanically, tomatoes would be categorized as fruits, but as this study has been performed from a consumer's point of view, they have been added to the vegetable juices group. The plant sterol concentrations measured were also more in line with the vegetable juices group than with the, generally higher in plant sterols, fruit juices group. Both mixed vegetable juices (a) and (b) also contained high concentrations of tomato juice (respectively 86% and 79.6% versus 99% in the tomato juice), which was reflected by the plant sterol concentrations measured in each of them. Surprisingly, vegetable juice (b) contained ergosterol (29 $\pm$ 4 µg per 100 mL), just like the pomegranate juice (17 $\pm$ 4 µg per 100 mL) (fruit juices group). The most plausible explanation for this is that the vegetables/fruits used for the production of these juices were contaminated with fungi. Parsi and Gorecki (2006) described how ergosterol could be used as an indicator for fungal biomass [36]. Upon visual fungal outgrowth they detected respectively 140 mg and 17 mg ergosterol per 100 g on moldy bread and maple leaves infected with powdery mildew, putting into perspective the concentrations measured here. Multiple authors have reported additional expectable concentrations of ergosterol per 100 g cells (DW) (Table 6) but cell mass estimations based upon concentrations of ergosterol detected will always be rough estimates, as the concentration of ergosterol present in fungal/yeast cells is dependent of light, age of the cell and growth conditions [37]. In any case, these very low concentrations of ergosterol measured did not contribute significantly to the overall intake of sterols.

Table 6. Concentrations of provitamine D$_2$ (ergosterol) measured in yeast and fungi (mg per 100 g dry weight, DW). Ranked according to concentration [36–39].

Species	Ergosterol (mg per 100 g DW)
Yeast	
Cryptococcus albidus	4200 $\pm$ 1200
Rhodotorulamucilaginosa	3700 $\pm$ 760
Rhodotorulaminuta	3700 $\pm$ 630
Saccharomycescerevisiae	400–2000
Fungi	
Acremoniumfurcatum	1400 $\pm$ 780
Stachybotryschartarum	1200 $\pm$ 520
Aspergillus versicolor	1100 $\pm$ 1500
Penicilliumbrevicompactum	580 $\pm$ 1300
Cladosporiumcladosporioides	560 $\pm$ 1100
Aureobasidiumpullulans	260 $\pm$ 1600

4.3. Plant-Based Milk Alternatives

High concentrations of BSS (up to 4 mg per 100 mL) and especially BSSG (up to 78 mg per 100 mL) were detected in the almond, oats and cashew base milk alternatives. The rice and rice-coconut based beverages, on the other hand, only contained low concentrations of plant sterols (<5 mg per mL in total). The soy based beverage contained higher concentrations of campesterol (1.3 $\pm$ 0.3 mg per 100 mL) and stigmasterol (0.9 $\pm$ 0.1 mg per 100 mL), and moderate concentrations of BSS and BSSG, respectively 2.5 $\pm$ 0.5 and 4.9 $\pm$ 1.9 mg per 100 mL. The high concentrations of campesterol and stigmasterol in soy are however in line with results obtained in a study by Yamaya et al. (2007) [40]. This study showed that the content of plant sterols ranged from 202 and 843 µg per g soy bean. The highest amounts were found in soybeans with high lipid content. BSS, campesterol, and stigmasterol were the main plant sterols found at the proportions of 43–67%, 17–34%, and 10–30%, respectively. The concentrations measured in the soy beverage are in line with these ranges, but at the higher end of the range for campesterol (respectively 52%, 27% and 21% in the soy based beverage). Another difference that immediately pops out of the list of results is the significant difference between the two almond based beverages. Almond beverage (a) contained particularly higher concentrations of BSSG (78 $\pm$ 14 mg per 100 mL) than almond beverage (b) (13 $\pm$ 2 mg per 100 mL), and lower concentrations of stigmasterol (<0.03 mg per 100 mL) versus (1.9 $\pm$ 0.1 mg per 100 mL). An important difference between these beverages however is that almond beverage (a) was based upon unroasted almonds, while for almond beverage (b) roasted almonds were used and beverage (a) was sweetened, while beverage (b) was not.

Brassicasterol is typically found in plants belonging to the Brassicaceae family. The family contains different edible plants such as *Brassica oleracea* (e.g., broccoli, cabbage and cauliflower),

Brassica nigra and *Sinapis alba* (black and white mustard seeds). Also part of this family are the canola oilseeds producing members of the species *Brassica rapa*, including *Brassica rapa* subspecies oleifera (field mustard) and *Brassica napus* (rapeseed), and the mustard subspecies of *Brassica juncea* (e.g., green and brown mustard). Canola oil producers claim that the total amount of free plant sterols in edible (low erucic acid) canola oils ranges from 0.63% to 0.71% with 10.8–16.2% brassicasterol, which would translate to 76–112 mg per 100 g for different cultivars (Canola Council of Canada, canola oil chemical properties, 2017). Mo et al. (2013) confirmed that canola oil can contain very high levels of brassicasterol, and other plant sterols, compared to other edible oils but they detected a more realistic concentration of 48.8 mg brassicasterol per 100 g [41]. Piironen et al. (2000) reported similar concentrations between 55 and 73 mg per 100 g [42]. Compared to that, concentrations of brassicasterol found in different vegetables such as cabbage, Brussels sprouts and broccoli are very low, ranging between 0.2 and 2.0 mg per 100 g [30]. Oat beverage (b), listing canola oil on its ingredient list (percentage used not listed), showed to contain 217 ± 12 µg brassicasterol per 100 mL. This concentration translates to 5 (or more) g canola oil per L oat beverage. The total fat percentage of the oat beverage is 1.5% (originating from the oats, 7–8% fat; and canola oil, 100% fat), proving that brassicasterol is a good indicator for the amount of canola oil used. The addition of canola oil is also reflected in the concentrations of other plant sterols found in oat beverage (b). Especially the high concentration of campesterol found in this beverage (1.10 ± 0.06 versus 0.48 ± 0.05 mg per 100 mL in oat beverage (a)) could be attributed to canola oil.

Interestingly, two other plant-based milk alternatives (soy and rice based) also contained traces of brassicasterol (respectively 10 ± 4 and 4.6 ± 0.4 µg per 100 mL), although they did not list canola oil as an ingredient. Given the low concentration of brassicasterol in the rice beverage it is most likely that sunflower oil, that is part of the rice beverage's ingredient list, (unintentionally) got mixed with canola/mustard seed oil (<1:50 ratio). The soy beverage result is even more intriguing, as no oil at all was mentioned in the ingredient list. The integrity of this beverage might be questionable. This suspicion is strengthened by the high concentration of campesterol and stigmasterol found in this soy beverage, suggesting that a (campesterol rich) oil might have been added after all. Sterol profiling has already been used to unravel adulteration of other (expensive) oils such as extra virgin olive oil with other cheaper oils [43–45], but these results show that with this sensitive method it is even possible to trace back the botanical origin of oils in processed end products such as beverages.

4.4. Gel, Sodas, Teas and Non-Alcoholic Malt-Based Drinks

Most of the teas, sodas, and (non-alcoholic) malt-based drinks contained only low concentrations of plant sterols (10 to >100-fold lower than the juices and plant-based milk alternatives discussed earlier) (Tables 4 and 5, orange color code). However, some exceptions should be noted. The *Aloe vera* gel–based drink showed to be moderately high in BSSG (17 ± 5 mg per 100 mL), yet low in the other plant sterols. The orange juice concentrate-based lemonade contained similar concentrations of plant sterols as the concentrate-based orange juice analyzed, illustrating the dilution effect and/or loss of plant sterols throughout both production processes. The other two malt-based (biolemonades) analyzed were slightly higher in plant sterols compared to other sodas (and teas/non-alcoholic beers/malt drinks) but still far less plant sterol rich than fruit and vegetable juices and plant-based milk alternatives.

4.5. Beers

The only available data on plant sterols in beer are results from Muller et al. (2007) and Rapota and Tyrsin (2015) [22,46]. Both indicated that BSS from malt and hop could compete with cholesterol for protein binding and uptake. Rapota and Tyrsin (2015) were able to prove the qualitative presence of plant sterols in malt and hop, but no quantitative data were reported [46]. Our own preliminary data showed that brewer's hop and malting barley contain, respectively, >140 and >50 mg free plant sterols per 100 g DW [23]. Muller et al. (2007) analyzed a few beer samples ($n = 4$), proving the presence of BSS in beer, but the results were not quantitative [22]. Throughout the current study, BSSG, BSS, campesterol, ergosterol, and stigmasterol could be detected and quantified in a variety of different beers (Table 5). In general, plant sterol concentrations in beer were very low (on average 10 times lower than concentrations in juices and milk alternatives). Nevertheless, these results did allow us to unravel correlations between the production process of the different beer types (technologies used) and the concentrations measured in the end beer.

The wheat beers ($n = 4$) contained the highest concentration of plant sterols, probably due to the lack of end filtration in this type of beer, which allows grain residues to remain in the final beer. This is also reflected by the turbidity of these beers compared to lagers and ales. The H90 EBC (European Brewery Convention units) turbidity, an indicator for the presence of sub 1 μm particles such as proteins ranged between 96 and >100 EBC in wheat beers, versus 12 ± 5 EBC and 0.55 ± 0.17 for ales ($n = 4$) and lagers ($n = 4$), respectively ($p < 0.001$). H25 EBC, indicative for larger particles such as yeast and diatomaceous earth, was 72 ± 14 EBC in wheat beers, versus 21 ± 12 EBC and 0.25 ± 0.05 EBC for lagers and ales, respectively ($p < 0.001$). One of the ales (ale (a)) was not filtered either, so this beer was excluded from the pool of ales. Its turbidity was indeed closer to the turbidity of the wheat beers (H90 47 ± 2 EBC and H25 71 ± 3 EBC). The opposite was true for ale (e), which includes very extensive removal of the cold break and end filtration in its production process. This is reflected by both the low turbidity (H90 9 ± 1 EBC, H25 13 ± 1 EBC) and low concentrations of plant sterols measured, three times lower than the other ales (Table 5). In general, however, top fermented ales contained higher concentrations of plant sterols compared to lager beers. This can be related to the higher original extract (16.4 ± 1.2 P), which is directly linked to the grain bill (amount of grain used), unless sugar or other carbon sources are being added (Supplementary Materials Table S1). The mean original extract was significantly lower in lagers (11.3 ± 0.4 P, $p < 0.001$) and wheat beers (10.3 ± 0.9 P, $p < 0.001$).

Interestingly, plant sterol concentrations measured in alcoholic beers and their non-alcoholic counterparts were significantly lower in the latter, suggesting that different production processes and less grain were used to produce the non-alcoholic alternatives, further reducing their plant sterol content. This is also reflected by the significantly lower mean original extract values measured in non-alcoholic beers compared to their alcoholic counterparts (6.9 ± 0.4 P versus 10.8 ± 0.6, $p < 0.001$). Ergosterol was only detected in the wheat beers and ales (with bottle refermentation), not in the non-alcoholic or lager beers. However, the concentrations were very low, showing that only very limited amounts of the yeast and its ergosterol end up in the glass. For ales with refermentation in the bottle, the yeast adheres to the bottle; therefore, ergosterol is not consumed.

4.6. Other Water-Soluble Glucose-Conjugated Plant Sterols

BSSG was the only conjugated plant sterol for which an analytical standard ($\geq$95% NMR purity) could be acquired. Nevertheless, this standard allowed understanding the fate of conjugated plant sterols in general. Due to the presence of the polar glucose conjugate the retention on the apolar column was less than for the free sterols (retention times for BSS and BSSG were 2.90 min and 1.80 min, respectively). A mean absolute retention time difference of 1.1 ± 0.1 min between both peaks could be determined. Glucose-conjugated plant sterols will thus arrive into the ionization source significantly earlier than their free counterparts. Upon ionization (APCI), the β-glycosidic bound is broken down; the main precursor ion measured in the first quadrupole (Q1) matches the precursor ion for free BSS. Upon Q2 fragmentation, the same product ions and product ion ratios could be found in Q3. Interestingly, when broadening the detection window, free campesterol was found to be proceeded by a second peak as well, at a very similar relative retention time difference (0.43 ± 0.01 for BSS and BSSG and 0.38 ± 0.01 for campesterol and "campesterol-glucoside"). Taking into account the mass spectral and product ion ratio match of this peak with campesterol precursor and product ions, it could be concluded that this peak is most likely campesterol-β-D-glucoside. In line with the results obtained for BSSG, the peak area of campesterol-β-D-glucoside is at least as high as the peak for free campesterol (Figure 2, top right campesterol-glucoside and campesterol, bottom right BSSG and BSS). This campesterol-β-D-glucoside peak was found in all beverages analyzed. It can be concluded that current methodologies to measure total plant sterol content underestimate the contribution of these glycosidic conjugates to the total plant sterol content.

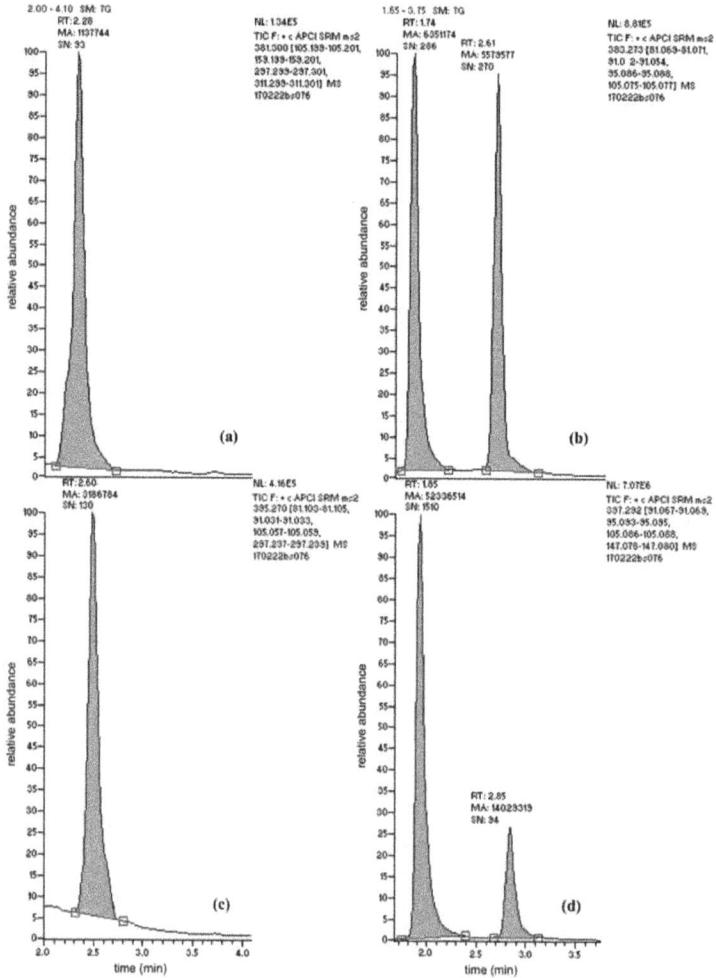

Figure 2. Chromatogram obtained using UPLC–MS/MS after the injection (10 μL) of a four times diluted organic oat beverage extract. This beverage contained 217 ± 12 μg brassicasterol (**a**), 1.1 ± 0.1 mg campesterol (**b**), <15 μg stigmasterol per 100 mL (**c**) and 3.9 ± 0.7 mg BSS and 33 ± 4 mg BSSG (**d**). Panel (**b**) also clearly illustrates the presence of high concentrations of campesterol-β-D-glucoside (retention time 1.74 min, m/z 383.3).

5. Conclusions

This study aimed to quantify free and conjugated plant sterols and ergosterol in a broad range of plant-based (health) drinks. Concentrations of water-soluble glycosidic phytosterols (e.g., BSSG) showed to be much higher than what could have been expected from concentrations previously (indirectly) determined in solid foods such as grains, fruits, and vegetables. Plant-based milk

Nutrients **2018**, *10*, 21

alternatives and fresh juices for example showed to contain up to 90 mg BSSG per 100 mL. Due to their water-soluble nature, these sterols may have been enriched throughout the liquid extraction process used to produce these beverages. Most concentrate based beverages and extracts on the other hand only contained low concentrations of plant sterols. In addition, previously used extraction and chemical hydrolysis protocols might not have sufficed to release all conjugated plant sterols from the matrix and complete hydrolysis of the β-glycosidic bound at the same time. In light of the ever-growing market of health-conscious consumers, one should be looking into more detail at production processes to increase enrichment of (conjugated) plant sterols were possible. Another possibility is to further expand the possibilities of the addition of water-soluble glycosylated plant sterols to low energy foods such as drinks instead of esterified plant sterols to fatty food matrices.

Supplementary Materials: The following are available online at www.mdpi.com/2072-6643/10/1/21/s1, Supplementary Materials Table S1: Detailed composition of the diverse beverages analyzed, including beverage category (group), beverage name, health claims listed, main ingredients, ingredients percentage, added sugars and/or sweeteners, vitamins, minerals, stabilizers and thickeners used, energy, fat, carbohydrates, fibers, proteins, salt content, and alcohol percentage. Upon request, the authors can also provide information on the producer and batch number of a beverage sample of interest.

Acknowledgments: This work was executed at the Laboratory of Chemical Analysis (Department of Veterinary Public Health and Food Safety, Faculty of Veterinary Medicine, Ghent University) and the Laboratorium of Biochemistry and Brewing (Campus Schoonmeersen, Association Ghent University). It was funded by both the Department of Applied Biosciences, Faculty of Biosciences Engineering, Ghent University, and the Laboratory of Chemical Analysis (Department of Veterinary Public Health and Food Safety, Faculty of Veterinary Medicine, Ghent University). Special thanks to the thesis students Bram Van Wesemael and Wouter Pyncket and colleagues Sylvie Vandoorne and Lieselot Hemeryck for their practical support.

Author Contributions: Anneleen Decloedt and Anita Van Landschoot conceived and designed the experiments; Anneleen Decloedt and Hellen Watson performed the experiments; Anneleen Decloedt and Hellen Watson analyzed the data; Lynn Vanhaecke, Dana Vanderputten, and Anita Van Landschoot contributed reagents, materials and analysis tools (a.o. UPLC-MS/MS analysis); Anneleen Decloedt wrote the paper, which was revised by all of the co-authors (Hellen Watson, Anita Van Landschoot, Dana Vanderputten, and Lynn Vanhaecke).

Conflicts of Interest: The authors declare no conflicts of interest. The founding sponsors had no role in the design of the study; in the collection, analyses, or interpretation of data; in the writing of the manuscript, and in the decision to publish the results.

References

1. Bradford, P.G.; Awad, A.B. Phytosterols as anticancer compounds. *Mol. Nutr. Food Res.* **2007**, *51*, 161–170. [CrossRef] [PubMed]
2. Ramprasath, V.R.; Awad, A.B. Role of Phytosterols in Cancer Prevention and Treatment. *J. AOAC Int.* **2015**, *98*, 735–738. [CrossRef] [PubMed]
3. Aldini, R.; Micucci, M.; Cevenini, M.; Fato, R.; Bergamini, C.; Nanni, C.; Cont, M.; Camborata, C.; Spinozzi, S.; Montagnani, M.; et al. Antiinflammatory effect of phytosterols in experimental murine colitis model: Prevention, induction, remission study. *PLoS ONE* **2014**, *9*, e108112. [CrossRef] [PubMed]
4. Ling, W.H.; Jones, P.J. Dietary phytosterols: A review of metabolism, benefits and side effects. *Life Sci.* **1995**, *57*, 195–206. [CrossRef]
5. Wang, T.; Hicks, K.B.; Moreau, R. Antioxidant activity of phytosterols, oryzanol, and other phytosterol conjugates. *J. Am. Oil Chem. Soc.* **2002**, *79*, 1201–1206. [CrossRef]
6. Woyengo, T.A.; Ramprasath, V.R.; Jones, P.J. Anticancer effects of phytosterols. *Eur. J. Clin. Nutr.* **2009**, *63*, 813–820. [CrossRef] [PubMed]
7. Moreau, R.A.; Whitaker, B.D.; Hicks, K.B. Phytosterols, phytostanols, and their conjugates in foods: Structural diversity, quantitative analysis, and health-promoting uses. *Prog. Lipid Res.* **2002**, *41*, 457–500. [CrossRef]
8. Phillips, K.M.; Ruggio, D.M.; Horst, R.L.; Minor, B.; Simon, R.R.; Feeney, M.J.; Byrdwell, W.C.; Haytowitz, D.B. Vitamin D and Sterol Composition of 10 Types of Mushrooms from Retail Suppliers in the United States. *J. Agric. Food Chem.* **2011**, *59*, 7841–7853. [CrossRef] [PubMed]
9. Hirsch, A.L. Vitamin D: Two-Volume Set. In *Industrial Aspects of Vitamin D*; Feldman, D., Pike, J.W., Adamn, J.S., Eds.; Academic Press: Cambridge, MA, USA, 2011; Chapter 6; pp. 73–93.

10. Brufau, G.; Canela, M.A.; Rafecas, M. Phytosterols: Physiologic and metabolic aspects related to cholesterol-lowering properties. *Nutr. Res.* **2008**, *28*, 217–225. [CrossRef] [PubMed]

11. Trautwein, E.A.; Duchateau, G.S.M.J.E.; Lin, Y.; Ntanios, F.Y. Proposed mechanisms of cholesterol-lowering action of plant sterols. *Eur. J. Lipid Sci. Technol.* **2003**, *105*, 171–185. [CrossRef]

12. Higdon, J.; Drake, V.; Higdon, J. *An Evidence-Based Approach to Phytochemicals and Other Dietary Factors*, 2nd ed.; Thieme: Stuttgart, Germany, 2013; p. 304.

13. Kritchevsky, D.; Chen, S.C. Phytosterols—Health benefits and potential concerns: A review. *Nutr. Res.* **2005**, *25*, 413–428. [CrossRef]

14. Abumweis, S.S.; Barake, R.; Jones, P.J. Plant sterols/stanols as cholesterol lowering agents: A meta-analysis of randomized controlled trials. *Food Nutr. Res.* **2008**, *52*. [CrossRef] [PubMed]

15. Ras, R.T.; Geleijnse, J.M.; Trautwein, E.A. LDL-cholesterol-lowering effect of plant sterols and stanols across different dose ranges: A meta-analysis of randomised controlled studies. *Br. J. Nutr.* **2014**, *112*, 214–219. [CrossRef] [PubMed]

16. Fernandes, P.; Cabral, J.M.S. Phytosterols: Applications and recovery methods. *Bioresour. Technol.* **2007**, *98*, 2335–2350. [CrossRef] [PubMed]

17. Quilez, J.; Garcia-Lorda, P.; Salas-Salvado, J. Potential uses and benefits of phytosterols in diet: Present situation and future directions. *Clin. Nutr.* **2003**, *22*, 343–351. [CrossRef]

18. Laitinen, K.; Gylling, H.; Kaipiainen, L.; Nissinen, M.J.; Simonen, P. Cholesterol lowering efficacy of plant stanol ester in a new type of product matrix, a chewable dietary supplement. *J. Funct. Foods* **2017**, *30*, 119–124. [CrossRef]

19. Lin, X.B.; Ma, L.; Racette, S.B.; Spearie, C.L.A.; Ostlund, R.E., Jr. Phytosterol glycosides reduce cholesterol absorption in humans. *Am. J. Physiol. Gastrointest. Liver Physiol.* **2009**, *296*, G931–G935. [CrossRef] [PubMed]

20. Racette, S.B.; Spearie, C.A.; Phillips, K.M.; Lin, X.; Ma, L.; Ostlund, R.E., Jr. Phytosterol-Deficient and High-Phytosterol Diets Developed for Controlled Feeding Studies. *J. Am. Diet. Assoc.* **2009**, *109*, 2043–2051. [CrossRef] [PubMed]

21. Phillips, K.M.; Ruggio, D.M.; Ashraf-Khorassani, M. Phytosterol composition of nuts and seeds commonly consumed in the United States. *J. Agric. Food Chem.* **2005**, *53*, 9436–9445. [CrossRef] [PubMed]

22. Muller, R.; Walker, S.; Brauer, J.; Junquera, M. Does beer contain compounds that might interfere with cholesterol metabolism? *J. Inst. Brew.* **2007**, *113*, 102–109. [CrossRef]

23. Decloedt, A.I.; van Landschoot, A.; Vanhaecke, L. Fractional factorial design-based optimisation and application of an extraction and UPLC-MS/MS detection method for the quantification of phytosterols in food, feed and beverages low in phytosterols. *Anal. Bioanal. Chem.* **2016**, *408*, 7731–7744. [CrossRef] [PubMed]

24. Nes, W.R.; Nes, W.D. *Lipids in Evolution*, 1st ed.; Plenum Press: New York, NY, USA; London, UK, 1980; p. 243.

25. Knapp, F.F.; Nicholas, H.J. Sterols and Triterpenes of Banana Pulp. *J. Food Sci.* **1969**, *34*, 584. [CrossRef]

26. Knapp, F.F.; Nicholas, H.J. Distribution of Sterols and Steryl Esters in Banana Plant. *Phytochemistry* **1969**, *8*, 2091. [CrossRef]

27. Ramu, R.; Shirahatti, P.S.; Zameer, F.; Prasad, N. Investigation of antihyperglycaemic activity of banana (Musa sp. var. Nanjangud rasa bale) pseudostem in normal and diabetic rats. *J. Sci. Food Agric.* **2015**, *95*, 165–173. [PubMed]

28. Abidi, S.L. Chromatographic analysis of plant sterols in foods and vegetable oils. *J. Chromatogr. A* **2001**, *935*, 173–201. [CrossRef]

29. Toivo, J.; Phillips, K.; Lampi, A.-M.; Piironen, V. Determination of sterols in foods: Recovery of free, esterified, and glycosidic sterols. *J. Food Compos. Anal.* **2001**, *14*, 631–643. [CrossRef]

30. Piironen, V.; Toivo, J.; Puupponen-Pimiä, R.; Lampi, A.M. Plant sterols in vegetables, fruits and berries. *J. Sci. Food Agric.* **2003**, *83*, 330–337. [CrossRef]

31. Normen, L.; Johnsson, M.; Andersson, H.; Van Gameren, Y.; Dutta, P. Plant sterols in vegetables and fruits commonly consumed in Sweden. *Eur. J. Nutr.* **1999**, *38*, 84–89. [CrossRef] [PubMed]

32. Gil-Izquierdo, A.; Gil, M.I.; Ferreres, F. Effect of processing techniques at industrial scale on orange juice antioxidant and beneficial health compounds. *J. Agric. Food Chem.* **2002**, *50*, 5107–5114. [CrossRef] [PubMed]

33. Spanos, G.A.; Wrolstad, R.E.; Heatherbell, D.A. Influence of Processing and Storage on the Phenolic Composition of Apple Juice. *J. Agric. Food Chem.* **1990**, *38*, 1572–1579. [CrossRef]

34. Demir, N.; Bahceci, K.S.; Acar, J. The effect of processing method on the characteristics of carrot juice. *J. Food Qual.* **2007**, *30*, 813–822. [CrossRef]

35. Clifford, T.; Howatson, G.; West, D.J.; Stevenson, E.J. The potential benefits of red beetroot supplementation in health and disease. *Nutrients* **2015**, *7*, 2801–2822. [CrossRef] [PubMed]

36. Parsi, Z.; Gorecki, T. Determination of ergosterol as an indicator of fungal biomass in various samples using non-discriminating flash pyrolysis. *J. Chromatogr. A* **2006**, *1130*, 145–150. [CrossRef] [PubMed]

37. Stuper-Szablewska, K.; Perkowski, J. Contamination of wheat grain with microscopic fungi and their metabolites in Poland in 2006-2009. *Ann. Agric. Environ. Med.* **2014**, *21*, 504–509. [CrossRef] [PubMed]

38. Arnezeder, C.; Koliander, W.; Hampel, W.A. Rapid-Determination of Ergosterol in Yeast-Cells. *Anal. Chim. Acta* **1989**, *225*, 129–136. [CrossRef]

39. Pasanen, A.L.; Yli-Pietilä, K.; Pasanen, P.; Kalliokoski, P.; Tarhanen, J. Ergosterol content in various fungal species and biocontaminated building materials. *Appl. Environ. Microbiol.* **1999**, *65*, 138–142. [PubMed]

40. Yamaya, A.; Endo, Y.; Fujimoto, K.; Kitamura, K. Effects of genetic variability and planting location on the phytosterols content and composition in soybean seeds. *Food Chem.* **2007**, *102*, 1071–1075. [CrossRef]

41. Mo, S.; Dong, L.; Hurst, W.J.; Van Breemen, R.B. Quantitative analysis of phytosterols in edible oils using APCI liquid chromatography-tandem mass spectrometry. *Lipids* **2013**, *48*, 949–956. [CrossRef] [PubMed]

42. Piironen, V.; Lindsay, D.G.; Miettinen, T.A.; Toivo, J.; Lampi, A.M. Plant sterols: Biosynthesis, biological function and their importance to human nutrition. *J. Sci. Food Agric.* **2000**, *80*, 939–966. [CrossRef]

43. Diaz, T.G.; Merás, I.D.; Casas, J.S.; Franco, M.A. Characterization of virgin olive oils according to its triglycerides and sterols composition by chemometric methods. *Food Control* **2005**, *16*, 339–347. [CrossRef]

44. Vrbkova, B.; Roblová, V.; Yeung, E.S.; Preisler, J. Determination of sterols using liquid chromatography with off-line surface-assisted laser desorption/ionization mass spectrometry. *J. Chromatogr. A* **2014**, *1358*, 102–109. [CrossRef] [PubMed]

45. Flakelar, C.L.; Prenzler, P.D.; Luckett, D.J.; Howitt, J.A.; Doran, G. A rapid method for the simultaneous quantification of the major tocopherols, carotenoids, free and esterified sterols in canola (*Brassica napus*) oil using normal phase liquid chromatography. *Food Chem.* **2017**, *214*, 147–155. [CrossRef] [PubMed]

46. Rapota, M.O.; Tyrsin, Y.A. Extraction of lipids from the raw materials for beer production and development of methods from phytosterols' determination by high performance liquid chromatography (HPLC). *Biol. Med.* **2015**, *7*, 5.

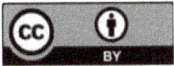

nutrients

MDPI

Article

Mothers' Perceptions of Toddler Beverages

Manuela Rigo [iD], **Jane Willcox, Alison Spence and Anthony Worsley** * [iD]

School of Exercise and Nutrition Sciences, Deakin University, 221 Burwood Highway, Burwood, VIC 3125, Australia; m.rigo@deakin.edu.au (M.R.); jwillcoxresearch @gmail.com (J.W.); a.spence@deakin.edu.au (A.S.)
* Correspondence: anthony.worsley@deakin.edu.au; Tel.: +61-03-9244-6743

Received: 12 February 2018; Accepted: 14 March 2018; Published: 19 March 2018

Abstract: Background: The prevalence of obesity among Australian pre-school children is a major concern with links to poor health outcomes. One contributing factor is excess energy intake. Sugar-sweetened beverages are energy-dense, nutrient-poor, readily available and have been implicated in the increasing prevalence of obesity. Furthermore, preschooler beverage consumption may develop into dietary habits that track into adulthood. There is little research on factors influencing parents' decision-making when serving beverages to their preschoolers, or on mothers' perceptions of preschooler's beverages. The aim of this study was to explore mothers' perceptions of commonly consumed preschooler beverages. Methods: The Repertory Grid Technique and the Laddering Technique methodologies were utilized in interviews with 28 mothers from Melbourne, Australia, to explore beverage perceptions. Results: A large number of diverse perceptual categories ('constructs') ($n = 22$) about beverages were elicited, demonstrating the complexity of mothers' perceptions when making beverage choices for their preschoolers. The five most common categories were related to health, sugar, dairy, packaging, and additives. Thematic analysis of responses from the laddering method identified three major themes: concerns about the types of beverages mothers would like to provide their preschoolers, the healthiness of a beverage, and the sugar content. Conclusions: Mothers' perceptions of beverages are sophisticated and need to be included in the design of health communication strategies by health promoters and government agencies to influence mothers' beverage selections for their preschoolers.

Keywords: toddlers; preschoolers; mothers; parents; sugar-sweetened beverages; Repertory Grid Technique; Laddering Technique; qualitative methods; Australia

---

1. Introduction

The high prevalence of overweight and obesity among young children is a major public health concern and is linked to poor health outcomes in childhood and adulthood, including non-communicable diseases such as Type 2 diabetes [1,2], sleep apnoea [3], and adverse mental health outcomes [4]. Poor diet quality, including excess energy, is associated with overweight and obesity in children including preschoolers [5]. Frequent and energy-dense, nutrient-poor beverage choices are indicators of overall poor diet quality [6], that may lead to excess energy intake and hence contribute to overweight and obesity. In addition, there is consistent evidence that dietary habits established in childhood track into adulthood [7,8]. Excess weight gain is difficult to reverse with interventions, thus early prevention is recommended [9,10].

Mothers are generally considered as the primary household gatekeepers [11]. They are typically primarily responsible for bringing beverages into the household and thus control their availability and accessibility [12]. They also influence beverage consumption through role modelling what, when and how to drink [13,14].

Mothers' perceptions or beliefs are likely to influence the types of beverages they provide for their preschoolers [15]. Unfortunately, there have been relatively few studies of mothers' perceptions of the beverages they provide for their preschoolers (or 'toddlers'), aged two to four years. Seven studies have examined mothers' perceptions of young children's beverages but four of them focused only on one attribute, health [16–19]. Two of the remaining three studies examined several attributes of beverages [20,21], although one of these examined only one beverage, chocolate-flavoured milk on six attributes [20]. In both these studies the researchers nominated the beverage characteristics that the respondents rated. Only one study in this area did not pre-empt mothers' perceptions of preschoolers' beverages and allowed them to identify attributes important to them [22].

More broadly, two studies of women's fruit and manufactured snack perceptions [23,24] are relevant here as they allowed participants to nominate their own food perceptions [25]. Both utilised the Repertory Grid Technique (RGT) to elicit perceptions of snacks compared to manufactured snack foods. Jack et al. [23] examined the self-elicited perceptions and the context of consumption of 15 snack foods, including sweet, savoury, fresh and processed in a sample of 12 friends and family members. These perceptions where then developed into a questionnaire which was administered to a sample of 51 women, aged 21–55 years, employed at a college in Edinburgh. They found that the women held a wide variety of perceptions, but these could be grouped into convenience and indulgence for manufactured snacks, whereas fruit was seen to be more suitable in certain contexts, e.g., for breakfast. Weston [24] examined mothers' perceptions, from 12 mothers, of six fruits and six manufactured, energy-dense and nutrient-poor, snacks commonly served to children aged two to five years in Australia. Again, a wide variety of perceptions were elicited. Subsequently these were incorporated in a questionnaire which was administered to 238 preschoolers' mothers. The results showed that mothers had four goals in mind when they fed snacks to their preschoolers: convenience, satiety, eating nutritious food and freedom from additives.

The present study was underpinned by the theoretical framework of the Food-Related Lifestyle Model [15]. This framework links lifestyle dimensions, such as beliefs about the concrete aspects of food and beverages (e.g., appearance, taste), higher order or quality attributed (e.g., nutritiousness), perceived consequences of consumption (e.g., health or mood effects), procedural scripts (shopping or meal-preparation skills), and personal values to food and beverage selection. The model has been validated in several countries and in cross-cultural settings [26–28].

In summary, there is a gap in the research literature in regards to mothers' perceptions of preschoolers' beverages. Therefore, the overall aim of this study was to investigate the beliefs and perceptions of commonly available preschoolers' beverages held by mothers in Melbourne, Australia.

2. Materials and Methods

2.1. Study Design

Two distinct methods were used in this study to provide a rich, in-depth exploration of the topic. The first method used was the RGT which is an established method based on Personal Construct Theory (PCT) [25,29–33]. PCT proposes that people understand or make sense of their world through their perceptions [30,32,33]. RGT is a semi-qualitative approach in which participants are asked multiple times to compare and contrast random sets of three 'elements' (in the present case: beverages), allowing the elicitation of bipolar 'constructs' (beliefs or perceptions) from the participant's reality [25,30,32], rather than the views of the researcher [34,35] .

The second method used in this study was "Laddering" [36]. It is based on means-end-chain theory [37] and allows the exploration of participants' motivations that underlie their beliefs or perceptions of objects such as children's beverages. It provides the link between the product attributes and the benefits of consumption and values of the consumer [36].

2.2. Study Participants

Mothers of children aged two to four years residing in two geographical areas in Melbourne, Australia were invited to participate in the study. The two areas were purposefully selected to represent different levels of socio-economic status according to the Australian Bureau of Statistics' Socio-Economic Indexes for Areas (SEIFA) [38]. We aimed to recruit approximately 15–20 participants based on the numbers involved in the qualitative portion of the study by Jack et al. [23] and Weston [24] of 12 participants. Flyers promoting the study were e-mailed to organizations that catered to young children, such as local swimming pools, crèches and libraries, to display to members. The senior author (MR) also visited some of these organizations to distribute the flyers in person. From details on the flyer, interested participants could contact the researcher via phone or e-mail for further information and a consent form. Mothers could arrange an interview at a time convenient to them and child and bring their children with them. Inclusion criteria included mothers with children aged two to four years and sufficient English to read the plain language statement. All participants received a $15 supermarket voucher in appreciation of their time, along with a unique summary of their perceptions derived from WebGrid Plus [39].

Ethics approval was obtained from the Human Research Ethics Committee at Deakin University, on the 10 April 2017, reference HEAG-H 35_2017.

2.3. Procedure

Consenting participants were invited to attend an interview at the recruitment venue or at Deakin University, and in-depth interviews were conducted. To review and streamline the procedure eight pilot interviews with mothers of preschoolers were conducted. These data were not used in the final analyses.

Each of the interviews were divided into two sections involving the administration of the RGT and then the Laddering Technique for the constructs that the participants considered important to them. Participant's socio-demographic characteristics were collected using a short questionnaire at the conclusion of the interview. These included maternal age, educational background, occupation, postcode, ethnicity, marital status, and whether the participant was the main shopper.

To determine the mothers' perceptions of children's' beverages, thirteen images of drinks commonly consumed by Australian preschoolers in the 2011–2012 National Nutrition and Physical Activity Survey (NNPAS) [40] were selected. Images were selected to represent a wide variety of products including different costs, nutritional values, and packaging types, with two featuring animated characters, given the appeal of animated characters to young children [41,42]. The interviews were audio-recorded and transcribed.

2.4. The Repertory Grid Technique

The beverage images were printed on A4 sized paper and presented in sets of three (triads). Mothers were asked which beverage was different from the other two and why. The mothers were advised that there were no incorrect or correct responses and that the researchers were only interested in the mother's own perceptions. The response to each triad (termed 'constructs' in PCT) were recorded in written form on five-point bi-polar scales (Figure 1). In judging the triads, the only caveat was that the participant could only use a construct once. Up to 12 sets of randomly pre-selected triads were presented to the mothers in the same order. Participants continued to judge new triads while they could provide a unique construct or until they had viewed all twelve triads. Once all the constructs had been elicited the mothers were asked to rate all 13 beverages according to the constructs that they had provided. For example, a construct might be 'milk-based versus non milk-based'; subsequently all the beverages would be rated on a five-point bi-polar scale with one anchor point being 'not milk-based' (scored as 1) and the opposite anchor point being 'most milk-based' (scored as 5).

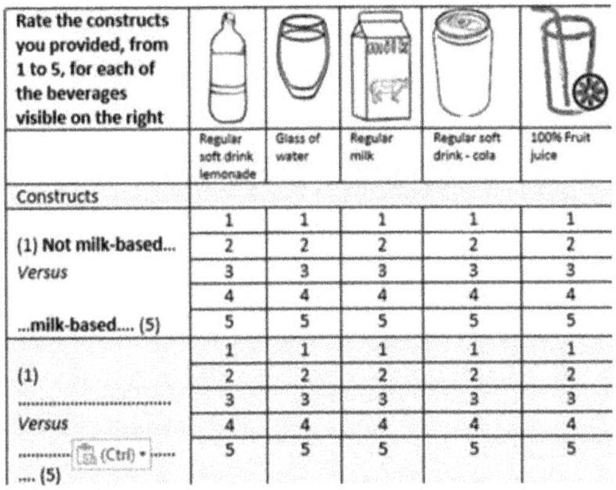

Rate the constructs you provided, from 1 to 5, for each of the beverages visible on the right					
	Regular soft drink lemonade	Glass of water	Regular milk	Regular soft drink - cola	100% Fruit juice
Constructs					
	1	1	1	1	1
(1) Not milk-based...	2	2	2	2	2
Versus	3	3	3	3	3
	4	4	4	4	4
...milk-based.... (5)	5	5	5	5	5
	1	1	1	1	1
(1)	2	2	2	2	2
....	3	3	3	3	3
Versus	4	4	4	4	4
.... (Ctrl) ▾ .... (5)	5	5	5	5	5

Figure 1. A portion of the bipolar scale on which constructs were recorded. Images have been changed to sketches to protect copyright.

2.5. The Laddering Technique

In the second part of the interview, the participants were asked if each of the constructs they had provided was important to them, and if so, why? Once the participant had provided a response, she was asked 'why?' again for further clarification. The laddering technique is qualitative in nature and the why questions are open-ended to explore the underlying motivations and values of the participants. Those participants who answered "no" to any constructs, i.e., they did not think it was important to them, were not asked the laddering questions for those constructs.

2.6. Data Analysis

Descriptive statistics were used to summarize the participants' socio-demographic characteristics (Table 1).

Table 1. Descriptive demographics of the sample.

Mothers	28
Age (years)	
25–29	3
30–34	8
35–39	12
≥40	5
Marital Status	
Married/De facto	27
Single/Divorced	1
Education	
Year 12 equivalent	4
TAFE [1] or trade qualification	5
University Degree or higher	19
Ethnicity	
Australian-born	17
Other nationality	11
Main Shopper in the household	
Yes	23
Shared the responsibility	4
No	1

Table 1. *Cont.*

Work Status	
On maternity leave	2
Employed full-time	3
Employed part-time/casual	12
Home duties/unemployed	7
Student	4
SEIFA [2] using Tertiles	
High SEIFA	17
Mid SEIFA	6
Low SEIFA	5
Mean Child Age (months) ± SD	38.68 ± 11.1 or (3.22 ± 0.93) years

[1] TAFE: vocational education for apprenticeships and traineeships. [2] SEIFA: socio-economic indexes for areas, a measure developed by the Australian Bureau of Statistics that ranks geographic areas in Australia according to relative socio-economic advantage and disadvantage [38].

2.7. Categorisation of Constructs

The constructs were grouped into similar categories according to the frequency of their key words (Table 2) [43,44]. The research team discussed and agreed on the categorization of these constructs.

Table 2. The six main categories of constructs elicited from the mothers.

Construct Categories	Number of Times the Participants Used the Construct
Health and Well-being e.g., Unhealthy/healthy *Hyperactivity* e.g., No effect on behaviour/can affect behaviour *Nutrition* e.g., Less nutrition for children/more nutrition for children; Contains no protein/contains protein *Satiety/Digestion* e.g., Does not keep him full/keeps him full *Teeth* e.g., Bad for teeth/better for teeth	41
Sugar—natural and artificial, intrinsic and extrinsic e.g., Contains no sugar/contains sugar; Natural sugar/artificial sugar;	33
Dairy e.g., Not milk-based/milk-based; No calcium/contains calcium	28
Packaging e.g., Not a plastic bottle/plastic bottle One time open/resealable	25
Additives e.g., Close to nature/contains additives	22
Pure, natural/man-made, artificial e.g., No or few natural ingredients/contains natural ingredients	19
Preparation e.g., Not ready-made/ready made	19

Table 2. *Cont.*

Fruit juice, fruit-based, made from real fruit e.g., Fruit-based/not fruit-based	17
Carbonation e.g., Not-carbonated/carbonated	15
Flavouring e.g., Natural flavour/artificial flavour	14
Soft Drink e.g., Not a soft-drink/soft drink	11
Diet Claims e.g., non diet/diet	9
Targeted to Children e.g., Not tailored to children/tailored to children	9
Real/Processed e.g., Not processed/processed	8
Miscellaneous e.g., Weak brand/strong brand Plant-based/animal-based Less tasty/more tasty Single serve/multiple serves	8
Water e.g., Little water concentration/essentially water	7
Caffeine e.g., No caffeine/contains caffeine	6
Organic e.g., Not organic/organic	6
Appearance e.g., Clear-opaque	5
Context e.g., Not a breakfast drink/breakfast drink Not a night-time drink-night time drink	4
Convenience/Cost Value e.g., Free, not-bought/must be purchased Have at home/have to buy	4
Origin/Environment e.g., Made in Australia/overseas owned Not environmentally friendly/environmentally friendly	3
Total	312

2.8. Analysis of Mothers' Repertory Grid Data

Each mother's ratings of all the beverages were analysed using WebGrid Plus [39]. In this program, participants' data were analysed by principal components analysis to derive 'perceptual maps' of each mother's perceptions of the beverages [31,45].

In the resulting perceptual maps, beverages that are in close proximity to a construct indicate that the participant perceived the beverage as having that particular attribute. Conversely, beverages that are far from a construct tend not to possess that construct in the mother's mind (Figure 2).

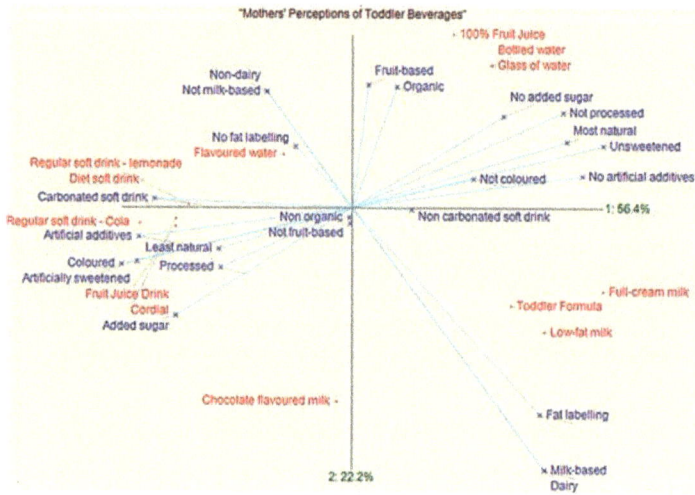

Figure 2. An example of a conceptual map of intermediate complexity.

2.9. Thematic Analysis of the Statements Derived from the Laddering Technique

The mothers' reasons for the importance of specific constructs, obtained from the laddering technique, were analysed via thematic analysis [34,35]. The statements were entered into Leximancer, an automatic thematic analysis software package. Leximancer uses statistical algorithms based on non-linear dynamics and machine learning to identify and group words or phrases according to their frequency and their co-occurrence [46]. These are termed 'concepts'. Concepts that cluster together form 'themes'. The themes are "heat mapped" according to the light spectrum; the red circle represents the strongest theme, and blue/violet is the weakest theme (Figure 3).

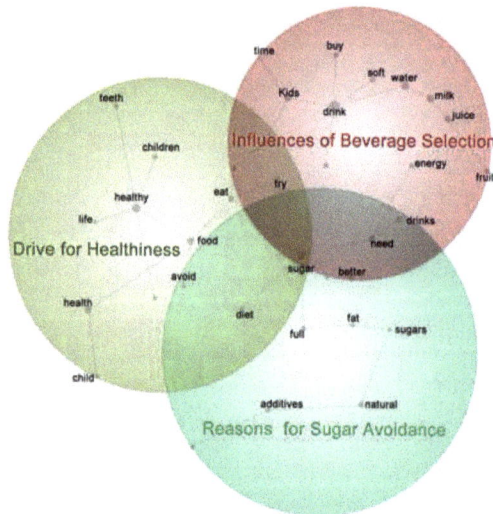

Figure 3. The themes derived from the laddering process. Theme size is set to 70%.

3. Results

Twenty-eight mothers of preschoolers aged two to four years participated in the interviews. Six further women who had expressed interest declined to participate for varying reasons (e.g., time constraints), and their demographics were not collected. The duration of the interviews was 20–55 min, with an average of 37 min.

The majority of the mothers (25/28) were aged over 30 years and all but one were married or in a de-facto relationship. Over two thirds (19/28) had a bachelor's degree or higher and 61% (17/28) were born in Australia with the remaining from ten different countries. Over four fifths (23/28) were primarily responsible for the procurement of foods for the household, and a further four participants shared this responsibility. Although mothers were recruited within organizations in the targeted area some lived in neighbouring suburbs of differing socio-economic position (SEP) based onSEIFA [38]. In total 17 mothers were in the high SEP, just over one fifth (6/28) were in the mid-SEP, and five were in the low SEP.

The number of constructs elicited per participant ranged from five to 12. The total, 28 participants provided a diverse range of 312 constructs about preschoolers' beverages. These were grouped into 22 categories (Table 2). The six most frequently mentioned perceptual categories accounted for 54% of all the constructs. Health and its sub-concepts, hyperactivity, nutrition, satiety, digestion, and oral health, were most frequently mentioned. In second place was sugar, in all its forms, from natural and artificial, intrinsic and extrinsic. The remaining top four construct categories were dairy, packaging type, and the presence or absence of 'additives'.

3.1. Perceptual Maps of Mothers' Constructs

Each mother's repertory grid data yielded a unique perceptual map of their constructs of the 13 beverages. There was great diversity within and between the maps. One example of a map of intermediate complexity is shown in Figure 2. Details of the other maps are available from the senior author. This mother perceived fruit juice drink and cordial as having similar attributes and she saw them low in "naturalness", processed, coloured and artificially sweetened.

3.2. Themes Derived from the Laddering Responses

Three main themes were identified, named as: 'Influences of beverage selection', 'Drive for healthiness' and 'Reasons for sugar avoidance' (Figure 2). Six minor themes included 'fruit', 'natural', 'body', 'teeth', 'time' and 'child'. There was some overlap of themes, for example many mothers mentioned 'sugar' and 'drink' in the same sentence.

3.2.1. Theme 1: Influences of Beverage Selection

The mothers were particularly concerned about the drinks their preschoolers consumed. All mothers considered certain beverages necessary or ideal for preschoolers such as water, milk and some mentioned juice, and they reasoned that these choices were important for health.

"The milk and some orange, like a fruit juice, they good because, and their taking. They need a water a little bit, but the cokes and other thing they not good for kids. Water is most important for them."

ID: 110, low SEP

There was also consideration of the purpose of the beverage by three mothers, of whether it quenched thirst or warded off hunger. Four mothers recognised that their children had limited appetites, or sometimes no appetite, and if a caloric beverage was provided, the child would not be able to consume a more nutritious food or beverage.

Four mothers mentioned their children's preferences, but most mothers decided they knew best. In an attempt to control consumption of undesirable beverages four mothers would ensure the beverage was inaccessible, for example supermarket shopping without her pre-schooler.

"I don't want the kids drink much soft drink although they really like it. So like if I take them to the supermarket and they see it and want to buy it. If I don't buy it they will not drink it. Usually I don't take them to the supermarket."

ID: 117, high SEP

In contrast, two mothers mentioned that their children influenced the beverage they received through their behavior.

"If she does not get juice when she asks for juice then the tantrum is not worth it."

ID: 106, high SEP

Eleven mothers acknowledged that the social and food context were considered when selecting a beverage for preschoolers. Therefore, a sugar-sweetened beverage might not be suitable for breakfast but acceptable for a birthday celebration.

"When we go to McDonalds we buy these things (pop-top fruit drink or soft drink). If we have a birthday or something."

ID: 127, low SEP

3.2.2. Theme 2: Drive for Healthiness

All the mothers wanted their children to have a good, disease-free, physically active and emotionally balanced life. Most acknowledged that both food and drink were important for good health, which included oral health, being physically fit and having strong disease immunity. Four mothers commented that it was important to develop habits that achieve healthy outcomes.

"I want him to grow healthy. I am trying to do everything I can in my power to make sure he has a healthy, well-balanced diet, to grow up healthy, and physically fit."

ID: 122, high SEP

Half of the mothers were also concerned about avoiding certain substances, like additives, or caffeine for health reasons, and the unknown consequences of these items.

" ... because the long-term effect of those additives on health are not always known and I think especially for young kids you don't want really want them consuming these artificial additives if you're not really sure how it will affect them short or long-term."

ID: 105, low SEP

3.2.3. Theme 3: 'Reasons for Sugar Avoidance'

Twenty-six mothers were concerned about sugar in their preschooler's diet. Generally, they felt their preschoolers consumed enough sugar in food, so additional sugar from drinks was excessive. One mother was concerned that sugar had worse consequences than fat in food.

"I think particularly for drinks, it should, it is always one of those areas where if you are going to cut down on sugar just not having sugary drinks is the one of the easiest ways to do that"

ID: 101, high SEP

Twenty-four of the mothers also worried about the short and long-term effects of sugary beverages causing conditions like hyperactivity, tooth decay, and diabetes. In contrast, two mothers believed that sugar was important and that it had a place in a child's diet.

"I think that sugar provides something to the body. I am not sure because I am not a doctor but I think that sugar still provides something to us, we need maybe a little bit because if we use too much we may be diabetes later. If you don't have sugar you will lack the nutrition or something like that."

ID: 117, low SEP

Three mothers differentiated between different types of sugars, for example: natural, added and artificial sugars.

"I prefer natural sugar because it is natural, you still have to keep track of how much she's having, but at least if it is natural it is better for you."

ID: 115, high SEP

4. Discussion

This study combined two methodologies, RGT and Laddering Technique, to provide rich data and in-depth exploration of mothers' perceptions of preschoolers' beverages. This is in contrast to most previous studies that have only focused on one attribute, health [16–19]. This study identified many unique and diverse perceptions of beverages commonly served to young children and also identified some of the motivations underlying their purchase and consumption.

The utility of the Food Related Lifestyle Model's was generally supported by the elicited perceptions which were complex and multi-faceted. For example, mothers mentioned their preference for serving milk over formula because of its convenience, a higher order attribute. Mentions of their preference for organic beverages because of their naturalness represent another higher order quality factor. References to lids on beverages are examples of concrete attributes that were linked to freshness and convenience (higher order quality factors). Similarly, references to the calcium content of milk can be seen as a concrete attribute but also as part of a shopping script: knowing and checking which beverages provided this nutrient. Finally, the avoidance of sugar-sweetened beverages to avoid child hyperactivity is a good example of a perceived consequence.

Multiple, Diverse, Perceptual Constructs

Although perceptual maps have been derived from previous studies of food perceptions [23,47] and preschoolers' snacks [24], to the best of the authors' knowledge, no other studies have used the RGT to examine mothers' perceptions of preschoolers' beverages. The perceptual maps of these beverages were unique to individual mothers and ranged from being very simple to highly complex. Nevertheless, almost 70% of all the constructs could be grouped into ten major categories, ranging from extrinsic concrete attributes, e.g., 'packaging', to abstract higher-order attributes, e.g. 'nutrition' and 'marketing to children'.

Some of the perceptual categories shown in Table 2 have been reported before. These include the various health-related constructs like hyperactivity, nutrition, satiety, digestion, dental health [16,21,22]; the mainly negative views of sugar and sugary beverages [16,17,20,22,48]; the benefits of milk [49], particularly for breakfast and at bedtime [21]; the concrete attributes of packaging such as lids to prevent spillage [19,22]; and the fear of additives [16,19]. The most novel feature of this study is the sheer diversity of the perceptions held by this small group of mothers and the complexity of the combinations of perceptions ('constructs') held by individual mothers. Whilst health related constructs were predominant, other aspects of beverages were also mentioned, such as their naturalness, content, appearance and suitability for children. Therefore, it cannot be assumed that one or two beverage attributes are important to mothers; intensive elicitation approaches are required to identify the main perceptions held within a population group.

The three major motivational themes derived from the thematic analysis of the laddering responses are consistent with previous research. The 'Influences on Beverage Selection' theme is about the contexts and maternal strategies that affect beverage purchasing and the control of the child's behavior by the mother or the child. These include the use of sugar-sweetened beverages as treats, the avoidance of situations such as supermarkets in which clashes between the mother's and child's purchase wishes might occur ('pester power') [50–55], and the provision of beverages such as sugar-sweetened beverages so mothers could avoid their tantrums (also reported in previous work [21,22]). This is similar to Weston's [24] findings that satisfying the child's demands and appetite were major considerations for mothers.

The 'Drive for Healthiness' theme highlights the nutritional trade-offs mothers may make between different beverages and foods according to their nutritional properties, for example, providing a chocolate-flavoured milk for its calcium content despite its sugar and additives. The theme is also linked to the development of healthy beverage preferences and life-long healthy habits [56–59]. Mother' beliefs in the importance of providing healthy drinks and setting up healthy habits concur with previous research that has shown that the early years are critical for gaining knowledge of which foods (and beverages) are suitable to eat (and drink) [55]. This highlights the importance of this research as mothers may provide a beverage to their preschoolers based on their perception of healthiness, but the beverage may not be recommended by dietary guidelines. Regularly supplying this beverage to the child may influence the child's preference and develop a habit or a 'junk food' dietary pattern with an excess of discretionary foods and beverages [6,57].

The 'Reasons for Sugar Avoidance' theme is topical, with over 200 articles in the "Newsbank" database of Australian newspapers [60] listed in the past 12 months and globally there has been an introduction of a sugar-tax on sugar-sweetened beverages in many countries [61,62]. The introduction of this tax has also been recommended by the Australian Medical Association [63]. This suggests that the perceptions identified in this study reflect recent shifts in public consciousness towards the dangers of excessive sugar consumption. This is a theme that is promoted by industry with increased production of low-sugar soft drinks [64] and health professionals, e.g., the dietary guidelines [65]. The increasing evidence of the effect of sugar-sweetened beverage consumption on the rising level of obesity in children [66,67] underscores the need for regular research in this area to gain insights on current beliefs that influence beverage consumption.

Some products' attributes such as taste and financial cost have been reported to be primary influences over adult food [67–70] and beverage selection [22,71,72] in many consumer research studies, but these were rarely mentioned by the mothers in the present study. Clearly, there are likely to be many differences between the context of this study of mothers' perceptions of preschoolers' beverages and adult food selection. As the laddering findings show, there are several higher order motivations underlying the mothers' selection of beverages for their children. Furthermore, the women in this study were relatively well educated and the majority were from mid to high SEP, which is associated with better diet quality [73,74] and fewer monetary constraints [75].

The present findings clearly show that preschoolers' mothers hold a great variety of perceptions about beverage attributes. When researchers pre-select certain perceptual attributes with little empirical foundation (e.g., cost and taste are commonly used), these may not reflect the diversity or priorities of perceptions and beliefs of the target population [76]. Any health promotion strategies, whether by health promoters, researchers or companies, should consider elicitation of perceptions as a first step. Such strategies are likely to be more effective if there is an understanding of the collective consciousness and individual interests of the target audience [77]. This would allow the creation of more tailored, and hopefully more effective, [78] health-focused strategies, consistent with the values and beliefs that are salient to the target population.

A limitation of the study was that the mothers were relatively well-educated and generally of high SEP so the findings may not reflect the socio-economic diversity of the Melbourne population. For example, mothers of low SEP may have perceived cost to be more important. However, the participants were ethnically diverse with 11 nationalities being represented and this allowed a broad range of perceptions to be elicited. The large number and variety of constructs identified in the study suggests that many perceptions of preschoolers' beverages important to the mothers were found. It remains for future research to examine the likely influences on these perceptions, for example, children's responses to beverages and mother's own preferences, and the extent to which they influence preschoolers' dietary behaviours.

5. Conclusions

Twenty-two categories of mothers' perceptions of young children's beverages were identified, indicating that mothers hold multiple, diverse perceptions. The perceptions ranged from 'concrete' attributes, e.g., packaging, to more abstract 'higher-order' perceptions, e.g., nutrition. These perceptions reflect the utility of the Food Related Lifestyle Model [15]. Thematic analysis revealed that the main motivational concerns for mothers were whether the type of beverage was suitable for their child in terms of context and behavioural control; the healthiness of the product in terms of nutritional trade-offs and long-term health habit formation; and the sugar content of the beverages. Future interventions to influence beverage consumption or research on beverage purchasing and perceptions and beliefs should include a perception elicitation component to determine the salient issues relevant to the target population. The findings could also inform interventions, planned for the near future, that educate parents of preschoolers about ways to determine the sugar concentration of beverages in order to make healthy choices.

Acknowledgments: Funding for this study was provided from HDR funding support from the School of Exercise and Nutrition Sciences, Faculty of Health, Deakin University.

Author Contributions: Anthony Worsley, Alison Spence and Manuela Rigo conceived and designed the experiments. Manuela Rigo conducted the pilot study and the interviews. Anthony Worsley, Manuela Rigo and Jane Willcox thematically analyzed the data and Manuela Rigo wrote the paper under supervision of Anthony Worsley, Jane Willcox and Alison Spence.

Conflicts of Interest: The authors declare no conflict of interest.

References

1. World Health Organization. *The Asia-Pacific Perspective: Redefining Obesity and Its Treatment*; International Diabetes Institiute: Brussels, Belgium, 2000.

2. Waters, E.; de Silva-Saanigorski, A.; Burford, B.J.; Brown, T.; Campbell, K.J.; Gao, Y.; Armstrong, R.; Prosser, L.; Summerbell, C.D. Interventions for preventing obesity in children. *Sao Paulo Med. J.* **2014**, *132*, 128–129. [CrossRef]

3. Beebe, D.W.; Lewin, D.; Zeller, M.; McCabe, M.; MacLeod, K.; Daniels, S.R.; Amin, R. Sleep in overweight adolescents: Shorter sleep, poorer sleep quality, sleepiness, and sleep-disordered breathing. *J. Pediatr. Psychol.* **2007**, *32*, 69–79. [CrossRef] [PubMed]

4. Dixon, J.B. The effect of obesity on health outcomes. *Mol. Cell. Endocrinol.* **2010**, *316*, 104–108. [CrossRef] [PubMed]

5. Ebbeling, C.B.; Pawlak, D.B.; Ludwig, D.S. Childhood obesity: Public-health crisis, common sense cure. *Lancet* **2002**, *360*, 473–482. [CrossRef]

6. Mrdjenovic, G.; Levitsky, D.A. Nutritional and energetic consequences of sweetened drink consumption in 6-to 13-year-old children. *J. Pediatr.* **2003**, *142*, 604–610. [CrossRef] [PubMed]

7. Mikkilä, V.; Räsänen, L.; Raitakari, O.T.; Pietinen, P. Consistent dietary patterns identified from childhood to adulthood: The cardiovascular risk in Young Finns Study. *Br. J. Nutr.* **2005**, *93*, 923–931. [CrossRef] [PubMed]

8. Golley, R.K.; Smithers, L.G.; Mittinty, M.N.; Emmett, P.; Northstone, K.; Lynch, J.W. Diet quality of UK infants is associated with dietary, adiposity, cardiovascular, and cognitive outcomes measured at 7–8 years of age. *J. Nutr.* **2013**, *143*, 1611–1617. [CrossRef] [PubMed]

9. Curioni, C.C.; Lourenço, P.M. Long-term weight loss after diet and exercise: A systematic review. *Int. J. Obes.* **2005**, *29*, 1168–1174. [CrossRef] [PubMed]

10. Kraschnewski, J.L.; Boan, J.; Sherwood, N.E.; Lehman, E.B.; Kephart, D.K.; Sciamanna, C.N. Long-term weight loss maintenance in the United States. *Int. J. Obes.* **2010**, *34*, 1644–1654. [CrossRef] [PubMed]

11. Reid, M.; Worsley, A.; Mavondo, F. The obesogenic household: Factors influencing dietary gatekeeper satisfaction with family diet. *Psychol. Mark.* **2015**, *32*, 544–557. [CrossRef]

12. Craigie, A.M.; Lake, A.A.; Kelly, S.A.; Adamson, A.J.; Mathers, J.C. Tracking of obesity-related behaviours from childhood to adulthood: A systematic review. *Maturitas* **2011**, *70*, 266–284. [CrossRef] [PubMed]

13. Scaglioni, S.; Salvioni, M.; Galimberti, C. Influence of parental attitudes in the development of children eating behaviour. *Br. J. Nutr.* **2008**, *99*, S22–S25. [CrossRef] [PubMed]

14. Peters, J.; Sinn, N.; Campbell, K.; Lynch, J. Parental influences on the diets of 2–5-year-old children: Systematic review of interventions. *Early Child Develop. Care* **2012**, *182*, 837–857. [CrossRef]

15. Grunert, K.G.; Brunsø, K.; Bisp, S. *Food-Related Life Style: Development of a Cross-Culturally Valid Instrument for Market Surveillance*; MAPP: Århus, Denmark, 1993; pp. 1–41.

16. Beck, A.L.; Takayama, J.I.; Halpern-Felsher, B.; Badiner, N.; Barker, J.C. Understanding how Latino parents choose beverages to serve to infants and toddlers. *Matern. Child Health J.* **2014**, *18*, 1308–1315. [CrossRef] [PubMed]

17. Hennessy, M.; Bleakley, A.; Piotrowski, J.T. Sugar-sweetened beverage consumption by adult caregivers and their children: The role of drink features and advertising exposure. *Health Edu. Behav.* **2015**, *42*, 677–686. [CrossRef] [PubMed]

18. McElligott, J.T.; Roberts, J.R.; Varadi, E.A.; O'Brien, E.S.; Freeland, K.D.; Basco, W.T., Jr. Variation in fruit juice consumption among infants and toddlers: Associations with WIC participation. *South Med. J.* **2012**, *105*, 364–369. [CrossRef] [PubMed]

19. Munsell, C.R.; Harris, J.L.; Sarda, V.; Schwartz, M.B. Parents' beliefs about the healthfulness of sugary drink options: Opportunities to address misperceptions. *Public Health Nutr.* **2015**, *19*, 46–54. [CrossRef] [PubMed]

20. Li, X.E.; Lopetcharat, K.; Drake, M. Extrinsic attributes that influence parents' purchase of chocolate milk for their children. *J. Food Sci.* **2014**, *79*, S1407–S1415. [CrossRef] [PubMed]

21. Mason, M.; Welch, S.B.; Morales, M. Hispanic caregiver perceptions of water intake recommendations for young children and their current beverage feeding practices. *J. Appl. Soc. Sci.* **2014**, *9*, 35–46. [CrossRef]

22. Tipton, J.A. Caregivers' psychosocial factors underlying sugar-sweetened beverage intake among non-Hispanic black preschoolers: An elicitation study. *J. Pediatr. Nurs.* **2014**, *29*, 47–57. [CrossRef] [PubMed]

23. Jack, F.; O'Neill, J.; Piacentini, M.G.; Schröder, M.J.A. Perception of fruit as a snack: A comparison with manufactured snack foods. *Food Qual. Pref.* **1997**, *8*, 175–182. [CrossRef]

24. Weston, C.V. The Role of Consumer Perceptions in Fruit and Energy-Dense Nutrient-Poor Snack Purchasing. Master's Thesis, University of Wollongong NSW, Wollongong, Australia, 2013.

25. Fransella, F.; Bell, R.; Bannister, D. *A Manual for Repertory Grid Technique*; John Wiley & Sons: Chichester, UK, 2004.

26. O'Sullivan, C.; Scholderer, J.; Cowan, C. Measurement equivalence of the food related lifestyle instrument (FRL) in Ireland and Great Britain. *Food Qual. Pref.* **2005**, *16*, 1–12. [CrossRef]

27. Grunert, K.G.; Perrea, T.; Zhou, Y.; Huang, G.; Sorenson, B.T. Is food-related lifestyle (FRL) able to reveal food consumption patterns in non-Western cultural environments? Its adaptation and application in urban China. *Appetite* **2011**, *56*, 357–367. [PubMed]

28. Brunsø, K.; Grunert, K.G. Development and testing of a cross-culturally valid instrument: Food-related life style. *Adv. Consum. Res.* **1995**, *22*, 475–480.

29. Fransella, F. *What Is a Personal Construct? In The Wiley Handbook of Personal Construct Psychology*; Winter, D.A., Reed, N., Eds.; John Wiley & Sons: West Sussex, UK, 2016; pp. 1–12.

30. Kelly, G.A. *The Psychology of Personal Constructs. Volume 1: A Theory of Personality*; WW Norton and Company: New York, NY, USA, 1955.

31. Shaw, M.L.; Gaines, B.R. On the Relationship between Repertory Grid and Term Subsumption Knowledge Structures: Theory, Practice and Tools. In *Research and Development in Expert Systems*; Bramer, M., Milne, R., Eds.; Cambridge University Press: Cambridge, UK, 1993; pp. 125–143.

32. Lexicon, F.T. Definition of Repertory Grid Technique. 2017. Available online: http://lexicon.ft.com/Term?term=repertory-grid-technique (accessed on 21 September 2017).

33. Jankowicz, D. *The Easy Guide to Repertory Grids*; John Wiley & Sons Ltd.: Chichester, UK, 2004.

34. Creswell, J.W.; Miller, D.L. Determining validity inquiry in qualitative. *Theory Pract.* **2000**, *39*, 124–130. [CrossRef]

35. Pillow, W. Confession, catharsis, or cure? Rethinking the uses of reflexivity as methodological power in qualitative research. *Int. J. Qual. Stud. Edu.* **2003**, *16*, 175–196. [CrossRef]

36. Gutman, J. A means-end chain model based on consumer categorization processes. *J. Mark.* **1982**, *16*, 60–72. [CrossRef]

37. Olson, J.C. Theoretical foundations of means-end chains. *Werbeforsch. Prax.* **1989**, *5*, 174–178.

38. Australian Bureau of Statistics. Socio-Economic Indexes for Areas. Available online: http://www.abs.gov.au/websitedbs/censushome.nsf/home/seifa (accessed on 21 December 2017).

39. Shaw, M.L.; Gaines, B. WebGrid Plus. 2016. Available online: http://webgrid.uvic.ca/ (accessed on 23 April 2017).

40. Australian Bureau of Statistics. *Australian Health Survey: First Results 2011–2012*; Australian Bureau of Statistics: Canberra, Australia, 2014. Available online: http://www.abs.gov.au/ausstats/abs@.nsf/Lookup/4364.0.55.007main+features12011-12 (accessed on 8 May 2016).

41. Kraak, V.I.; Story, M. Influence of food companies' brand mascots and entertainment companies' cartoon media characters on children's diet and health: A systematic review and research needs. *Obes. Rev.* **2015**, *16*, 107–126. [CrossRef] [PubMed]

42. Roberto, C.A.; Baik, J.; Harris, J.L.; Brownell, K.D. Influence of licensed characters on children's taste and snack preferences. *Pediatrics* **2010**, *126*, 88–93. [CrossRef] [PubMed]

43. Hsieh, H.F.; Shannon, S.E. Three approaches to qualitative content analysis. *Qual. Health Res.* **2005**, *15*, 1277–1288. [CrossRef] [PubMed]

44. Bryman, A.; Bell, E. *Business Research Methods*; Oxford University Press: New York, NY, USA, 2011.

45. Shaw, M.L. The analysis of a repertory grid. *Br. J. Med. Psychol.* **1980**, *53*, 117–126. [CrossRef] [PubMed]

46. Smith, A.E.; Humphreys, M.S. Evaluation of unsupervised semantic mapping of natural language with Leximancer concept mapping. *Behav. Res. Methods* **2006**, *38*, 262–279. [CrossRef] [PubMed]

47. Jack, F.R.; Piacentini, M.G.; Schröder, M.J.A. Perception and role of fruit in the workday diets of Scottish lorry drivers. *Appetite* **1998**, *30*, 139–149. [CrossRef] [PubMed]

48. Bucher, T.; Siegrist, M. Children's and parents' health perception of different soft drinks. *Br. J. Nutr.* **2015**, *113*, 526–535. [CrossRef] [PubMed]

49. Greer, F.R.; Krebs, N.F. Optimizing bone health and calcium intakes of infants, children, and adolescents. *Pediatrics* **2006**, *117*, 578–585. [CrossRef] [PubMed]

50. Miller, K.E.; Ginter, J.L. An investigation of situational variation in brand choice behavior and attitude. *J. Mark. Res.* **1979**, *16*, 111–123. [CrossRef]

51. Suwandinata, H. Children's Influence on the Family Decision-Making Process in Food Buying and Consumption: An Empirical Study of Children Influence in Jakarta-Indonesia. Ph.D. Thesis, Universitätsbibliothek, Gießen, Germany, 2012.

52. Haselhoff, V.; Faupel, U.; Holzmüller, H. Strategies of children and parents during shopping for groceries. *Young Consum.* **2014**, *15*, 17–36. [CrossRef]

53. Nicholls, A.J.; Cullen, P. The child–parent purchase relationship: 'Pester power', human rights and retail ethics. *J. Retail. Consum. Serv.* **2004**, *11*, 75–86. [CrossRef]

54. Russell, C.G.; Worsley, A. Why don't they like that? And can I do anything about it? The nature and correlates of parents' attributions and self-efficacy beliefs about preschool children's food preferences. *Appetite* **2013**, *66*, 34–43. [CrossRef] [PubMed]

55. Cashdan, E. A sensitive period for learning about food. *Hum. Nat.* **1994**, *5*, 279–291. [CrossRef] [PubMed]

56. Köster, E.P. Diversity in the determinants of food choice: A psychological perspective. *Food Qual. Pref.* **2009**, *20*, 70–82. [CrossRef]

57. Lanigan, J.; Singhal, A. Early nutrition and long-term health: A practical approach: Symposium on 'Early nutrition and later disease: Current concepts, research and implications'. *Proc. Nutr. Soc.* **2009**, *68*, 422–429. [CrossRef] [PubMed]

58. Birch, L.L. Development of food preferences. *Annu. Rev. Nutr.* **1999**, *19*, 41–62. [CrossRef] [PubMed]

59. Leung, C.W.; DiMatteo, S.G.; Gosliner, W.A.; Ritchie, L.D. Sugar-sweetened beverage and water intake in relation to diet quality in U.S. Children. *Am. J. Prev. Med.* **2018**, *54*, 394–402. [CrossRef] [PubMed]

60. Newsbank Newspapers. *Newsbank Newspapers—Australia and the World, 2016–2017*; Newsbank Newspapers: Naples, FL, USA.

61. Colchero, M.A.; Popkin, B.M.; Rivera, J.A.; Ng, S.W. Beverage purchases from stores in Mexico under the excise tax on sugar sweetened beverages: Observational study. *BMJ* **2016**, *352*, h6704. [CrossRef] [PubMed]

62. Berardi, N.; Sevestre, P.; Tepaut, M.; Vigneronm, A. The impact of a 'soda tax' on prices: Evidence from French micro data. *Appl. Econ.* **2016**, *18*, 3976–3994. [CrossRef]

63. Australian Medical Association Position Statement. Nutrtion—2018, AMA Recommendations. 2018. Available online: https://ama.com.au/position-statement/nutrition-2018 (accessed on 16 January 2018).

64. Levy, G.; Tapsell, L. Shifts in purchasing patterns of non-alcoholic, water-based beverages in Australia, 1997–2006. *Nutr. Diet.* **2007**, *64*, 268–279. [CrossRef]

65. NHMRC. Australian Dietary Guidelines. 2013. Available online: https://www.nhmrc.gov.au/guidelines/publications/n55 (accessed on 16 March 2017).

66. Vartanian, L.R.; Herman, C.P.; Wansink, B. Are we aware of the external factors that influence our food intake? *Health Psychol.* **2008**, *27*, 533. [CrossRef] [PubMed]

67. Anderson, P.M.; Butcher, K.F. Childhood obesity: Trends and potential causes. *Future Child* **2006**, *16*, 19–45. [CrossRef] [PubMed]

68. Furst, T.; Connors, M.; Bisogni, C.A.; Sobal, J.; Falk, L.W. Food choice: A conceptual model of the process. *Appetite* **1996**, *26*, 247–266. [CrossRef] [PubMed]

69. Drewnowski, A. Taste preferences and food intake. *Annu. Rev. Nutr.* **1997**, *17*, 237–253. [CrossRef] [PubMed]

70. Glanz, K.; Basil, M.; Maibach, E.W.; Snyder, D. Why Americans eat what they do: Taste, nutrition, cost, convenience, and weight control concerns as influences on food consumption. *J. Am. Diet. Assoc.* **1998**, *98*, 1118–1126. [CrossRef]

71. Lewis, C.J.; Sims, L.S.; Shannon, B. Examination of specific nutrition/health behaviors using a social cognitive model. *J. Am. Diet. Assoc.* **1989**, *89*, 194–202. [PubMed]

72. Zoellner, J.; Krzeski, M.S.; Harden, S.; Cook, E.; Allen, K.; Estabrooks, P.A. Qualitative application of the theory of planned behavior to understand beverage consumption behaviors among adults. *J. Acad. Nutr. Diet.* **2012**, *112*, 1774–1784. [CrossRef] [PubMed]

73. Brady, C.F. Making Health a Priority: Constrained Choices at the Grocery Store. Ph.D. Thesis, University of Kentucky, Lexington, KY, USA, 2016.

74. Zanoli, R.; Naspetti, S. Consumer motivations in the purchase of organic food: A means-end approach. *Br. Food J.* **2002**, *104*, 643–653. [CrossRef]

75. Turrell, G.; Kavanagh, A.M. Socio-economic pathways to diet: Modelling the association between socio-economic position and food purchasing behaviour. *Public Health Nutr.* **2006**, *9*, 375–383. [CrossRef] [PubMed]

76. Grunert, K.G.; Bech-Larsen, T. Explaining choice option attractiveness by beliefs elicited by the laddering method. *J. Econ. Psychol.* **2005**, *26*, 223–241. [CrossRef]

77. Andreasen, A.R. Marketing social marketing in the social change marketplace. *J. Public Policy Mark.* **2002**, *21*, 3–13. [CrossRef]

78. Rimer, B.K.; Kreuter, M.W. Advancing tailored health communication: A persuasion and message effects perspective. *J. Commun.* **2006**, *56*, S184–S201. [CrossRef]

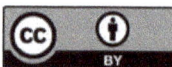

nutrients

MDPI

Article

The Impact of Caloric and Non-Caloric Sweeteners on Food Intake and Brain Responses to Food: A Randomized Crossover Controlled Trial in Healthy Humans

Camille Crézé [1], Laura Candal [1], Jérémy Cros [1], Jean-François Knebel [2,3], Kevin Seyssel [1], Nathalie Stefanoni [1], Philippe Schneiter [1], Micah M. Murray [2,3,4,5], Luc Tappy [1,6] and Ulrike Toepel [2,3,*]

[1] Department of Physiology, Faculty of Biology and Medicine, University of Lausanne, 1005 Lausanne, Switzerland; crezecamille@gmail.com (C.C.); candlau@gmail.com (L.C.); jeremy.cros@unil.ch (J.C.); kevin.seyssel@unil.ch (K.S.); nathalie.stefanoni@unil.ch (N.S.); philippe.schneiter@unil.ch (P.S.); luc.tappy@unil.ch (L.T.)
[2] The Laboratory for Investigative Neurophysiology (The LINE), Departments of Radiology and Clinical Neurosciences, University of Lausanne and Lausanne University Hospital, 1011 Lausanne, Switzerland; jean.francois.knebel@gmail.com (J.-F.K.); micah.murray@chuv.ch (M.M.M.)
[3] Electroencephalography Brain Mapping Core, Center for Biomedical Imaging (CIBM) of Lausanne and Geneva, 1015 Lausanne, Switzerland
[4] Department of Hearing and Speech Sciences, Vanderbilt University, Nashville, TN 37232, USA
[5] Department of Ophthalmology, Jules Gonin Eye Hospital, 1004 Lausanne, Switzerland
[6] Metabolic Center, Hôpital Intercantonal de la Broye, 1470 Estavayer-le-Lac, Switzerland
* Correspondence: ulrike.toepel@unil.ch; Tel.: +41-(0)21-314-13-17

Received: 12 April 2018; Accepted: 10 May 2018; Published: 15 May 2018

Abstract: Whether non-nutritive sweetener (NNS) consumption impacts food intake behavior in humans is still unclear. Discrepant sensory and metabolic signals are proposed to mislead brain regulatory centers, in turn promoting maladaptive food choices favoring weight gain. We aimed to assess whether ingestion of sucrose- and NNS-sweetened drinks would differently alter brain responses to food viewing and food intake. Eighteen normal-weight men were studied in a fasted condition and after consumption of a standardized meal accompanied by either a NNS-sweetened (NNS), or a sucrose-sweetened (SUC) drink, or water (WAT). Their brain responses to visual food cues were assessed by means of electroencephalography (EEG) before and 45 min after meal ingestion. Four hours after meal ingestion, spontaneous food intake was monitored during an ad libitum buffet. With WAT, meal intake led to increased neural activity in the dorsal prefrontal cortex and the insula, areas linked to cognitive control and interoception. With SUC, neural activity in the insula increased as well, but decreased in temporal regions linked to food categorization, and remained unchanged in dorsal prefrontal areas. The latter modulations were associated with a significantly lower total energy intake at buffet (mean kcal ± SEM; 791 ± 62) as compared to WAT (942 ± 71) and NNS (917 ± 70). In contrast to WAT and SUC, NNS consumption did not impact activity in the insula, but led to increased neural activity in ventrolateral prefrontal regions linked to the inhibition of reward. Total energy intake at the buffet was not significantly different between WAT and NNS. Our findings highlight the differential impact of caloric and non-caloric sweeteners on subsequent brain responses to visual food cues and energy intake. These variations may reflect an initial stage of adaptation to taste-calorie uncoupling, and could be indicative of longer-term consequences of repeated NNS consumption on food intake behavior.

Keywords: electroencephalography; non-nutritive sweeteners; sweet taste; visual food cues; food intake; ad libitum buffet

1. Introduction

Excess sugar consumption, in particular in the form of sugar-sweetened beverages (SSBs), has been repeatedly identified as a major factor contributing to weight gain, overweight and obesity prevalence as well as associated metabolic disorders [1–3]. In order to fight increasing rates of overweight and obesity and help body weight management, many non-caloric molecules with a high sweetening power, called non-caloric or non-nutritive sweeteners (NNS), were developed and introduced into our daily diet. That is, hedonic properties of sweet taste can be enjoyed without consuming excess liquid calories. Yet, epidemiological studies have shown a link between NNS consumption and an increased prevalence of overweight and obesity risk on the long-run [4–6]. Although risks of reverse causality cannot be excluded when interpreting the results of observational cohort studies, one other reason for such a link could be functional properties of the central food intake regulation system discussed below.

In healthy humans, food intake is regulated by a fine-tuned balance between drives towards palatable items ('hedonic' processing and reward valuation), physiological needs ('homeostatic' processing), and inhibitory control. While inhibitory control is supported by brain areas of the executive function network, i.e., dorsal, ventrolateral prefrontal and parietal regions [7], reward valuation is assisted by cortico-limbic networks comprising basal ganglia, the anterior cingulate and orbitofrontal cortices [8]. Reward is integrated with homeostatic signals in the hypothalamus and insula. Gastro-intestinal hormones secreted before (e.g., ghrelin) and after a meal (e.g., insulin), nervous afferents as well as sweet taste receptor activation in the mouth (and possibly along the digestive track) all provide feedbacks to the brain and thereby inform these networks on physiological states and consequences of food ingestion [9–11]. This regulatory system likely evolved with a caloric value assigned to sweet taste, as naturally occurring sweeteners generally contain about 4 kcal/g. Due to their sweet but non-caloric properties NNS might thus provide erroneous information to the food intake regulatory system, potentially inducing maladaptive food choices as compensatory mechanism [12,13].

In animals, findings support this hypothesis by showing detrimental effects of NNS consumption on food intake behavior and increased adiposity and body weight longitudinally [14,15]. So far, the impact of NNS consumption on food choices and body weight control in humans remains controversial, showing either beneficial, detrimental, or no effects [16–19]. From a neurophysiological perspective, some studies have shown differences in the cerebral processing of taste information between NNS and sucrose stimuli of equal sweetness intensity, highlighting the capacity of the human brain to readily discriminate between caloric and non-caloric sweet taste [20–22]. However, these studies assessed immediate gustatory responses and neural activity, but not subsequent food cravings and intake of excess solid calories.

Neuroimaging studies in humans have further shown that food cravings and choices often result from exposure to visual food cues [23,24]. However, only one study, to our knowledge, has investigated brain response modulations to food cue exposure following NNS consumption in humans, i.e., in the context of a 3-month replacement of sucrose-sweetened beverages by artificially sweetened equivalents [25]. This former study of our group highlighted the potential implication of central cognitive control mechanisms in weight loss failure. However, that study did not directly compare the impact of consuming caloric vs. non-caloric sweeteners on responses. Further, participants had not been blinded to the type of beverage they consumed. Thus, how NNS influence subsequent drives towards certain types of foods (in particular sweet foods) and how this relates to modulations in food intake behavior remains largely unknown.

The goal of our current study was thus to investigate whether, as compared to water consumption, activation of sweet taste receptors with NNS or with sucrose, as part of a standardized meal, exert different acute effects on (a) postprandial brain responses to food viewing, (b) postprandial gastro-intestinal hormone secretion known to impact hunger and satiety feelings and (c) subsequent food intake behavior, both in terms of quantity and quality of choices (ad libitum buffet).

2. Materials and Methods

2.1. Participants

Eighteen healthy, normal-weight men were recruited. All volunteers used to drink on average ≥3 cans of 33 cL of SSBs per week. None of the participants had current, prior, or family history of diabetes, cardiovascular, kidney, hepatic, neurological or psychiatric disease. Further exclusion criteria were color blindness, particular diets (e.g., vegetarianism), any food intolerance or allergy, arterial blood pressure > 140/90 mmHg at rest, exercising for more than 3 h per week, current medication, drug-taking or smoking habits, and consuming more than 10 g of alcohol per day. Only infrequent consumers of NNS-sweetened beverages (≤1 can of 33 cL per week) were included. All volunteers were weight-stable, right-handed according to the Edinburgh Handedness Inventory [26], and had normal or corrected-to-normal vision. To ensure medical safety, volunteers were not included when hemoglobin and ferritin levels were below 13.5 g/L and 50 μg/L respectively, when weighing less than 50 kg, and when having donated blood or participated to another clinical trial in the prior three months.

Recruitment was done by means of advertising at local university campuses. Recruitment, screening, and follow-up of participants is shown in Figure 1A. Potential participants were first screened by email and then invited to a screening visit. Nineteen volunteers met all eligibility criteria and were enrolled in the study. One participant had to be excluded due to medical discomfort during the first test day; so that 18 volunteers completed the entire protocol.

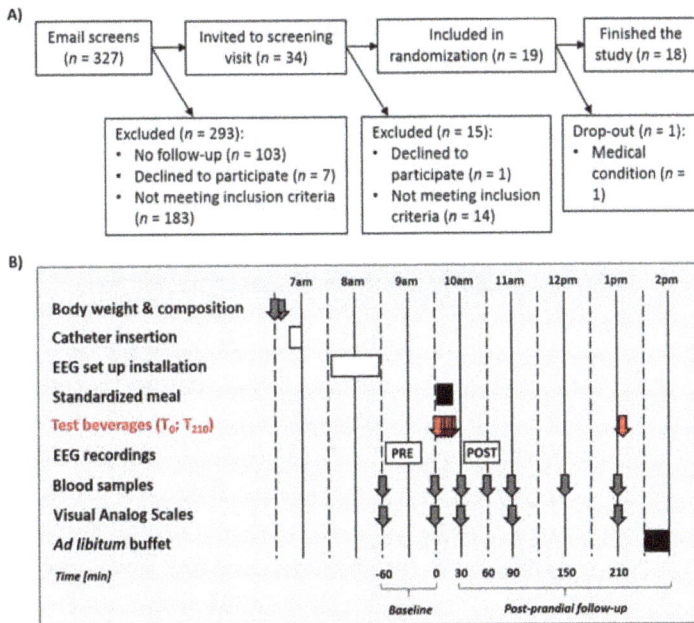

Figure 1. (**A**) Flow diagram for study participants' eligibility, enrollment, and follow-up. (**B**) Detailed protocol of the in-center test days. Identical procedures were used on the three test days. Test beverages (WAT, SUC, NNS) were ingested at $T = 0$ min (350 mL; five 70 mL-glasses every 5 min) and at $T = 210$ min (one 200 mL glass). EEG: electroencephalographic recording session.

2.2. General Procedure

The study consisted of three in-center test days for each volunteer, on which one of the three beverage conditions (i.e., Water, Sucrose, and NNS consumption, further referred to as WAT, SUC, and

NNS) was tested in a randomized crossover controlled design. The beverage conditions were separated by a wash-out period of three weeks. Each test day was preceded by a 5-day nutritional and lifestyle recommendation period followed by a 2-day run-in period. During this run-in period, volunteers received a controlled weight-maintenance diet (55% carbohydrates (including 10% as sugars), 30% lipids and 15% proteins) calculated from the Harris–Benedict equation with a physical activity factor set at 1.5. Participants were instructed to consume all meals and snacks at specified times of the day (7 a.m., 10 a.m., 12 a.m., 3 p.m., 7 p.m.), and to drink only water.

Detailed procedures for the in-center test days are provided in Figure 1B. On each test day, volunteers reported to the Metabolism, Nutrition, and Physical Activity unit from the Clinical Research Center of the Lausanne University Hospital at 6.30 a.m. They were fasting since 10 p.m. the evening before the test. They were asked to void, and body weight was measured thereafter (Seca 708, Seca GmbH, Hamburg, Germany). Body composition was assessed using bio-electrical impedancemetry (Biacorpus, Medical Healthcare GmbH, Germany). Each volunteer was then placed in a bed, and a catheter was inserted into an antecubital vein of the left forearm to allow for repeated blood collection throughout the test day. The venous path was kept open with a slow perfusion of saline solution (NaCl 0.9%). Two blood samples were collected in fasted state at $T = -60$ and 0 min before standardized meal and beverage ingestion. At those time points, participants were also asked to fill visual analog scales (VAS; 0–100) for hunger, thirst, and satiety levels as well as a Likert scale (LS; 1–9) for taste cravings. Each volunteer was then accompanied to a light-proof room where the electroencephalographic (EEG) recording system was installed. A cap with 64 active electrodes was placed on the participants' head and prepared so that electrical impedance between electrical sensor and scalp were kept below 40 kΩ. A first EEG recording took place between $T = -60$ and 0 min (i.e., further referred to as the pre-prandial recording session), while participants completed an online continuous recognition task. The EEG recording procedure, as well as visual stimuli and task used are detailed below (Section 2.8). At $T = 0$ min, a standardized meal and the 350 mL test drink (T_0-beverage; WAT, SUC, or NNS) were given to each volunteer. Five blood samples were collected over the post-prandial period, at $T = 30, 60, 90, 150$ and 210 min after meal and beverage consumption had started. At $T = 30, 60$ and 210 min, participants also filled VAS and LS for hunger, thirst, satiety, and taste cravings. A second EEG recording took place 45 min after meal and beverage ingestion (i.e., further referred to as the post-prandial recording session), that followed the same procedure as the pre-prandial session. In order to avoid ceiling effects and further strengthen the impact of beverage type on spontaneous food intake, participants received a 200 mL pre-buffet drink 210 min after the meal ingestion (T_{210}-beverage; SUC, WAT or NNS), its composition repeating the beverage condition. This drink served as a preload for further quantitative and qualitative assessments of spontaneous food intake at an ad libitum buffet taking place 20 min after the preload ingestion.

The primary study outcomes were pre- to post-prandial changes in brain responses to food viewing across beverage conditions. All behavioral and physiological parameters were considered as secondary outcomes. Study sample size was determined by assuming the same effect size on the spatio-temporal brain dynamics as in [25] $(1 - \beta$: 80%; α: 5%). The randomization sequence of treatment allocation was determined before the start of recruitment by random generation of blocks using the R software version 3.3.1 (R Foundation for Statistical Computing, Vienna, Austria). To ensure double-blinding of both participants and experimenters to the beverage condition, a third person (J.C.) prepared the beverages. The experimental protocol was conducted according to the Declaration of Helsinki and was approved by the Ethics Committee of the Canton de Vaud in September 2015 (protocol number 353/15). The protocol is registered in the international and national registers for clinical trials (clinicaltrials.gov: NCT02853773 and kofam.ch: SNCTP000001882). Participants were enrolled between February 2016 and April 2017. All test days were performed between March 2016 and July 2017. All experimental visits took place in the Metabolism, Nutrition and Physical Activity unit from the Center for Clinical Research of the Lausanne University Hospital. All volunteers were informed about the procedures during the screening visit and signed a written consent.

2.3. Meal and Test Beverage Composition

The T_0-beverage consisted of five 70 mL-glasses (i.e., 350 mL in total) corresponding to one of the three beverage conditions (WAT, SUC, NNS). Beverage composition was based on commercialized concentrations, as determined by Ordoñez and colleagues [27]. The SUC T_0-beverage provided 149 kcal (37.1 g of sucrose). The WAT and NNS T_0-beverages provided 0 kcal, with 137.2 mg cyclamate, 63.35 mg acesulfame K and 40.6 mg aspartame for the NNS. The standardized meal provided at $T = 0$ min was identical for all three beverage conditions. It corresponded to 30% of the estimated individual 24-h energy requirements calculated from the Harris–Benedict equation, and was low in sugars and sweet taste (55% carbohydrates (2% sugars), 30% lipids and 15% proteins). Participants were asked to drink one 70 mL-glass every five minutes and consumed the provided meal in-between, i.e., starting and ending the meal with the consumption of a 70 mL-glass. To maximize the sweet taste receptor stimulation by sucrose or NNS, each mouthful of liquid was to be kept in the mouth for ten seconds before swallowing. The T_{210}-beverage was of the same composition as the T_0-beverages. The SUC T_{210}-beverage thus provided 85 kcal (21.2 g of sucrose). The WAT and NNS T_{210}-beverages provided 0 kcal, with 78.4 mg cyclamate, 36.2 mg acesulfame K and 23.2 mg aspartame for the NNS. All beverages were provided at room temperature.

2.4. Qualitative and Quantitative Assessments of Spontaneous Food Intake

The ad libitum buffet presented at the end of the test day comprised 12 snacks, subdivided into 4 categories (3 snacks each) based on the fat content and taste quality of the foods provided, i.e., Low Fat/Non-Sweet (LF/NSW), Low Fat/Sweet (LF/SW), High Fat/Non-Sweet (HF/NSW), and High Fat/Sweet (HF/SW). The threshold for Low-Fat/High-Fat and Non-Sweet/Sweet subdivisions was set at 10 g of lipids/sugars per 100 g of food based on the nutritional information available on the packaging. The textures were matched as much as possible between food categories. The presentation context was kept as identical as possible between all beverage conditions, and always took place in the kitchen of the Clinical Research Center. Snacks were consistently prepared by the same experimenters (C.C. and L.C.), weighed and presented following the same protocol, and served on identical white dishes. Each snack was available in larger quantity than the expected average intake. The environment was kept neutral (e.g., no visible food packaging and no particular odor), and each participant was either accompanied by the experimenter or left alone for periods of five minutes. Participants remained uninformed of their food intake being measured, and were told to eat until feeling comfortably sated. Questions regarding food type were answered, but no nutritional information was given. Water was provided ad libitum with the snacks. All snack leftovers were carefully weighed after consumption. Total energy intake and energy intake per food category was calculated based on the nutritional information available on the packaging.

2.5. Analytical Procedures for Plasma Samples

Plasma was separated from blood cells immediately after sampling by centrifugation during 10 min at 4 °C and 3500 rotations per minute. Aliquots of plasma were stored at −20 °C until analysis. Plasma glucose concentrations were measured by enzymatic methods (Randox Laboratories Ltd., Crumlin, UK). Plasma insulin and ghrelin concentrations were determined by radioimmunoassay (Merck Millipore Merck KGaA, Darmstadt, Germany).

2.6. Behavioral Ratings

VAS for hunger, thirst, and satiety consisted of 15-cm long lines with '0' and '100' anchored to the left and right side, respectively, presented with the written indication *"Please indicate how hungry/thirsty/satiated you are at present by drawing a point on the line below"*. Individuals' responses were converted to % of the scale maximum. Taste cravings were assessed with a 9-point LS with 'salty' and 'sweet' anchored to the left and right side, presented with the written indication *"Please indicate how much you crave for a rather salty or sweet food item at present by ticking the correct box on the scale below"*.

2.7. Statistical Analyses of Food Intake, Behavioral Ratings and Plasmatic Parameters

Data distribution was controlled for normality and homoscedasticity using the Shapiro–Wilk and Bartlett tests, respectively. Data that were not normally distributed were transformed using the BoxCox algorithm. All anthropometric parameters (body weight, body mass index (BMI), and body composition), plasma concentrations and behavioral parameters (VAS and LS ratings) were tested for differences between beverage condition baselines with a one-way repeated-measure ANOVA including the independent within-subject factor of Beverage (three levels: WAT, SUC, and NNS). The impact of beverage type on food intake at the ad libitum buffet (total energy intake) was investigated first by a one-way repeated-measure ANOVA with the within-subject factor of Beverage. In a second step, the impact of the beverage type was detailed for food categories ingested by a two-way repeated-measure ANOVA with the within-subject factors of Beverage and Food category (four levels: LF/NSW, LF/SW, HF/NSW and HF/SW). Whenever a significant main effect of Beverage or an interaction Beverage × Food category was found, post-hoc paired *t*-tests (two-tailed) were conducted between Beverage conditions and/or Food categories. The effect of beverage type on the kinetics of plasma concentrations and behavioral scales was assessed using two-way repeated-measure ANOVAs with the within-subject factors of Beverage and Time. Whenever an interaction Beverage × Time was found, post-hoc paired *t*-tests (two-tailed) were conducted between Beverage conditions at each time point. Further, one-way repeated-measure ANOVAs with the within-subject factor of Beverage were conducted on plasma concentrations and behavioral scales at $T = 210$ min, irrespective of the kinetic results, to investigate the pre-buffet state. Whenever a main effect of Beverage was found, post-hoc paired *t*-tests (two-tailed) were conducted between beverage conditions. All data are expressed as mean ± SEM (standard error of mean). All analyses were performed with R version 3.3.1 (R Foundation for Statistical Computing, Vienna, Austria), and *p*-values ≤ 0.05 were considered as significant.

2.8. Electroencephalography (EEG) Stimuli Presentation Procedure, EEG Acquisition and Preprocessing

During both EEG recording sessions, color photographs showing foods that differed in fat content and in taste quality were presented to participants. This image database (240 items) has been used in several studies investigating food perception [25,28–30] and pictures were controlled for low-level visual features [31]. Stimulus presentation took place in a light-proof room, using the E-prime 2 software (Psychology Software Tools, Inc., Pittsburgh, PA, USA). Images were presented centrally for 500 ms each on a 19″ computer screen, in 3 consecutive blocks lasting 5 min. Each block contained 120 items, i.e., 80 initial encounters and 40 repeated items. Participants were asked to categorize initial from repeated image encounters via button-press. This behavioral task served to ensure participants' attention to food images, and they were instructed to perform as quickly and accurately as possible. Following participants' button press, the Inter-Trial-Interval (ITI) randomly varied between 250 and 750 ms to avoid anticipatory responses. During the ITI, a fixation cross was centrally displayed on screen to avoid eye movements. Number of trials between initial and repeated items were controlled across blocks and recording sessions to ensure similar difficulty of the recognition task.

Continuous EEG was recorded while participants viewed the images and performed the online recognition task. EEG was acquired at a sampling rate of 500 Hz using a 64-channel BrainProducts ActiCAP system. Details of the electrode montage can be found on the BrainProducts website (http://www.brainproducts.com/products_apps.php). All pre-processing analyses were performed using the CarTool software version 3.51 (2268) (https://sites.google.com/site/fbmlab/cartool). Only the responses to initially encountered images were used to compute visual evoked potentials (VEPs). VEPs were computed over the period from −100 ms to +500 ms peri-stimulus epoch for each image. During single subject averaging, EEG epochs were cleaned from artifacts with a semi-automatic procedure using a 80 μV rejection criterion and visual trial-by-trial inspection. Epochs containing eye blinks or other motor artifacts were manually removed. During averaging, baseline correction was applied on the peri-stimulus period (i.e., −100 ms to +500 ms), and data was band-pass filtered at 0.1–30 Hz. An additional notch filter of 50 Hz was applied. First, VEPs were averaged for each single subject, recording session (Pre- and Post-prandial) and beverage condition (WAT, SUC, and NNS). Electrodes with artefactual signals were then interpolated [32]. In a second step, group-average VEPs were calculated for each session and beverage condition, while baseline-correcting over the pre-stimulus period and recalculating the VEPs to an average reference [33].

2.9. EEG Analyses and Estimations of Neural Source Activity

Time windows of interest in brain responses to food viewing in the SUC, WAT, and NNS conditions were determined around GFP peaks in the group-average Global Field Power (GFP) waveform. The GFP is a reference-independent measure of the global amplitude of the electric field (VEPs), i.e., calculated as the standard deviation of the electric field amplitude across all 64 electrodes at a given time point [34]. These peak periods in the GFP represent the time windows of highest synchronized neural activity underlying distinct steps in sensory and cognitive processes, and thus served as a rationale for further investigation of beverage type-induced modulations in source activity [25,35]. The center and width of each time windows of interest were determined by the average peak timing and the standard deviation across participants' individual GFP peaks, across sessions and beverage conditions.

Over each time window of interest, we estimated the neural source activity based on the head-surface recorded VEPs using a local autoregressive average (LAURA) distributed a linear inverse solution [36]. That is, mean amplitudes of neural activity were calculated for each of the 4350 solution points of an inverse solution matrix based on a realistic 3D head model. The output of this algorithm is one scalar value ($\mu A/mm^3$) per solution point, per viewing condition and time window. As the goal of our study was to investigate the differential effects of three beverages on the meal-induced modulations in brain responses to food viewing, we focused our analyses on the relative change in neural activity from pre- to post-prandial recording sessions [25].

For each time window of interest, statistical analyses first comprised of whole-brain repeated-measure one-way ANOVAs with the within-subject factor of Beverage, computed on the % neural activity change from pre- to post-prandial session on each node of the 4350 solution point matrix. Only regions showing a significant main effect of Beverage in a cluster of ≥10 neighboring nodes were considered for post-hoc region-of-interest (ROI) analyses. Results of these analyses were rendered on the Montreal Institute template brain (MNI) and Talairach coordinates of the node showing the maximal statistical difference between beverage conditions are given for each statistically determined brain region. In each ROI showing a significant main effect of Beverage, neural activity of the source node revealing maximal statistical differences plus the 6 neighboring nodes was extracted and averaged in each individuals' data, for each beverage condition. These results are visualized as bar plots, indicating pre-to-post changes in neural activity to food viewing. Statistical outliers (< or >3 standard deviations from the mean) were removed from further analyses. Post-hoc paired *t*-tests (two-tailed) were then conducted on the respective pre-to-post change in neural activity (in %) between beverage conditions. Additionally, orthogonal one-sample *t*-tests (two-tailed) assessed, within each ROI and in each beverage condition, whether the relative pre-to-post % change in signal significantly differed from baseline (i.e., pre-prandial activity; [25]). Overall, only results with $p \leq 0.05$ were considered significant. All analyses were conducted using customized Python scripts, the software R version 3.3.1, and the STEN toolbox version 2.0 developed by Jean-François Knebel and Michael Notter (http://doi.org/10.5281/zenodo.1164038).

3. Results

Participants' body weight, BMI, body composition, plasma concentrations of glucose, insulin and ghrelin and behavioral ratings for hunger, thirst, satiety, and taste cravings are shown in Table 1 for each beverage condition. None of the parameters showed differences between beverage conditions at baseline (all p = ns).

Table 1. Study participants' anthropometric, metabolic, and behavioral characteristics at baseline.

	Beverage Condition			One-Way ANOVA	
	WAT	**SUC**	**NNS**	**F-Value**	**p-Value**
Body weight [kg]	66.6 ± 1.2	66.5 ± 1.2	66.5 ± 1.1	0.39	0.68
BMI [kg/m^2]	21.4 ± 0.4	21.4 ± 0.4	21.3 ± 0.4	0.12	0.89
Body fat mass [kg]	12.3 ± 1.2	12.2 ± 0.9	12.2 ± 1.1	0.04	0.97
Plasma glucose [mmol/L]	4.9 ± 0.1	4.8 ± 0.1	4.9 ± 0.1	1.23	0.31
Plasma insulin [µU/mL]	10.3 ± 0.7	9.8 ± 0.5	9.5 ± 0.7	2.33	0.11
Plasma ghrelin [pg/mL]	984.8 ± 94.1	925.7 ± 70.4	963.3 ± 94.1	0.90	0.41
Hunger level [%]	71.4 ± 5.1	73.3 ± 4.4	72.6 ± 4.7	0.12	0.89
Thirst level [%]	55.7 ± 5.5	67.1 ± 3.8	61.5 ± 5.1	2.38	0.11
Satiety level [%]	21.7 ± 4.2	23.6 ± 4.8	20.4 ± 3.4	0.25	0.78
Taste cravings (1–9)	5.4 ± 0.4	5.6 ± 0.5	5.8 ± 0.5	0.30	0.75

Data are expressed as mean ± SEM (standard error of mean). WAT, SUC, NNS: Water-, Sucrose-, NNS-beverage conditions. BMI: body mass index.

3.1. Spontaneous Food Intake at the Ad Libitum Buffet

Total energy intake and energy intake by food category at the ad libitum buffet are shown in Table 2. Regarding total energy intake, we observed a main effect of Beverage ($F_{2,17}$ = 3.62; p < 0.05), i.e., participants on average ingested significantly less energy in SUC than in WAT (Δ = −151 ± 59 kcal; t_{17} = −2.58; p < 0.05) and NNS (Δ = −126 ± 56 kcal; t_{17} = −2.26; p < 0.05). However, no significant difference was observed between WAT and NNS (Δ = 25 ± 66 kcal; t_{17} = 0.38; p = ns). Further analyses on energy intake segregated by food categories did not show an interaction between Beverage × Food category ($F_{2,17}$ = 0.54; p = ns), i.e., participants did not modify their food choice pattern as a function of the beverage type ingested.

Table 2. Spontaneous food intake at the ad libitum buffet.

	Beverage Condition		
	WAT	**SUC**	**NNS**
Total energy intake [kcal]	942 ± 71	791 ± 62 [a,b]	917 ± 70
Energy intake from LF/NSW foods [kcal]	142 ± 28	141 ± 29	167 ± 37
Energy intake from LF/SW foods [kcal]	77 ± 22	62 ± 15	78 ± 20
Energy intake from HF/NSW foods [kcal]	515 ± 74	428 ± 50	449 ± 56
Energy intake from HF/SW foods [kcal]	209 ± 36	161 ± 24	224 ± 35

Data are expressed as mean ± SEM. WAT, SUC, NNS: Water-, Sucrose-, NNS-beverage conditions. LF, HF: low-, high-fat. NSW, SW: Non-sweet, sweet. [a] p < 0.05 for post-hoc paired t-test (two-tailed) between SUC and WAT. [b] p < 0.05 for post-hoc paired t-test (two-tailed) between SUC and NNS.

3.2. Plasma Concentrations of Metabolites and Gastro-Intestinal Hormones

Plasma concentrations of glucose, insulin, and ghrelin in response to meal and test beverage ingestion are shown in Figure 2. The main effect of Beverage was significant for insulin (Figure 2B; $F_{2,17}$ = 8.29; p < 0.05; i.e., plasma insulin yielded overall higher values in SUC as compared with both WAT and NNS) and ghrelin (Figure 2C; $F_{2,15}$ = 4.56; p < 0.05; i.e., plasma ghrelin yielded overall lower values in SUC as compared with both WAT and NNS), but not for plasma glucose (Figure 2A; $F_{2,17}$ = 0.15; p = ns). More importantly, a significant interaction between Beverage × Time was observed for all parameters (glucose: $F_{2,17}$ = 2.83; insulin: $F_{2,17}$ = 5.31; ghrelin: $F_{2,15}$ = 2.41; all p < 0.05). Plasma glucose and insulin concentrations were significantly higher in SUC at T = 30 min (glucose: t_{17} = −3.77 and t_{17}= −2.46; insulin: t_{17} = −3.94 and t_{17} = −5.11; all p < 0.05) as compared to WAT and NNS, respectively. Plasma ghrelin concentration, on the other hand, was significantly lower in SUC, as compared to WAT; this difference being significant at T = 30 min (t_{15} = −2.77; p < 0.05) and

$T = 60$ min ($t_{15} = -2.48$; $p < 0.05$). No differences were observed between WAT and NNS for any of the parameter kinetics.

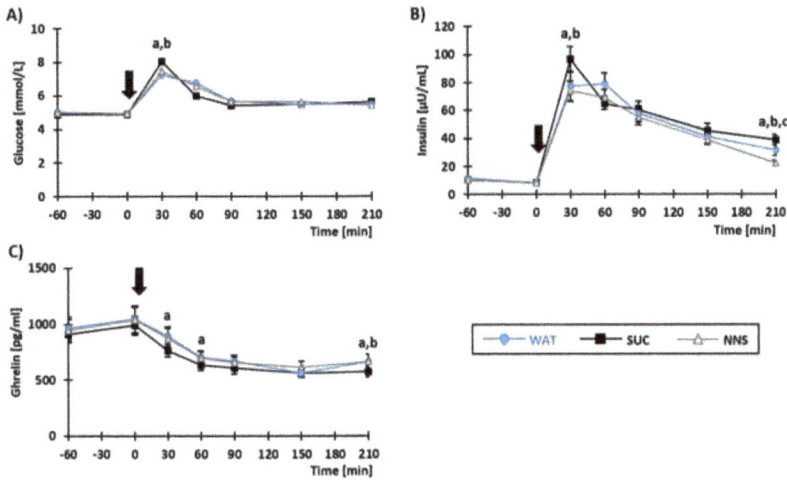

Figure 2. Plasma concentrations of glucose (**A**), insulin (**B**), and ghrelin (**C**) in response to beverage and concomitant meal ingestion at $T = 0$ min, indicated by a black arrow. Data are presented as mean ± SEM. [a,b,c]: $p < 0.05$ for post-hoc paired *t*-tests (two-tailed), respectively between SUC-WAT, SUC-NNS, and WAT-NNS. WAT, SUC, NNS: Water-, Sucrose-, NNS-beverage conditions.

Before the buffet ($T = 210$ min), plasma glucose concentrations were similar in all beverage conditions ($F_{2,17} = 0.70$; $p = $ ns). By contrast, a significant main effect of Beverage was observed for plasma insulin ($F_{2,17} = 13.04$; $p < 0.05$) and ghrelin concentrations ($F_{2,16} = 9.44$; $p < 0.05$). Plasma insulin concentration was most elevated in SUC ($t_{17} = 2.55$ and $t_{17} = 4.77$; both $p < 0.05$ against WAT and NNS, respectively), and the lowest in NNS ($t_{17} = 2.74$; $p < 0.05$ against WAT). Plasma ghrelin concentration was lower in SUC as compared with WAT ($t_{17} = 2.88$; $p < 0.05$) and NNS ($t_{17} = 3.89$; $p < 0.05$), but there was no difference between WAT and NNS ($t_{17} = 0.81$; $p = $ ns).

3.3. Results of Behavioral Ratings

No main effect of Beverage nor interaction between Beverage × Time were observed for any of the parameter kinetics (Supplementary Figure S1A–D for hunger, satiety, thirst ratings and taste cravings).

Before the buffet ($T = 210$ min), a significant main effect of Beverage was found on hunger ratings ($F_{2,17} = 5.68$; $p < 0.05$). Hunger ratings were lower in SUC as compared with WAT ($t_{17} = -2.71$; $p < 0.05$) and NNS ($t_{17} = -2.66$; $p < 0.05$). No difference in hunger ratings was found between WAT and NNS ($t_{17} = 0.28$; $p = $ ns). No significant main effect of Beverage was found for thirst ratings ($F_{2,17} = 0.07$), satiety ratings ($F_{2,17} = 1.10$) and taste cravings ($F_{2,17} = 0.37$; all $p = $ ns).

3.4. Pre- to Post-Prandial Changes in Neural Source Activity To Food Viewing

Two time periods of interest were defined around the peaks of the group-average GFP waveform. A first period of interest ranged from 120 to 150 ms, and a second period of interest ranged from 250 to 320 ms after image onset (Figure 3A).

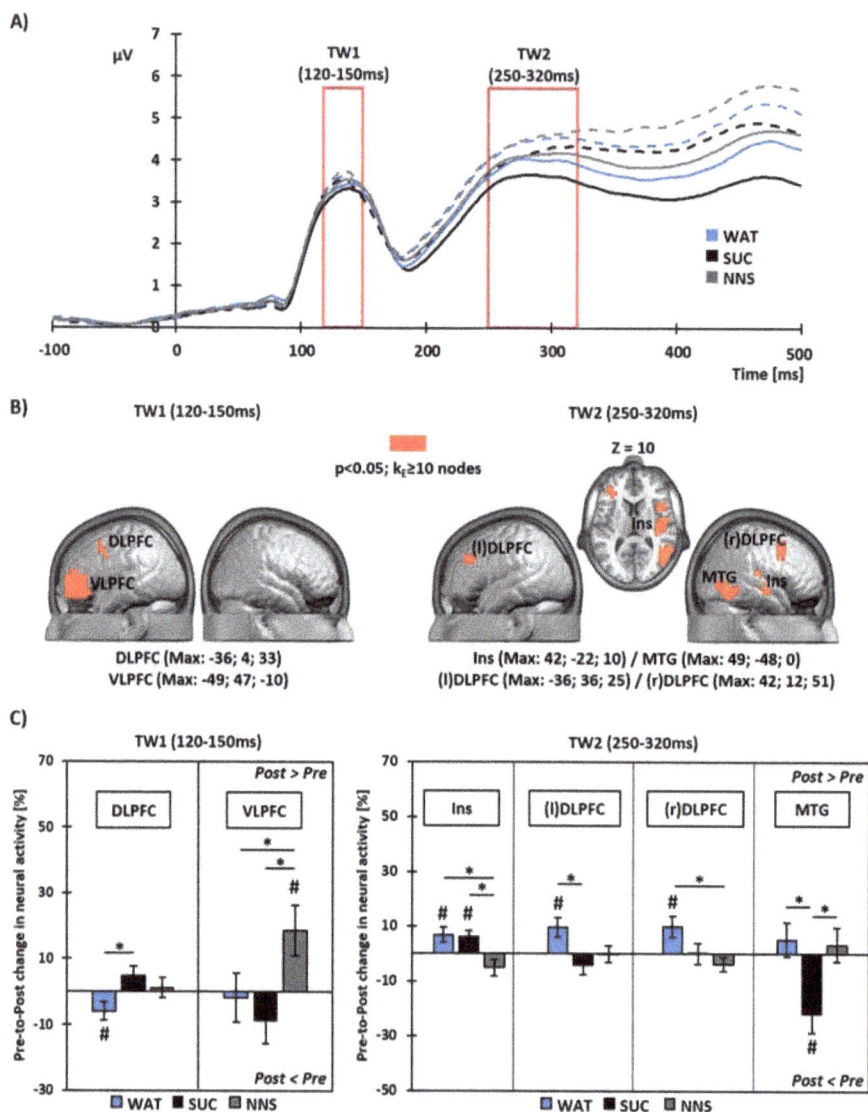

Figure 3. (**A**) Group-average Global Field Power (GFP) waveform over the peri-stimulus period (−100 to +500 ms from image onset). Red borders indicate the time windows of interest (TW) for subsequent neural source analyses. Solid lines illustrate the GFP during the pre-prandial recording session and dotted lines show GFP during the post-prandial recording session. (**B**) Visualization of brain regions showing a main effect of Beverage in the whole brain analyses on pre- to post-prandial changes in neural activity. Talairach coordinates (*x*, *y*, *z*) indicate the position of the source node showing maximal statistical differences. (**C**) Results of post-hoc analyses on changes in neural activity within each region of interest. Bar plots detail the direction of changes in each region of (**B**) and for each Beverage condition. Data are shown as mean (±SEM). *: $p < 0.05$ for paired *t*-tests (two-tailed) between Beverage conditions. #: $p < 0.05$ for one-sample *t*-tests vs baseline (pre-prandial). VLPFC: ventrolateral prefrontal cortex. Ins: insula. (l)- & (r)DLPFC: left & right dorsolateral prefrontal cortex. MTG: Middle Temporal Gyrus. WAT, SUC, NNS: Water-, Sucrose-, NNS-beverage conditions.

Over the first time window of interest (TW1: 120–150 ms post-image onset), whole brain analyses revealed a main effect of Beverage on the pre- to post-prandial % change in neural activity in the left dorsolateral prefrontal cortex (DLPFC; Max: $x = -36$, $y = 4$, $z = 33$) and in the left ventrolateral prefrontal cortex (VLPFC; Max: $x = -49$, $y = 47$, $z = -10$). That is, the beverage type differentially modulated the neural activity to food viewing within these brain areas (Figure 3B, left panel).

With WAT, meal intake led to decreased neural activity within the DLPFC ($t_{16} = -2.16$; $p < 0.05$ for t-test against baseline), but did not impact neural activity within the VLPFC ($t_{17} = -0.25$; $p =$ ns for t-test against baseline) (Figure 3C, left panel). Unlike WAT, there was no modulation in the neural response within the DLPFC with SUC ($t_{16} = 1.66$; $p =$ ns for t-test against baseline; $t_{16} = 3.31$; $p < 0.05$ for paired t-test between WAT and SUC responses). Like WAT however, SUC did not lead to modulated neural activity within the VLPFC ($t_{17} = -1.22$; $p =$ ns for t-test against baseline). NNS also did not impact neural activity within the DLPFC ($t_{16} = 0.39$; $p =$ ns). Yet, in contrast to WAT and SUC, NNS led to increased neural activity within the VLPFC ($t_{17} = 2.42$; $p < 0.05$ for t-test against baseline; $t_{17} = -3.20$ and $t_{17} = -4.19$; both $p < 0.05$ for paired t-tests between NNS-WAT and NNS-SUC, respectively).

Over the second time window of interest (250–320 ms post-image onset), a main effect of Beverage on the pre- to post-prandial % change in neural activity was observed in the right insula (Ins; Max: $x = 42$, $y = -22$, $z = 10$), in the left (l) and right (r) DLPFC ((l)DLPFC Max: $x = -36$, $y = 36$, $z = 25$ and (r)DLPFC Max: $x = 42$, $y = 12$, $z = 51$), and in the right middle temporal gyrus (MTG; Max; $x = 49$, $y = -48$, $z = 0$) (Figure 3B, right panel).

With WAT, meal intake led to increased neural activity within the insula ($t_{17} = 2.55$; $p < 0.05$), (l)DLPFC ($t_{17} = 2.82$; $p < 0.05$) and (r)DLPFC ($t_{16} = 2.60$; $p < 0.05$), but did not impact neural activity within the MTG ($t_{16} = 0.85$; $p =$ ns; all t-tests against baseline) (Figure 3C, right panel). Like WAT, SUC also led to increased neural activity within the insula ($t_{17} = 2.48$; $p < 0.05$ for t-test against baseline). Unlike WAT however, there were no pre-to-post changes in neural activity in SUC in the (l)DLPFC ($t_{17} = -1.09$; $p =$ ns for t-test against baseline; $t_{17} = -4.94$; $p < 0.05$ for paired t-test between SUC and WAT) and the (r)DLPFC ($t_{16} = 0.04$; $p =$ ns for t-test against baseline). In addition, SUC led to decreased neural activity within the MTG ($t_{16} = -3.21$; $p < 0.05$ for t-test against baseline; $t_{16} = -3.74$; $p < 0.05$ for paired t-test between SUC and WAT). In contrast to WAT and SUC, NNS did not impact neural activity within the insula ($t_{17} = -1.72$; $p =$ ns for t-test against baseline; $t_{17} = 3.11$ and $t_{17} = 2.86$; both $p < 0.05$ for paired t-tests between NNS-WAT and NNS-SUC, respectively). Like in SUC, there were no pre-to-post changes in neural activity in NNS within the (l)DLPFC ($t_{17} = -0.01$; $p =$ ns for t-test against baseline) and the (r)DLPFC ($t_{16} = -1.49$; $p =$ ns for t-test against baseline; $t_{16} = 2.56$; $p < 0.05$ for paired t-test between NNS and WAT). Like WAT, but unlike SUC, NNS consumption did not impact neural activity within the MTG ($t_{16} = 0.55$; $p =$ ns for t-test against baseline; $t_{16} = -2.46$; $p < 0.05$ for paired t-test between NNS and SUC).

4. Discussion

Our study aimed at investigating the acute impact of consuming caloric (sucrose) and non-caloric sweeteners (NNS), as compared to water, on the subsequent brain responses to visual food cues and spontaneous food intake behavior. As expected, we found neurophysiological and physiological markers of satiety following the ingestion of the standardized meal with water. We further observed that sucrose consumption impacted the responses in brain areas associated with cognitive control (prefrontal cortices) and food categorization (temporal cortices), and led to decreased subsequent food intake, indicating an adequate compensatory behavior. In contrast, NNS consumption did not alter spontaneous food intake when compared to water, but altered postprandial brain responses to visual food cues, most pronounced in prefrontal areas and in the insula.

4.1. Brain Responses to Food Viewing Following Water or Sucrose Consumption

Meal ingestion combined with water (i.e., control beverage condition lacking sweet taste and caloric load) impacted brain responses to visual food cues in bilateral dorsal prefrontal areas and in the right insula. The neural activity in dorsal prefrontal areas has long been linked with the capacity to exert cognitive control over food intake when exposed to palatable food cues, as part of the executive function network. Tataranni and colleagues [37] were the first to highlight differences in brain responses between hunger and satiety beyond hypothalamic areas using functional neuroimaging, and found increased neural activity in the dorsolateral prefrontal cortex. Since then, many other studies have found dorsolateral prefrontal regions to be involved in top-down cognitive control over food intake [38–40]. A study of Camus and colleagues [41] could even attest causality in the role of dorsolateral prefrontal regions in control and decision-making using transcranial magnetic stimulation. Using the high temporal resolution of EEG, Harris and colleagues [42] were able to provide further insights on the dual role of DLPFC in cognitive control, showing that early response modulations (around 150 ms post-stimulus onset) were associated with top-down filtering of sensory input, whereas later ones (from 450 ms post-stimulus onset) were associated with reward value modulation. In our study, we observed decreased activity in the left dorsal prefrontal region over an early time window following food viewing (120–150 ms) and increased activity in the bilateral dorsal prefrontal region over later timing (250–320 ms). Our findings thus likely reflect elevated cognitive control following meal ingestion, which is rather due to value integration than to response modulation by the sensory input per se.

We also observed increases in neural activity in the insula following meal ingestion accompanied by water. Insular responses to visual food cues have consistently been associated with interoception, i.e., awareness of bodily energy states. Also, the insula does contain molecular receptors for several gastro-intestinal hormones relaying this peripheral information to central nervous responses [11,43,44]. Furthermore, other studies have found increased insular activity subsequent to PYY infusion mimicking satiety [45], to mouth rinsing with a glucose drink mimicking food intake anticipation [46], but also in response to calorie ingestion as such [20,47]. The insula, being a hub between salience, homeostatic and control networks, is generally involved in signal integration, and thought to perform flavor-nutrient conditioning, too [48]. In accordance with these findings, we also found a higher postprandial insular activity following sucrose ingestion. Altogether, increases in insular activity both in the sucrose and water conditions thus likely reflect the adequate adaptation of participants' responses as a function of the beverage consumed when taste properties and caloric load were congruent.

Sucrose drinking (i.e., the beverage condition combining sweet taste and caloric load) elicited partially different modulations in brain responses to visual food cues as compared to meal ingestion with water. In particular, the postprandial response to visual food cues in cognitive control related areas was found blunted in the sucrose condition. Sucrose consumption also led to markedly decreased neural activity in the middle temporal lobe. This brain area is involved in the categorization and optimization of visual stimulus processing by attention [49], and is generally more active when participants are exposed to palatable food over neutral stimuli [50], as well as when responses to food are compared between hunger and satiety [24,51]. These differential patterns of brain responses to food cues following sucrose *vs.* water ingestion likely show that when sweet taste is coupled to a caloric load, brain responses shift from a rather reflective (usually involving prefrontal brain areas) to a more reflexive processing of food cues [52].

4.2. Brain Responses to Food Viewing Following NNS Consumption

NNS consumption (i.e., the beverage condition with discrepant sweet taste and caloric load) also yielded differential neural activity in response to subsequent exposure to visual food cues. In contrast to the ingestion of the meal with water or a sucrose drink, we observed early enhanced ventrolateral prefrontal cortex activity (120–150 ms after food image onset), but no changes in insular activity to food viewing over the later time window of interest (250–320 ms).

Increases in neural activity following NNS tasting in ventrolateral prefrontal cortices has been highlighted in gustatory processing when neural responses were assessed at the time of or immediately after tasting. For instance, Smeets and colleagues [53] have shown greater activation of the ventrolateral prefrontal cortex directly after the ingestion of an artificially sweetened beverage as compared to sucrose. Ventral prefrontal regions have been widely associated with hedonic integration and reward valuation of (visually) perceived stimuli, including food cues [54–56]. However, these functions were mostly attributed to medial parts of the ventral prefrontal cortex, whereas we show enhanced activity within the ventrolateral prefrontal cortex in response to visual cues following NNS consumption. Ventrolateral regions of the prefrontal cortex are part of the executive function circuitry, supporting decision-making adjustments, in particular related to motor response inhibition when exposed to cues associated with high reward, as well as targeting attention to behaviorally significant stimuli (reviewed in [57]). Thus, this area is proposed to be responsible for altering behavior as a function of estimated changes in the reward value of (viewed) stimuli. Our results show increased neural activity to visual food cues within the ventrolateral prefrontal area, likely related to greater (need for) impulse retaining and control over anticipated food intake. Although no study so far investigated the impact of NNS consumption on brain responses to food cues longitudinally, research in the gustatory modality showed differences in neural activation to NNS tasting between non-diet soda drinkers and frequent consumers of diet soda [58]. The study of Green & Murphy found increased responses to saccharin vs. sucrose in the ventrolateral prefrontal cortex in non-diet soda drinkers, whereas this difference was absent in frequent diet soda drinkers. These findings were interpreted as reflecting 'fading' neural activity in this region with repeated consumption of NNS, impacting impulse control over time. In line, we previously found decreased activity in the more posterior part of the ventrolateral prefrontal cortex following a 3-month replacement of SSBs by non-calorically sweetened equivalents [25]. Our current results thus provide additional evidence as to a target region for future longitudinal studies on the longer-term impact of sweet taste stimulation by NNS, and on responses to tempting visual food cues following NNS ingestion.

With NNS consumption, on the other hand, we did not observe pre-to postprandial changes in insular activity. This suggests that congruent caloric and taste signaling is required to elicit adequate response adaptation to food cues, and that incongruences between taste information and caloric load may impair nutrient-flavor conditioning [48]. Rudenga and Small [59] have further shown that the neural response to sucrose tasting in the insula (and also in the amygdala) decreased as a function of NNS consumption habits of participants, implying that this region might be more vulnerable to chronic dissociations between sweet taste signaling and metabolic consequences.

4.3. Integration of Postprandial Brain Responses to Food Viewing with Gastro-Intestinal Hormone Secretion and Food Intake Behavior

Sucrose drinking during meal ingestion, as compared to water, led to subsequent decreased food intake at the ad libitum buffet indicative of a compensatory food intake behavior. In parallel, we observed elevated plasma concentrations of insulin (an anorexigenic hormone) and decreased plasma concentrations of ghrelin (an orexigenic hormone), likely promoting some of the brain response alterations. Thus, the effects of sucrose intake may be related to hormonal signaling and/or to sweet taste receptor activation coupled with other peripheral satiety signals (e.g., vagal afferents). Yet, whether the observed differences are sucrose-specific effects or more general ones driven by an extra caloric load cannot be concluded from our current study, as there was no condition with a caloric load from another nutrient source (e.g., maltodextrin or fat).

NNS consumption did not lead to pronounced modulations of glucose, insulin, and ghrelin concentrations, nor to higher caloric consumption or variation of the food choice pattern at the ad libitum buffet. Thus, the observed changes in brain activity to food viewing post-meal and food intake pattern cannot be attributed solely to differential signaling of gastro-intestinal mediators. Although we did not measure other anorexigenic hormones such as leptin or PYY, the observed differences in brain responses between the water and NNS condition are congruent with the idea that discrepant information between sweet taste receptor activation and gastrointestinal hormone signaling leads to changes in brain response patterns [12].

4.4. Limitations

Several limitations of our work need to be considered. First, the study design likely pronounces the impact of the meal ingestion stronger than the impact of the test beverage. However, we aimed at designing this study with the highest ecological validity, i.e., having volunteers consuming standard amounts of beverages concomitant with a meal (quantity close to a commercially available can size). For this reason, we cannot exclude that the design was not sensitive enough to detect all secondary outcome differences, especially between the water and NNS conditions, and in terms of qualitative analyses on food choice patterns. Second, while we used a double-blinded design, participants could still detect the absence of sweet taste in the water condition, as opposed to both sweet taste conditions. Thus, some differences in brain response patterns might have arisen from these perceptual properties [60]. Finally, using electroencephalographic recording and electrical neuroimaging analyses, we are not able to detect deeper activity changes, e.g., in the basal ganglia (dopaminergic origin of the reward system), that might occur together with response modulations in cortices associated with higher-level functions.

5. Conclusions

To our knowledge, this is the first study to assess the impact of NNS consumption on neural activity to food viewing, and the relationship with food intake behavior. We did not observe an acute effect of NNS consumption on immediate food intake in humans who are not frequently drinking NNS beverages. Yet, we observed imminent changes in brain response patterns in brain areas that are key players in food intake regulation. The responsiveness of these brain areas to sweet taste has been shown to 'fade' as a function of longer-term NNS consumption [58,59]. Thus, it remains to be investigated whether such longer-term brain response alterations can also be observed to visual food cues, often mediating pre-ingestive food choices. Given such longer-term alterations, the brain response modulations observed under the NNS condition in our study might reflect an initial stage of adaptation to taste-calorie uncoupling, possibly indicating that longer-term alterations of food intake regulation (via responses to tempting visual cues) take place when NNS are repeatedly consumed over time. Our study thus provides first insights linking neuroimaging research in the gustatory modality and behavioral research on the impact of non-caloric sweetener consumption on food intake, by investigating the neural correlates of drives towards visually conveyed food cues.

Supplementary Materials: The following materials are available online at http://www.mdpi.com/2072-6643/10/5/615/s1. Figure S1: Behavioral ratings for hunger, satiety, thirst, and taste cravings in response to drink and concomitant meal ingestion.

Author Contributions: C.C., L.T. and U.T. conceived and designed the experiments; C.C. and L.C. enrolled participants; J.C. generated and assigned participants to allocation sequence, and carried out beverage preparation; C.C. collected the electroencephalographic data. C.C., L.C., J.C., K.S., P.S. and U.T. performed the metabolic tests; C.C., L.C., N.S. and J.-F.K. analyzed the data; M.M.M. and J.-F.K. contributed with materials and analysis tools; C.C., L.T. and U.T. wrote the manuscript. All authors had final approval of the submitted version.

Funding: The research was funded by a grant from the Swiss National Science Foundation (Grant number 32002B_156167) attributed to Luc Tappy. Micah M. Murray is supported by the Swiss National Science Foundation (Grant number 320030_169206) and by a generous grantor advised by CARIGEST SA for research unrelated to this work. The Cartool software used for EEG data analysis has been programmed by Denis Brunet (Functional Brain Mapping Laboratory, Geneva) and is supported by the Center for Biomedical Imaging (CIBM) of Geneva and Lausanne. The STEN toolbox (http://doi.org/10.5281/zenodo.1164038) has been programmed by Jean-François Knebel and Michael Notter, from the Laboratory for Investigative Neurophysiology (the LINE), Lausanne, Switzerland, and is supported by the Center for Biomedical Imaging (CIBM) of Geneva and Lausanne and by National Center of Competence in Research project "SYNAPSY—The Synaptic Bases of Mental Disease"; project no. 51AU40_125759.

Acknowledgments: The authors would like to warmly thank all the participants and Françoise Secretan, Christiane Pellet, Laura Pezzi and Anamelba Peceros Mendoza from the Clinical Research Center of the Lausanne University Hospital for their contribution to this study, Evrim Jaccard and Christel Tran for their availabilities on medical assistance, as well as Michael Notter from the Laboratory of Investigative Neurophysiology for his help with programming the behavioral paradigm used during EEG recording sessions. We further thank two anonymous reviewers for valuable comments on the manuscript.

Conflicts of Interest: L.T. has received speaker's honoraria from Nestlé, Switzerland; Soremartec srl, Italy; and the Gatorade Sport Science Institute, USA. The other authors have no conflict of interest to disclose. The funding sponsors had no role in the design of the study; in the collection, analyses, or interpretation of data; in the writing of the manuscript, and in the decision to publish the results.

References

1. DiMeglio, D.P.; Mattes, R.D. Liquid versus solid carbohydrate: Effects on food intake and body weight. *Int. J. Obes. Relat. Metab. Disord.* **2000**, *24*, 794–800. [CrossRef] [PubMed]
2. Malik, V.S.; Popkin, B.M.; Bray, G.A.; Després, J.P.; Hu, F.B. Sugar-sweetened beverages, obesity, type 2 diabetes mellitus, and cardiovascular disease risk. *Circulation* **2010**, *121*, 1356–1364. [CrossRef] [PubMed]
3. Vartanian, L.R.; Schwartz, M.B.; Brownell, K.D. Effects of soft drink consumption on nutrition and health: A systematic review and meta-analysis. *Am. J. Public Health* **2007**, *97*, 667–675. [CrossRef] [PubMed]
4. Dhingra, R.; Sullivan, L.; Jacques, P.F.; Wang, T.J.; Fox, C.S.; Meigs, J.B.; D'Agostino, R.B.; Gaziano, J.M.; Vasan, R.S. Soft drink consumption and risk of developing cardiometabolic risk factors and the metabolic syndrome in middle-aged adults in the community. *Circulation* **2007**, *116*, 480–488. [CrossRef] [PubMed]
5. Fowler, S.P.; Williams, K.; Resendez, R.G.; Hunt, K.J.; Hazuda, H.P.; Stern, M.P. Fueling the obesity epidemic? Artificially sweetened beverage use and long-term weight gain. *Obesity* **2008**, *16*, 1894–1900. [CrossRef] [PubMed]
6. Stellman, S.D.; Garfinkel, L. Patterns of artificial sweetener use and weight change in an american cancer society prospective study. *Appetite* **1988**, *11* (Suppl. 1), 85–91. [CrossRef]
7. Seeley, W.W.; Menon, V.; Schatzberg, A.F.; Keller, J.; Glover, G.H.; Kenna, H.; Reiss, A.L.; Greicius, M.D. Dissociable intrinsic connectivity networks for salience processing and executive control. *J. Neurosci.* **2007**, *27*, 2349–2356. [CrossRef] [PubMed]
8. Berthoud, H.R. Metabolic and hedonic drives in the neural control of appetite: Who is the boss? *Curr. Opin. Neurobiol.* **2011**, *21*, 888–896. [CrossRef] [PubMed]
9. Laffitte, A.; Neiers, F.; Briand, L. Functional roles of the sweet taste receptor in oral and extraoral tissues. *Curr. Opin. Clin. Nutr. Metab. Care* **2014**, *17*, 379–385. [CrossRef] [PubMed]
10. Peng, Y.; Gillis-Smith, S.; Jin, H.; Tränkner, D.; Ryba, N.J.; Zuker, C.S. Sweet and bitter taste in the brain of awake behaving animals. *Nature* **2015**, *527*, 512–515. [CrossRef] [PubMed]
11. Schloegl, H.; Percik, R.; Horstmann, A.; Villringer, A.; Stumvoll, M. Peptide hormones regulating appetite–focus on neuroimaging studies in humans. *Diabetes Metab. Res. Rev.* **2011**, *27*, 104–112. [CrossRef] [PubMed]
12. Burke, M.V.; Small, D.M. Physiological mechanisms by which non-nutritive sweeteners may impact body weight and metabolism. *Physiol. Behav.* **2015**, *152*, 381–388. [CrossRef] [PubMed]
13. Swithers, S.E. Artificial sweeteners produce the counterintuitive effect of inducing metabolic derangements. *Trends Endocrinol. Metab.* **2013**, *24*, 431–441. [CrossRef] [PubMed]
14. Davidson, T.L.; Martin, A.A.; Clark, K.; Swithers, S.E. Intake of high-intensity sweeteners alters the ability of sweet taste to signal caloric consequences: Implications for the learned control of energy and body weight regulation. *Q. J. Exp. Psychol.* **2011**, *64*, 1430–1441. [CrossRef] [PubMed]
15. Wang, Q.P.; Lin, Y.Q.; Zhang, L.; Wilson, Y.A.; Oyston, L.J.; Cotterell, J.; Qi, Y.; Khuong, T.M.; Bakhshi, N.; Planchenault, Y.; et al. Sucralose promotes food intake through npy and a neuronal fasting response. *Cell Metab.* **2016**, *24*, 75–90. [CrossRef] [PubMed]
16. Bruyère, O.; Ahmed, S.H.; Atlan, C.; Belegaud, J.; Bortolotti, M.; Canivenc-Lavier, M.C.; Charrière, S.; Girardet, J.P.; Houdart, S.; Kalonji, E.; et al. Review of the nutritional benefits and risks related to intense sweeteners. *Arch. Public Health* **2015**, *73*, 41. [CrossRef] [PubMed]
17. Bruyère, O.; Ahmed, S.H.; Atlan, C.; Belegaud, J.; Bortolotti, M.; Canivenc-Lavier, M.C.; Charrière, S.; Girardet, J.P.; Houdart, S.; Kalonji, E.; et al. Erratum to: Review of the nutritional benefits and risks related to intense sweeteners. *Arch. Public Health* **2015**, *73*, 49. [CrossRef] [PubMed]
18. Renwick, A.G.; Molinary, S.V. Sweet-taste receptors, low-energy sweeteners, glucose absorption and insulin release. *Br. J. Nutr.* **2010**, *104*, 1415–1420. [CrossRef] [PubMed]

19. Shankar, P.; Ahuja, S.; Sriram, K. Non-nutritive sweeteners: Review and update. *Nutrition* **2013**, *29*, 1293–1299. [CrossRef] [PubMed]

20. Frank, G.K.; Oberndorfer, T.A.; Simmons, A.N.; Paulus, M.P.; Fudge, J.L.; Yang, T.T.; Kaye, W.H. Sucrose activates human taste pathways differently from artificial sweetener. *Neuroimage* **2008**, *39*, 1559–1569. [CrossRef] [PubMed]

21. Kilpatrick, L.A.; Coveleskie, K.; Connolly, L.; Labus, J.S.; Ebrat, B.; Stains, J.; Jiang, Z.; Suyenobu, B.Y.; Raybould, H.E.; Tillisch, K.; et al. Influence of sucrose ingestion on brainstem and hypothalamic intrinsic oscillations in lean and obese women. *Gastroenterology* **2014**, *146*, 1212–1221. [CrossRef] [PubMed]

22. Ginieis, R.; Franz, E.A.; Oey, I.; Peng, M. The "Sweet" Effect: Comparative assessments of dietary sugars on cognitive performance. *Physiol. Behav.* **2018**, *184*, 242–247. [CrossRef] [PubMed]

23. Dagher, A. Functional brain imaging of appetite. *Trends Endocrinol. Metab.* **2012**, *23*, 250–260. [CrossRef] [PubMed]

24. Van der Laan, L.N.; de Ridder, D.T.; Viergever, M.A.; Smeets, P.A. The first taste is always with the eyes: A meta-analysis on the neural correlates of processing visual food cues. *Neuroimage* **2011**, *55*, 296–303. [CrossRef] [PubMed]

25. Crézé, C.; Notter-Bielser, M.L.; Knebel, J.F.; Campos, V.; Tappy, L.; Murray, M.; Toepel, U. The impact of replacing sugar- by artificially-sweetened beverages on brain and behavioral responses to food viewing—An exploratory study. *Appetite* **2018**, *123*, 160–168. [CrossRef] [PubMed]

26. Oldfield, R.C. The assessment and analysis of handedness: The edinburgh inventory. *Neuropsychologia* **1971**, *9*, 97–113. [CrossRef]

27. Ordoñez, E.Y.; Rodil, R.; Quintana, J.B.; Cela, R. Determination of artificial sweeteners in beverages with green mobile phases and high temperature liquid chromatography-tandem mass spectrometry. *Food Chem.* **2015**, *169*, 162–168. [CrossRef] [PubMed]

28. Lietti, C.V.; Murray, M.M.; Hudry, J.; le Coutre, J.; Toepel, U. The role of energetic value in dynamic brain response adaptation during repeated food image viewing. *Appetite* **2012**, *58*, 11–18. [CrossRef] [PubMed]

29. Toepel, U.; Knebel, J.F.; Hudry, J.; le Coutre, J.; Murray, M.M. The brain tracks the energetic value in food images. *Neuroimage* **2009**, *44*, 967–974. [CrossRef] [PubMed]

30. Toepel, U.; Ohla, K.; Hudry, J.; le Coutre, J.; Murray, M.M. Verbal labels selectively bias brain responses to high-energy foods. *Neuroimage* **2014**, *87*, 154–163. [CrossRef] [PubMed]

31. Knebel, J.F.; Toepel, U.; Hudry, J.; le Coutre, J.; Murray, M.M. Generating controlled image sets in cognitive neuroscience research. *Brain Topogr.* **2008**, *20*, 284–289. [CrossRef] [PubMed]

32. Perrin, F.; Pernier, J.; Bertrand, O.; Giard, M.H.; Echallier, J.F. Mapping of scalp potentials by surface spline interpolation. *Electroencephalogr. Clin. Neurophysiol.* **1987**, *66*, 75–81. [CrossRef]

33. Murray, M.M.; Brunet, D.; Michel, C.M. Topographic erp analyses: A step-by-step tutorial review. *Brain Topogr.* **2008**, *20*, 249–264. [CrossRef] [PubMed]

34. Lehmann, D.; Skrandies, W. Reference-free identification of components of checkerboard-evoked multichannel potential fields. *Electroencephalogr. Clin. Neurophysiol.* **1980**, *48*, 609–621. [CrossRef]

35. Toepel, U.; Bielser, M.L.; Forde, C.; Martin, N.; Voirin, A.; le Coutre, J.; Murray, M.M.; Hudry, J. Brain dynamics of meal size selection in humans. *Neuroimage* **2015**, *113*, 133–142. [CrossRef] [PubMed]

36. Michel, C.M.; Murray, M.M.; Lantz, G.; Gonzalez, S.; Spinelli, L.; Grave de Peralta, R. Eeg source imaging. *Clin. Neurophysiol.* **2004**, *115*, 2195–2222. [CrossRef] [PubMed]

37. Tataranni, P.A.; Gautier, J.F.; Chen, K.; Uecker, A.; Bandy, D.; Salbe, A.D.; Pratley, R.E.; Lawson, M.; Reiman, E.M.; Ravussin, E. Neuroanatomical correlates of hunger and satiation in humans using positron emission tomography. *Proc. Natl. Acad. Sci. USA* **1999**, *96*, 4569–4574. [CrossRef] [PubMed]

38. Jastreboff, A.M.; Sinha, R.; Arora, J.; Giannini, C.; Kubat, J.; Malik, S.; Van Name, M.A.; Santoro, N.; Savoye, M.; Duran, E.J.; et al. Altered brain response to drinking glucose and fructose in obese adolescents. *Diabetes* **2016**, *65*, 1929–1939. [CrossRef] [PubMed]

39. Weygandt, M.; Mai, K.; Dommes, E.; Leupelt, V.; Hackmack, K.; Kahnt, T.; Rothemund, Y.; Spranger, J.; Haynes, J.D. The role of neural impulse control mechanisms for dietary success in obesity. *Neuroimage* **2013**, *83*, 669–678. [CrossRef] [PubMed]

40. Lavagnino, L.; Arnone, D.; Cao, B.; Soares, J.C.; Selvaraj, S. Inhibitory control in obesity and binge eating disorder: A systematic review and meta-analysis of neurocognitive and neuroimaging studies. *Neurosci. Biobehav. Rev.* **2016**, *68*, 714–726. [CrossRef] [PubMed]

41. Camus, M.; Halelamien, N.; Plassmann, H.; Shimojo, S.; O'Doherty, J.; Camerer, C.; Rangel, A. Repetitive transcranial magnetic stimulation over the right dorsolateral prefrontal cortex decreases valuations during food choices. *Eur. J. Neurosci.* **2009**, *30*, 1980–1988. [CrossRef] [PubMed]

42. Harris, A.; Hare, T.; Rangel, A. Temporally dissociable mechanisms of self-control: Early attentional filtering versus late value modulation. *J. Neurosci.* **2013**, *33*, 18917–18931. [CrossRef] [PubMed]

43. Critchley, H.D.; Wiens, S.; Rotshtein, P.; Ohman, A.; Dolan, R.J. Neural systems supporting interoceptive awareness. *Nat. Neurosci.* **2004**, *7*, 189–195. [CrossRef] [PubMed]

44. Menon, V.; Uddin, L.Q. Saliency, switching, attention and control: A network model of insula function. *Brain Struct. Funct.* **2010**, *214*, 655–667. [CrossRef] [PubMed]

45. Batterham, R.L.; ffytche, D.H.; Rosenthal, J.M.; Zelaya, F.O.; Barker, G.J.; Withers, D.J.; Williams, S.C. Pyy modulation of cortical and hypothalamic brain areas predicts feeding behaviour in humans. *Nature* **2007**, *450*, 106–109. [CrossRef] [PubMed]

46. Chambers, E.S.; Bridge, M.W.; Jones, D.A. Carbohydrate sensing in the human mouth: Effects on exercise performance and brain activity. *J. Physiol.* **2009**, *587*, 1779–1794. [CrossRef] [PubMed]

47. Connolly, L.; Coveleskie, K.; Kilpatrick, L.A.; Labus, J.S.; Ebrat, B.; Stains, J.; Jiang, Z.; Tillisch, K.; Raybould, H.E.; Mayer, E.A. Differences in brain responses between lean and obese women to a sweetened drink. *Neurogastroenterol. Motil.* **2013**, *25*, 579-e460. [CrossRef] [PubMed]

48. Small, D.M. Flavor is in the brain. *Physiol. Behav.* **2012**, *107*, 540–552. [CrossRef] [PubMed]

49. Hopfinger, J.B.; Buonocore, M.H.; Mangun, G.R. The neural mechanisms of top-down attentional control. *Nat. Neurosci.* **2000**, *3*, 284–291. [CrossRef] [PubMed]

50. Killgore, W.D.; Young, A.D.; Femia, L.A.; Bogorodzki, P.; Rogowska, J.; Yurgelun-Todd, D.A. Cortical and limbic activation during viewing of high- versus low-calorie foods. *Neuroimage* **2003**, *19*, 1381–1394. [CrossRef]

51. Führer, D.; Zysset, S.; Stumvoll, M. Brain activity in hunger and satiety: An exploratory visually stimulated fmri study. *Obesity* **2008**, *16*, 945–950. [CrossRef] [PubMed]

52. Alonso-Alonso, M.; Pascual-Leone, A. The right brain hypothesis for obesity. *JAMA* **2007**, *297*, 1819–1822. [CrossRef] [PubMed]

53. Smeets, P.A.; Weijzen, P.; de Graaf, C.; Viergever, M.A. Consumption of caloric and non-caloric versions of a soft drink differentially affects brain activation during tasting. *Neuroimage* **2011**, *54*, 1367–1374. [CrossRef] [PubMed]

54. Berthoud, H.R. The neurobiology of food intake in an obesogenic environment. *Proc. Nutr. Soc.* **2012**, *71*, 478–487. [CrossRef] [PubMed]

55. Berridge, K.C. 'liking' and 'wanting' food rewards: Brain substrates and roles in eating disorders. *Physiol. Behav.* **2009**, *97*, 537–550. [CrossRef] [PubMed]

56. Kringelbach, M.L. The human orbitofrontal cortex: Linking reward to hedonic experience. *Nat. Rev. Neurosci.* **2005**, *6*, 691–702. [CrossRef] [PubMed]

57. Mitchell, D.G. The nexus between decision making and emotion regulation: A review of convergent neurocognitive substrates. *Behav. Brain Res.* **2011**, *217*, 215–231. [CrossRef] [PubMed]

58. Green, E.; Murphy, C. Altered processing of sweet taste in the brain of diet soda drinkers. *Physiol. Behav.* **2012**, *107*, 560–567. [CrossRef] [PubMed]

59. Rudenga, K.J.; Small, D.M. Amygdala response to sucrose consumption is inversely related to artificial sweetener use. *Appetite* **2012**, *58*, 504–507. [CrossRef] [PubMed]

60. Verhagen, J.V. The neurocognitive bases of human multimodal food perception: Consciousness. *Brain Res. Rev.* **2007**, *53*, 271–286. [CrossRef] [PubMed]

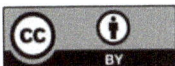

nutrients

MDPI

Article

Gain-Framed Messages Were Related to Higher Motivation Scores for Sugar-Sweetened Beverage Parenting Practices than Loss-Framed Messages

Arwa Zahid and Marla Reicks * [iD]

Department of Food Science and Nutrition, University of Minnesota, St. Paul, MN 55108, USA; zahid001@umn.edu

* Correspondence: mreicks@umn.edu; Tel.: +1-612-624-4735

Received: 11 April 2018; Accepted: 12 May 2018; Published: 16 May 2018

Abstract: Parents play an important role in promoting healthy beverage intake among children. Message-framing approaches, where outcomes are described as positive (gain) or negative (loss) results, can be used to encourage parenting practices that promote healthy beverage intakes. This study tested the effectiveness of message framing on motivation for parenting practices targeting reductions in child sugar-sweetened beverage (SSB) intake (controlling availability, role modeling) and dispositional factors moderating effectiveness. Parents ($n = 380$) completed a survey to assess motivation after viewing gain- and loss-framed messages to engage in parenting practices, usual beverage intake, and home beverage availability. Paired t-tests were used to examine differences in motivation scores after viewing gain- vs. loss-framed messages for all parents and by subgroups according to low vs. high SSB intake and home availability, and weight status. Gain- versus loss-framed messages were related to higher motivation scores for both parenting practices for all parents ($n = 380$, $p < 0.01$) and most subgroups. No differences were observed by message frame for parents in low home SSB availability or normal and overweight BMI subgroups for controlling availability. Gain- versus loss-framed messages were related to higher motivation scores, therefore gain-framed messages are recommended for parent interventions intended to decrease child intake of SSBs.

Keywords: parenting practices; sugar-sweetened beverages; gain- and loss-framed messages

---

1. Introduction

Consumption of sugar-sweetened beverages (SSBs) by children in the United States (U.S.) is a concern because of high intake [1,2] and associated health problems [3–6]. National consumption data (2011–2014) showed that 62.9% youth aged 2–19 years in the U.S. consumed at least one SSB on a given day [2]. A recent review found consistent evidence for negative effects of SSB consumption on the health of children and adolescents, with strongest evidence for risk of overweight or obesity and dental caries [6]. Parenting practices, such as role modeling and controlling beverage availability are considered part of the social and physical environment which can be manipulated by parents to change SSB intake behaviors of children under the organizing framework of Social Cognitive Theory [7,8].

Message framing is a common method used to promote health behavior change [9,10]. Gain-framed messages (where outcomes are described in positive terms) have been found to be more effective for prevention behaviors (sunscreen use and exercise) whereas, loss-framed messages (where outcomes are described in negative terms) were more effective for detection behaviors (breast self-exams) [11,12]. In addition, a recent review suggested that gain-framed messages were more effective when the individual had a low level of involvement or interest in the issue, the outcome of the behavior was certain, and the behavior helped individuals avoid risk [10]. Another review found additional dispositional factors that consistently moderated motivation based on gain and loss framing of health messages including self-efficacy beliefs and ambivalence [13]. The frequency of SSB parenting practices, such as role modeling intake and controlling beverage availability, and weight status may reflect dispositional factors such as self-efficacy beliefs, level of involvement, or risk aversion. The limited number of studies that tested message framing to promote healthy dietary behaviors supported the effectiveness of gain- vs. loss-framed messaging but few studies examined the effects of various dispositional factors [14–17].

Studies involving message framing to change dietary behaviors have primarily focused on messages that target behaviors of the person receiving the messages [14–16]. Few studies have investigated how message framing might be used to promote behaviors aimed at the health of someone other than the person receiving the messages (proxy) [18]. For example, parenting practices that affect the diet of children are completed by parents to directly benefit the health of their child. Having healthy children translates into benefits for parents such as limiting future healthcare costs and enhancing peace of mind [19], therefore message framing may produce similar results when the benefits directly impact the child and indirectly benefit the parent. Furthermore, few studies have examined the effectiveness of message framing to promote different behaviors that could achieve the same outcome [20]. For example, a variety of parenting practices can be used to promote the same healthy dietary behavior and health outcomes for children [20].

The purpose of this study was to test the hypothesis that exposure to gain-framed messages would result in greater intention (measured as motivation scores) for parents of children (6–12 years) for two different behaviors (role modeling intake and controlling home availability of SSBs) compared to exposure to loss-framed messages. Additionally, the effectiveness of gain- and loss-framed messages were tested among parents grouped by low and high scores on home availability of SSBs, low and high SSB intake, and normal, overweight, and obese weight status.

2. Materials and Methods

Parents/caregivers attending the Minnesota State Fair in 2015 were recruited to complete a questionnaire in a building specifically designed for research studies (Driven to Discover building) through a website providing study information. Parents were eligible if they had a child (6–12 years), had primary responsibility for food acquisition and preparation, and could complete the survey in English. The University Institutional Review Board approved the study with consent procedures. After participation, parents were given $5 in cash and a backpack.

Gain- and loss-framed messages were developed for parents promoting two parenting practices that addressed a single overall health outcome for children—role modeling intake and controlling home availability of beverages to limit SSB intake and improve diet quality and health (Table 1). Message phrasing was based on recent examples where gain-framed messages focused on benefits of engaging in the behavior and loss-framed messages focused on the costs of not engaging in the behavior [10,21,22]. For example, Churchill and Pavey [22] used the following gain- and loss-framed messages to promote fruit and vegetable intake, respectively: "Evidence suggests that people who eat enough fruit and vegetables, compared to those that do not, are at lower risk of many serious life-threatening diseases and gain several potential health benefits." and "Evidence suggests that people who do not eat enough fruits and vegetables, compared to those that do, are at higher risk of many serious life-threatening diseases and lose several potential health benefits".

An initial set of PowerPoint slides was developed presenting facts about the usual daily calories children consumed from added sugars (>10%), the relationship between high intake of sugary drinks and overweight or obesity, health risks associated with overweight or obesity, and prevalence of childhood obesity. For parents, sugary drinks were defined as sodas, fruit drinks, and fruit punch. These slides were followed by slides including the gain- and loss-framed messages for role modeling and controlling home beverage availability. The slides were transformed into short YouTube videos, tested with a small group of parents (*n* = 8) for clarity and comprehension, and revised accordingly prior to implementation with the large group.

For implementation, the revised slides were embedded as still images as part of a Qualtrics survey platform. The messages developed for each parenting practice are presented in Table 1. The order of the messages was randomized within the Qualtrics survey so different parents viewed the gain- vs. loss-framed messages in different order. Parents viewed the still images and then immediately reported behavioral intention (measured as motivation scores).

Table 1. Gain- and Loss-Framed Messages.

Parenting Practice	Messages
Controlling Availability Gain-framed	Parents who do not make sugary drinks available in their home are more likely to have children who do not drink sugary drinks.
Controlling Availability Loss-framed	Parents who make sugary drinks available in their home are more likely to have children who drink sugary drinks.
Role Modeling Gain-framed	Parents who set a good example by not drinking sugary drinks are more likely to have children who do not drink sugary drinks.
Role Modeling Loss-framed	Parents who do not set a good example by drinking sugary drinks are more likely to have children who drink sugary drinks.

Questions to evaluate behavioral intention with respect to controlling availability of beverages and role modeling included: How much would this message motivate you to have healthy beverages at home for your child to drink (controlling home beverage availability)? and How much would this message motivate you to set a good example for your child by drinking healthy beverages (role modeling beverage intake)? Response options (motivation scores) were 1 = not at all—4 = a lot. These questions were similar to those used in another study evaluating motivation to engage in parenting practices based on messaging [23].

A subset of parents (*n* = 75) were asked if they perceived the messages to be framed according to the intended valence. Parents were asked whether the consequences of the parenting practices were described in a positive or negative way, which was a similar approach used in another study [24]. Response options were positive, negative, and I do not know.

Home availability of beverages was measured with nine questions based on a similar questioning framework for foods available at home that had been used with parents of adolescents in a previous study [25]. The questions asked parents how often milk, soft drinks, fruit drinks, fruit juice, and water were available in their home with response options of never = 1—always = 4. Two items were grouped to construct a variable to assess the availability of sugar-sweetened beverages (regular soda pop and fruit drinks).

Usual beverage intake was assessed using a 15-item beverage questionnaire previously evaluated for validity and reliability as an indication of modeling beverage intakes [26]. Hedrick et al. [26] found that beverage intake measured with the 15-item beverage questionnaire was significantly correlated with intake measured with three 24-h dietary recalls (SSB R^2 = 0.69), but not with whole milk. Various beverage items were included (dairy, sugar-sweetened, caffeinated, and energy beverages). Respondents were asked to indicate their usual intake over the past month by indicating how often they consumed the beverage (never or less than 1 per week, 1/week, 2–3/week, 4–6/week, 1/day 2+/day, 3+/day) and how much they consumed (less than 6 oz., 8 oz., 12 oz., more than 12 oz.). Items were grouped to construct variables to assess daily intake of SSBs including soft drinks, sweetened juice, sweetened tea, tea or coffee with cream and/or sugar, and energy drinks.

Parents answered questions assessing demographic and physical characteristics for themselves (age, sex, ethnicity, education, employment, food assistance, self-reported height and weight) and for their child (age, sex). Surveys were completed on iPads using a Qualtrics survey platform in about 10 min per participant. Parents first answered questions about home availability and usual beverage intake, followed by questions to evaluate behavioral intention based on viewing the gain-and loss-framed messages, and finally questions about demographic and physical characteristics.

For categorical variables, frequency counts were calculated. For continuous variables, means and standard deviations were computed. BMI (kg/m^2) was calculated for parents from self-reported height and weight. Parents were divided into subgroups based on weight status (normal weight: BMI < 25, n = 130, overweight: BMI $\geq$ 25 and <30, n = 115, obese: BMI $\geq$ 30, n = 86); low and high home availability of SSBs based on summing ratings for two items, regular soda pop and fruit drinks, (below or above an availability rating of 5 (n = 170 and 210, respectively); and intake of SSBs (below or above median intake (n = 191 and 189, respectively). Paired t-tests were used to determine differences in behavioral intention (motivation scores) by type of message framing among all parents and within parent subgroups. Statistical significance was assessed at the p = 0.05 level. ANOVA models were used to assess between group differences in mean behavioral intention differences for each subgroup analysis. For the weight group comparisons, the Tukey adjustment for multiple comparisons was used to identify significant between group differences while preserving the overall alpha significance level at 0.05. Statistical Analysis System software (SAS; version 9.4, Cary, NC, USA) was used to analyze data.

3. Results

Three-hundred and eighty parents completed the survey; an additional 7 parents provided consent but did not complete the survey. The majority were white (90.8%), women (79.7%), employed full time (72.9%), and had a 4-year college degree (70.5%); mean age was 42.0 years and mean BMI was 27.3 (Table 2). Twenty-eight percent of children were 6–8 years old, 72% were 9–12 years old and 50% were girls.

Table 2. Demographic Characteristics of Parent Survey Respondents.

Characteristic	Mean (SD)
Age (n = 380)	42.0 (6.6)
Body Mass Index (n = 331) [1]	27.3 (6.0)
	N (%) [1]
Sex	
Female	303 (79.7)
Male	77 (20.3)
Education	
High school diploma	21 (5.5)
Some college or technical school	91 (24.0)
4-year college, advanced degree	268 (70.5)
Ethnicity	
Hispanic or Latino	7 (1.8)
Asian	26 (6.8)
White/Caucasian	338 (88.9)
American Indian/Black/multi-ethnicity	9 (2.4)
Food Assistance Programs	
None	343 (90.3)
SNAP/WIC/Free or reduced price school meals) [2]	50 (13.2)

[1] BMI data are missing from 49; [2] SNAP—Supplemental Nutrition Assistance Program, WIC—Women's, Infants and Children Supplemental Assistance Program. Participants could check all that apply.

The manipulation check with 75 parents showed that a majority perceived the messages to be framed according to the intended valence. For the behavior of controlling availability of beverages for children, 85% of parents perceived the gain-framed message as positive; and 56% of parents perceived the loss-framed message as negative. For the behavior of role modeling beverage intake, 87% of parents perceived the gain-framed message as positive; and 76% of parents perceived the loss-framed message as negative.

A greater number of parents indicated that the gain-framed versus the loss-framed messages would motivate them (some and a lot) to control beverage availability at home (73.2% vs. 65.8%) and to role model beverage intake for their children (76.1% vs. 64.0%). Mean intention to control beverage availability in the home was greater ($p = 0.002$) after exposure to the gain-framed message (M = 3.06, SD = 0.90) compared to the loss-framed message (M = 2.93, SD = 0.96). Mean intention was also greater for role modeling beverage intake for children after exposure to the gain-framed message (M = 3.10, SD = 0.85) ($p <0.001$) compared to the loss-framed message (M = 2.81, SD = 1.03).

In the group with high availability of SSBs at home, exposure to the gain-framed message resulted in a higher mean intention to control availability of beverages at home ($p < 0.010$) compared to parents exposed to the loss-framed message (Table 3). However, in the group with low availability of SSBs at home, intention was not different after exposure to either the gain or loss framed message ($p = 0.068$). For parents consuming either a low or high amount of SSBs, intention to role model beverage intake was greater after exposure to the gain vs. the loss framed messages ($p = 0.001$) (Table 3). No differences were observed between low and high availability groups for intention to control availability of SSBs or between low and high SSB intake groups for intention to role model beverage intake (Table 3).

Table 3. Behavioral Intention[1] for Parenting Practices Based on Message Valence by SSB[2] Availability and SSB Intake.

Parenting Practice	Gain-Framed Mean (SD)	Loss-Framed Mean (SD)	p-Value [3]	Gain-Framed Mean (SD)	Loss-Framed Mean (SD)	p-Value [3]	p-Value [4]
	Low Availability SSB ($n = 170$)			High Availability SSB ($n = 210$)			
Controlling availability	3.01 (0.90)	2.90 (0.98)	0.068	3.12 (0.90)	2.98 (0.96)	0.010	0.296
	Low SSB Intake ($n = 191$)			High SSB Intake ($n = 189$)			
Role Modeling	3.21 (0.85)	2.86 (1.10)	0.0001	2.96 (0.83)	2.75 (0.95)	0.0005	0.125

[1] Mean of response options 1–4, where 1 = not at all—4 = a lot; [2] SSB—sugar-sweetened beverages, [3] p-value based on paired *t*-test for differences in mean intention scores within groups, [4] p-value based on ANOVA F-test for between group differences in mean intention score differences.

For both normal and overweight subgroups, no significant differences were observed in mean intention to control beverage availability at home after viewing the gain- and loss-framed messages ($p = 0.066$ and 0.668, respectively) (Table 4). For obese parents, the gain-framed message was more motivating than the loss-framed message regarding controlling availability. For all weight subgroups, gain-framed messages resulted in higher mean intention to role model beverage intake ($p = 0.001$) compared to loss-framed messages. No differences were observed in intention score differences to control availability of SSBs or role model SSB intake by weight subgroups.

Table 4. Behavioral Intention [1] for Parenting Practices Based on Message Valence by Weight Status.

	Normal Weight ($n = 130$)	Overweight ($n = 115$)	Obese ($n = 86$)	ANOVA p-Value [3]
Controlling Availability	Mean (SD)	Mean (SD)	Mean (SD)	0.325
Gain-framed	3.19 (0.86)	3.03 (0.96)	3.05 (0.82)	
Loss-framed	3.06 (0.95)	2.99 (0.98)	2.84 (0.93)	
t-test p-Value [2]	0.066	0.668	0.019	
Role Modeling	Mean (SD)	Mean (SD)	Mean (SD)	0.756
Gain-framed	3.17 (0.82)	3.19 (0.87)	3.06 (0.78)	
Loss-framed	2.93 (1.07)	2.85 (1.05)	2.72 (0.89)	
t-test p-Value [2]	0.001	<0.0001	0.001	

[1] Mean of response options 1–4, where 1 = not at all—4 = a lot; [2] p-value based on paired *t*-tests for differences in mean intention scores within weight subgroups, [3] p-value based on ANOVA F-test for between weight group differences in mean intention score differences.

4. Discussion

For all parents and within most parent subgroups, findings from the current study showed that gain-framed messages were related to greater motivation than loss-framed messages for both SSB parenting practices aimed at achieving the same outcome and focusing on behaviors that produced indirect benefits for the message recipient. Therefore the general principle that gain-framed messages are more effective than loss-framed messages in promoting prevention behaviors like healthy eating as shown in several reviews [10,18] is also likely to be applicable to messages targeting multiple parenting practices to improve diet and health of children.

Self-efficacy has been tested as a dispositional factor hypothesized to moderate the effectiveness of gain- or loss-framed health messages with inconclusive results [13]. Parent self-efficacy regarding SSB intake among youth has been addressed in previous studies [27–29]. Self-efficacy of parents was associated with SSB intake among young children in an observational study [27]. Self-efficacy was proposed as a control belief for serving SSBs to children by parents in a qualitative study [28]. Self-efficacy was also addressed through motivational interviewing as an intervention target to help parents control child SSB intake [29]. In the current study, the subgroup of parents with low home SSB availability may have been intentionally not keeping SSBs in the home to limit child intake based on strong self-efficacy for this parenting practice (although self-efficacy was not assessed). For these parents, no differences were observed in motivation based on gain- or loss-framed messages, thus the relationship between a potentially high level of confidence in limiting home availability of SSBs and a particular message valence remains unclear. Additional studies are needed to determine how self-efficacy affects motivation based on gain- or loss-framed messages promoting positive parenting practices.

Level of involvement in a specific health issue is another dispositional factor that has been reviewed regarding effectiveness of gain- or loss-framed health messages [10,11,13]. For individuals with low involvement, gain-framed messages were generally more effective than loss-framed messages [10,13]. For the subgroup of parents in the current study with high availability of SSBs at home, involvement in controlling beverage availability for children may be low, consistent with the finding that gain-framed messages were more effective than loss-framed messages in improving motivation.

In the current study, gain-framed compared to loss-framed messages resulted in greater motivation for role modeling beverage intake by all parents, and subgroups by SSB intake and weight status. However, parent beverage intake was assessed as an indication of role modeling and not measured with a general scaled variable. This approach was similar to that used in another recent study [30] and consistent with observed associations between parent and adolescent SSB intakes [31]. Therefore results based on subgroups by SSB intake may not be consistent with tests of the effectiveness of gain- vs. loss-framed messaging based on other measures of role modeling.

Parental obesity has been associated with child obesity [32], increased likelihood that children and adolescents are less physically active [33], and a less supportive home food and physical activity environment [34]. Therefore, level of involvement in SSB parenting practices was expected to be low among the overweight/obese subgroup, indicating that gain-framed messages may have been more influential than loss-framed messages. This was the case for role modeling, where the gain-framed message was related to higher motivation scores versus the loss-framed message. However, no differences in effectiveness of message type were observed between normal and overweight parents for controlling availability.

A strength of the current study was the novelty of testing effectiveness of gain- vs. loss-framed health messages to promote multiple behaviors that would benefit someone other than the message recipient. A limitation was that only a slight majority (56%) of parents perceived the loss-framed message as negative for controlling home beverage availability. Thus, caution should be used in interpreting the results regarding controlling home beverage availability. In addition, exposure to the messages was immediately followed by assessment of outcomes, whereas some parents may need time to process the information to influence behavior. Also, parents self-reported their height and weight, which could have led to over- or underestimation of the real values. Most parents were white, did not use food assistance programs and were well-educated women, thus limiting the ability to examine findings by ethnicity, food assistance, sex or education or to apply the findings to the broader population.

In summary, given the positive findings regarding gain-framed messages and previous research on framing effects in nutrition education [10], future parent intervention programs may benefit from using gain-framed messages to promote parenting practices aimed at decreasing SSB intake by children. Further studies are needed to determine whether gain- compared to loss-framed messages are more effective in influencing actual change in SSB parenting practices and ultimately, child SSB intake and health outcomes.

5. Conclusions

Gain-framed messages promoting the SSB parenting practices of role modeling healthy beverage intake and making healthy beverages available were related to greater motivation scores than loss-framed messages for all parents. Within most parent subgroups based on low or high availability of SSBs, low or high SSB intake, and weight subgroups, gain- versus loss-framed messages were also related to higher motivation scores. Therefore gain-framed messages are recommended for parent interventions intended to decrease child intake of SSBs.

Author Contributions: A.Z. and M.R. conceived and designed the experiments; A.Z. and M.R. performed the experiments; A.Z. and M.R. analyzed the data; A.Z. and M.R. wrote the paper.

Conflicts of Interest: The authors declare no conflict of interest.

References

1. U.S. Department of Health and Human Services and U.S. Department of Agriculture. *2015–2020 Dietary Guidelines for Americans*, 8th ed.; U.S. Department of Health and Human Services and U.S. Department of Agriculture: Washington, DC, USA, 2015. Available online: http://health.gov/dietaryguidelines/2015/guidelines/ (accessed on 9 March 2018).
2. Rosinger, A.; Herrick, K.; Gahche, J.; Park, S. Sugar-sweetened beverage consumption among US youth, 2011–2014. *NCHS Data Brief* **2017**, *271*, 1–8.
3. Malik, V.S.V.; Pan, A.; Willett, W.C.; Hu, F.B.F. Sugar-sweetened beverages and weight gain in children and adults: A systematic review and meta-analysis. *Am. J. Clin. Nutr.* **2013**, *98*, 1084–1102. [CrossRef] [PubMed]
4. Berkey, C.; Rockett, H.; Field, A. Sugar-added beverages and adolescent weight change. *Obesity* **2004**, *12*, 778–788. [CrossRef] [PubMed]
5. Ambrosini, G.L.; Oddy, W.H.; Huang, R.C.; Mori, T.A.; Beilin, L.J.; Jebb, S.A. Prospective associations between sugar-sweetened beverage intakes and cardiometabolic risk factors in adolescents. *Am. J. Clin. Nutr.* **2013**, *93*, 327–334. [CrossRef] [PubMed]
6. Bleich, S.N.; Vercammen, K.A. The negative impact of sugar-sweetened beverages on children's health: An update of the literature. *BMC Obes.* **2018**, *5*, 6. [CrossRef] [PubMed]
7. Vaughn, A.E.; Dearth-Wesley, T.; Tabak, R.G.; Bryant, M.; Ward, D.S. Development of a comprehensive assessment of food parenting practices: The home self-administered tool for Environmental Assessment of Activity and Diet Family Food Practices Survey. *J. Acad. Nutr. Diet.* **2017**, *117*, 214–227. [CrossRef] [PubMed]
8. Vereecken, C.; Keukelier, E.; Maes, L. Influence of mother's educational level on food parenting practices and food habits of young children. *Appetite* **2004**, *43*, 93–103. [CrossRef] [PubMed]
9. Akl, E.A.; Oxman, A.D.; Herrin, J.; Vist, G.E.; Terrenato, I.; Sperati, F.; Costiniuk, C.; Blank, D.; Schünemann, H. Framing of health information messages. *Cochrane Database Syst. Rev.* **2011**, *12*. [CrossRef] [PubMed]
10. Wansink, B.; Pope, L. When do gain-framed health messages work better than fear appeals? *Nutr. Rev.* **2015**, *73*, 4–11. [CrossRef] [PubMed]
11. Rothman, A.J.; Salovey, P. Shaping perceptions to motivate healthy behavior: The role of message framing. *Psychol. Bull.* **1997**, *121*, 3–19. [CrossRef] [PubMed]

12. Rothman, A.J.; Martino, S.C.; Bedell, B.T.; Detweiler, J.B.; Salovey, P. The systematic influence of gain-and loss-framed messages on interest in and use of different types of health behavior. *Pers. Soc. Psychol. Bull.* **1999**, *25*, 1355–1369. [CrossRef]

13. Covey, J. The role of dispositional factors in moderating message framing effects. *Health Psychol.* **2014**, *33*, 52–65. [CrossRef] [PubMed]

14. Bannon, K.; Schwartz, M. Impact of nutrition messages on children's food choice: Pilot study. *Appetite* **2006**, *46*, 124–129. [CrossRef] [PubMed]

15. Satia, J.; Barlow, J.; Armstrong-Brown, J. A qualitative study to explore Prospect theory and message framing and diet and cancer prevention-related issues among African American adolescents. *Cancer Nurs.* **2010**, *33*, 102–109. [CrossRef] [PubMed]

16. Wirtz, J.; Kulpavaropas, S. The effects of narrative and message framing on engagement and eating intention among a sample of adult Hispanics. *J. Nutr. Educ. Behav.* **2014**, *46*, 396–400. [CrossRef] [PubMed]

17. Latimer, A.; Brawley, L. A systematic review of three approaches for constructing physical activity messages: What messages work and what improvements are needed? *Int. J. Behav. Nutr. Phys. Act.* **2010**, *7*. [CrossRef] [PubMed]

18. Gallagher, K.M.; Updegraff, J.A. Health message framing effects on attitudes, intentions, and behavior: A meta-analytic review. *Ann. Behav. Med.* **2012**, *43*, 101–116. [CrossRef] [PubMed]

19. Richards, R.; Reicks, M.; Wong, S.S.; Gunther, C.; Cluskey, M.; Ballejos, M.S.; Bruhn, C.; Johnston, N.P.; Misner, S.; Watters, C. Perceptions of how parents of early adolescents will personally benefit from calcium-rich food and beverage parenting practices. *J. Nutr. Educ. Behav.* **2014**, *46*, 595–601. [CrossRef] [PubMed]

20. Vaughn, A.E.; Ward, D.S.; Fisher, J.O.; Faith, M.S.; Hughes, S.O.; Kremers, S.O.; Kremers, S.P.; Musher-Eizenman, D.R.; O'Connor, T.M.; Patrick, H.; et al. Fundamental constructs in food parenting practices: A content map to guide future research. *Nutr. Rev.* **2016**, *74*, 98–117. [CrossRef] [PubMed]

21. Gerend, M.A.; Maner, J.K. Fear, anger, fruits, and veggies: Interactive effects of emotion and message framing on health behavior. *Health Psychol.* **2011**, *30*, 420–423. [CrossRef] [PubMed]

22. Churchill, S.; Pavey, L. Promoting fruit and vegetable consumption: The role of message framing and autonomy. *Br. J. Health Psychol.* **2013**, *18*, 610–622. [CrossRef] [PubMed]

23. Banna, J.C.; Reicks, M.; Gunther, C.; Richards, R.; Bruhn, C.; Cluskey, M.; Wong, S.S.; Misner, S.; Hongu, N.; Johnston, N.P. Evaluation of emotion-based messages designed to motivate Hispanic and Asian parents of early adolescents to engage in calcium-rich food and beverage parenting practices. *Nutr. Res. Pract.* **2016**, *10*, 456–463. [CrossRef] [PubMed]

24. Ferguson, E.; Gallagher, L. Message framing with respect to decisions about vaccination: The roles of frame valence, frame method and perceived risk. *Br. J. Health Psychol.* **2007**, *98*, 667–680. [CrossRef] [PubMed]

25. Neumark-Sztainer, D.; Wall, M.; Perry, C.; Story, M. Correlates of fruit and vegetable intake among adolescents: Findings from Project EAT. *Prev. Med.* **2003**, *37*, 198–208. [CrossRef]

26. Hedrick, V.; Savla, J.; Comber, D.; Flack, K. Development of a brief questionnaire to assess habitual beverage intake (BEVQ-15): Sugar-sweetened beverages and total beverage energy intake. *J. Acad. Nutr. Diet.* **2012**, *112*, 840–849. [CrossRef] [PubMed]

27. Nickelson, J.; Lawrence, J.C.; Parton, J.M.; Knowlden, A.P.; McDermott, R.J. What proportion of preschool-aged children consume sweetened beverages? *J. Sch. Health* **2014**, *84*, 185–194. [CrossRef] [PubMed]

28. Tipton, J.A. Caregivers' psychosocial factors underlying sugar-sweetened beverage intake among non-Hispanic Black preschoolers: An elicitation study. *J. Pediatr. Nurs.* **2014**, *29*, 47–57. [CrossRef] [PubMed]

29. Taveras, E.M.; Gortmaker, S.L.; Hohman, K.H.; Horan, C.M.; Kleinman, K.P.; Mitchell, K.; Price, S.; Prosser, L.A.; Rifas-Shiman, S.L.; Gillman, M.W. A randomized controlled trial to improve primary care to present and manage childhood obesity: The high five for kids study. *Arch. Pediatr. Adolesc. Med.* **2011**, *165*, 714–722. [CrossRef] [PubMed]

30. Heredia, N.I.; Ranjit, N.; Warren, J.L.; Evans, A.E. Association of parental social support with energy balance-related behaviors in low-income and ethnically diverse children: A cross-sectional study. *BMC Public Health* **2016**, *16*. [CrossRef] [PubMed]

31. Lundeen, E.A.; Park, S.; Onufrak, S.; Cunningham, S.; Blanck, H.M. Adolescent sugar-sweetened beverage intake is associated with parent intake, not knowledge of health risks. *Am. J. Health Promot.* **2018**. [CrossRef] [PubMed]

32. Bushnik, T.; Garriguet, D.; Colley, R. Parent-child association in weight status. *Health Rep.* **2017**, *28*, 12–19. [PubMed]

33. Angoorani, P.; Heshmat, R.; Ejtahed, H.S.; Motlagh, M.E.; Ziaodini, H.; Taheri, M.; Hminaee, T.; Shafiee, G.; Godarzi, A.; Qorbani, M.; et al. The association of parental obesity with physical activity and sedentary behaviors of their children: The CASPIAN-V study. *J. Pediatr.* **2017**. [CrossRef] [PubMed]

34. Williams, J.E.; Helsel, B.; Griffin, S.F.; Liang, J. Associations between parental BMI and the family nutrition and physical activity environment in a community sample. *J. Commun. Health* **2017**, *42*, 1233–1239. [CrossRef] [PubMed]

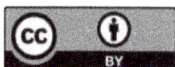

nutrients

MDPI

Article

Predicting Athletes' Pre-Exercise Fluid Intake: A Theoretical Integration Approach

Chunxiao Li [1],*,[†] , Feng-Hua Sun [1],[†] , Liancheng Zhang [2] and Derwin King Chung Chan [3]

[1] Department of Health and Physical Education, The Education University of Hong Kong, Hong Kong, China; fhsun@eduhk.hk

[2] Key Laboratory of Competitive Sport Psychological and Physiological Regulation, Tianjin University of Sport, Tianjin 301617, China; zlc-hhht@163.com

[3] School of Public Health, Li Ka Shing Faculty of Medicine, The University of Hong Kong, Hong Kong, China; derwin.chan@hku.hk

* Correspondence: cxlilee@gmail.com; Tel.: +852-55739596

† Co-first authors.

Received: 14 April 2018; Accepted: 16 May 2018; Published: 21 May 2018

Abstract: Pre-exercise fluid intake is an important healthy behavior for maintaining athletes' sports performances and health. However, athletes' behavioral adherence to fluid intake and its underlying psychological mechanisms have not been investigated. This prospective study aimed to use a health psychology model that integrates the self-determination theory and the theory of planned behavior for understanding pre-exercise fluid intake among athletes. Participants ($n = 179$) were athletes from college sport teams who completed surveys at two time points. Baseline (Time 1) assessment comprised psychological variables of the integrated model (i.e., autonomous and controlled motivation, attitude, subjective norm, perceived behavioral control, and intention) and fluid intake (i.e., behavior) was measured prospectively at one month (Time 2). Path analysis showed that the positive association between autonomous motivation and intention was mediated by subjective norm and perceived behavioral control. Controlled motivation positively predicted the subjective norm. Intentions positively predicted pre-exercise fluid intake behavior. Overall, the pattern of results was generally consistent with the integrated model, and it was suggested that athletes' pre-exercise fluid intake behaviors were associated with the motivational and social cognitive factors of the model. The research findings could be informative for coaches and sport scientists to promote athletes' pre-exercise fluid intake behaviors.

Keywords: self-determination; planned behavior; intention; beverage consumption; sport

1. Introduction

Exercise is defined as a planned, structured, and repetitive physical activity for improving or maintaining physical fitness [1]. To start the exercise with a normal state of body water content, athletes should drink enough fluid or should be well hydrated prior to exercise [2]. The goal of pre-exercise fluid intake is critical for decreasing the risk of dehydration (loss of body water) and its negative health consequences (e.g., heart disease), and maintaining exercise performance [3]. Sawka et al. [3] proposed an evidence-based guideline of pre-exercise fluid intake. In particular, athletes are advised to slowly intake fluid (e.g., 5–7 mL/kg per body weight) at least four hours prior to exercise, and the fluid intake should be increased (e.g., 3–5 mL/kg per body weight) and be taken about two hours before exercise when athletes are dehydrated (i.e., dehydration is indicated by having no urine or highly concentrated urine). Many athletes seem to not be committed to this recommended behavior [4]. Although pre-exercise fluid intake could be facilitated by increasing drinking-water facilities and improving the convenience of executing the behavior, the actual pre-exercise fluid intake is also highly dependent on decision making factors, motivation, and commitment [5,6].

It is, therefore, valuable to understand the underlying psychological mechanisms of pre-exercise fluid intake and the results might be important to explain why some athletes are not committed to this advisory behavior. The present study aims to apply a unified health psychology model that integrates self-determination theory (SDT) [7] and the theory of planned behavior (TPB) [8] in order to understand athletes' pre-exercise fluid intake.

It is conceptualized in the integrated model that human health behaviors are governed by distal motivational factors from SDT and proximal decision-making factors from TPB [9]. According to SDT, there are two broad forms of motivation behind human actions, including autonomous motivation and controlled motivation [10]. *Autonomous motivation* reflects those motivational behaviors that are consistent with a sense of volition and choice. In contrast, *controlled motivation* is concerned with those motivational behaviors that are regulated by external contingencies, such as rewards/punishment and internal pressure to avoid feelings of guilt and shame [10]. As compared to controlled motivation, autonomous motivation is considered to be more adaptive [10], and it is more likely to lead to behavioral persistence and psychological well-being. However, it is postulated in the integrated model that the relationship between motivations and behavior is not direct, but it is mediated by the decision-making factors from the TPB [9].

The TPB is a social-cognitive model [8], in which the intention is regarded as the central predictor of one's behavior (e.g., fluid intake behavior). According to the TPB [8], three sets of social cognitive variables (i.e., attitude, subjective norm, and perceived behavioral control [PBC]) positively predict behavior via intention. PBC is also proposed to directly predict behavior. *Attitude* concerns one's overall subjective evaluation towards the target behavior. *Subjective norm* reflects one's perception of how the behavior is regarded as being socially appropriate. *PBC* summarizes one's personal judgement on capacity of engaging in the target behavior [8].

The theoretical components of SDT and TPB are merged into the integrated model, such that autonomous motivation (rather than controlled motivation) from SDT is speculated to positively predict attitude, subjective norm, and PBC from the TPB. These three social-cognitive variables further link intention and behavior according to the tenets of the TPB [9]. Integrating these two theoretical frameworks may bring forth a more comprehensive understanding towards health behaviors because the theoretical integration combines the merits and it resolves the limitations of the theories. Specifically, SDT supplements the TPB by providing the superordinate motivational antecedents that account for the origin of the social cognitive process. On the other hand, the TPB accounts for the proximal belief-oriented decision-making process [9].

The integration of SDT and the TPB has been successfully applied in fields, such as anti-doping [11], physical activity [12], prevention and rehabilitation of injury [13], myopia prevention [14], and sleep hygiene [15]. Early studies that are guided by the integrated framework generally indicated that autonomous motivation positively predicted attitude, subjective norm, and PBC, while controlled motivation typically exerted either small or no effects on these three belief-based TPB constructs [12,14]. More recent research findings began to reveal a positive relationship between controlled motivation and subjective norms [11,13]. This is because social approval, external pressure, and recognition of behavior could be regarded as externally referenced motives, and they may be also closely linked to individuals' normative beliefs [11,13]. In addition, the three TPB constructs had a positive effect on healthy behaviors through intention [9,14,15]. Although the utility of the integrated framework in explaining fluid intake behaviors has not been explored, studies applying either SDT or the TPB alone have been conducted in the context of healthy diets. Findings of these early studies could somewhat provide information about the potential application of the integrated model into fluid intake behavior [16,17].

For instance, a few empirical studies that are based on SDT found that autonomous motivation promoted adoption of healthy eating behaviors and controlled motivation showed no or little effect on healthy diets [16,18]. A recent meta-analysis summarizing the findings of 34 studies about the TPB and dietary behaviors among youth showed that the relationship between the three social cognitive factors, intention, and dietary behavior agreed with the tenets of the TPB [17]. Although these studies only focused on a healthy diet, given pre-exercise fluid intake is also a self-regulatory dietary behavior specifically for athletes and physically active individuals, the findings of SDT and the TPB on healthy diets lead to speculation that the integration of both the theories could be useful in explaining athletes' pre-exercise fluid intake behavior.

Although there is an evidence-based guideline for pre-exercise fluid intake, little is known about the underlying psychological mechanisms for this healthy behavior among athletes. From a practical perspective, understanding the underlying mechanisms will help practitioners (e.g., coaches and trainers) and researchers to establish evidence-based intervention programs to promote healthy pre-exercise fluid intake behaviors. Therefore, this two-wave prospective research was undertaken in order to test the utility of the integrated framework consisting of SDT and the TPB in predicting pre-exercise fluid intake among university athletes (see Figure 1). According to our literature review above [8,9,17], it was hypothesized that:

(H1) Autonomous motivation would be a positive predictor of the three social cognitive variables (i.e., attitude, subjective norm, and PBC).

(H2) Controlled motivation would be positively related to subjective norm, but its effect on attitude and PBC would be either small or insignificant.

(H3) Autonomous motivation and the three social cognitive variables were expected to positively predict intention.

(H4) Intention would positively predict pre-exercise fluid intake behavior.

(H5) The three social cognitive variables were proposed to mediate the predictive effects of autonomous/controlled motivation on intention.

(H6) Intention was expected to mediate the relationship between the three social cognitive variables and pre-exercise fluid intake behavior (i.e., full mediation for attitude, subjective norm, and partial mediation for PBC).

(H7) Autonomous/controlled motivation would have an indirect effect on the fluid intake behavior via the three social cognitive variables and intention.

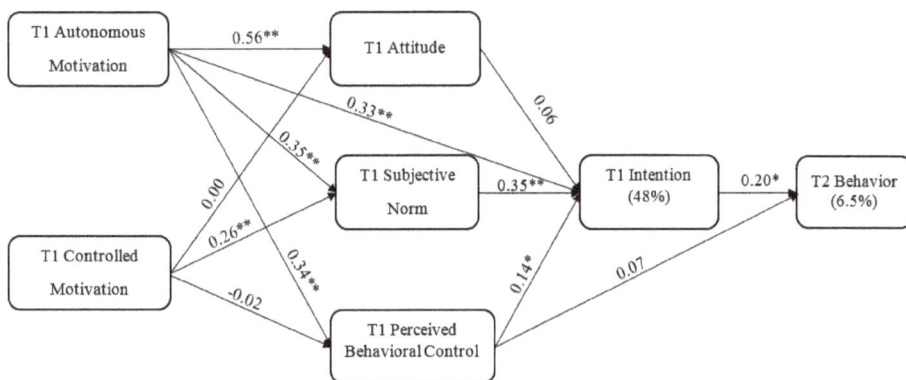

Figure 1. Path estimates of the model. T1 = baseline; T2 = one-month after the baseline; * $p < 0.05$; ** $p < 0.01$. For clarity, correlations between gender and major study variables are omitted.

2. Materials and Methods

A two-wave prospective survey design with a one-month interval between the baseline assessment and the prospective follow-up was used in the current research.

2.1. Participants

A sample of university athletes (*n* = 182) was recruited from three public universities in China. Participants had a mean age of 20.75 (*SD* = 2.24) and 66.5% of them were male. The participants were from a wide range of sports (*n* = 13), such as badminton, soccer, and volleyball. On average, they received training for 5.51 (*SD* = 3.40) years and trained 9.28 h per week (*SD* = 5.39).

2.2. Measures

2.2.1. Autonomous and Controlled Motivation

We adapted 12 items from the Chinese version of the Treatment Self-Regulation Questionnaire for assessing the autonomous and controlled motivation (see Table S1) [13]. The scale has been used for measuring motivation of the integrated model in various behavioral contexts that are related to the prevention or management of injury or illnesses [11,14]. There are six items for evaluating each broad form of motivation including autonomous motivation (e.g., "I want to intake sufficient fluid before exercise because it is consistent with my life goals") and controlled motivation (e.g., "I want to intake sufficient fluid before exercise because I would feel ashamed of myself if I did not"). Participants gave responses on seven-point Likert scales, ranging from *"not at all true"* (1) to *"very true"* (7).

2.2.2. Social Cognitive Constructs and Intention

Items measuring attitude, subjective norm, PBC, and intention were again adapted from the Chinese version of the TPB scale that was developed and used in prior studies of the integrated model conducted in China (see Table S1) [11,14]. The common stem ("Intake sufficient fluid before exercise is … ") was employed to assess participants' attitude, and they made responses on five seven-point semantic differential scales, which included "valuable–worthless", "beneficial–harmful", "pleasant–unpleasant", "enjoyable–unenjoyable", and "good–bad". Measures of subjective norm (three items; e.g., "The people in my life whose opinions I value would approve of me consuming sufficient fluid before exercise in the forthcoming month"), PBC (four items; e.g., "I have complete control over consuming sufficient fluid before exercise in the forthcoming month"), and intention (three items; e.g., "I intend to consume sufficient fluid before exercise in the forthcoming month") were rated on seven-point Likert scales that were anchored from *"strongly disagree"* (1) to *"strongly agree"* (7).

2.2.3. Pre-Exercise Fluid Intake Behavior

Since the required amount of pre-exercise fluid intake is determined by a number of factors (e.g., the type of fluid, individual differences, sport type, temperature, and humidity) [3], measuring the exact amount of pre-exercise fluid intake might not necessarily indicate the hydration status of the athletes. The study, therefore, aims to examine the behavioral adherence that athletes apply toward maintaining an optimal hydration status before exercise, and it requires a self-regulatory effort in monitoring the hydration status and intake fluid when necessary (e.g., monitor one's weight). With the input from one sport physiologist and two sport psychologists, four items (e.g., "I will observe my urine color three to four hours prior to exercise") were developed to measure behavioral adherence to pre-exercise fluid intake, according to the guidelines of Sawka et al. (see Table S1) [3]. Pilot testing with 10 athletes indicated that no item revisions were necessary. Participants rated on the items using five-point Likert scales, which ranged from *"almost never"* (1) and *"almost always"* (5). Since this is a newly developed scale, we conducted an exploratory factor analysis to examine its underlying structure. The results supported the one-factor model of the scale (Eigenvalue = 2.14), and the four items explained 53.6% of the total variance in pre-exercise fluid intake.

2.3. Procedures

The Human Research Ethics Committee of The Education University of Hong Kong granted ethical approval of this research on 20 May 2016 (ref. No. 15216). The first author contacted course lecturers from three public universities located in Southeastern and Northern China to invite the university team athletes to participate in this research. The course lecturers then invited their athletes to participate in this survey through a social media platform. Upon obtaining participants' informed consent, the survey form was distributed to them during their scheduled lecture hours in quiet classrooms (Time 1). A follow-up behavioral measure (i.e., fluid intake behavior) was taken one month later (Time 2) in the same class. The one-month interval between the two measurement points has been recommended [19]. For both administration occasions, participants were under supervision of researchers and were encouraged to provide honest responses. Special emphasis was placed on confidentiality and no mandatory participation. Of 200 athletes invited, 182 (91%) agreed to participate and filled out the survey form at Time 1 and 179 completed the survey at Time 2 (response rate at follow-up = 98.4%).

2.4. Data Analyses

Since there was only a small amount of missing values (0.4%) among study variables, the missing values were imputed through variable means in SPSS 21 (IBM, Armonk, NY, USA) [20]. Cronbach's alphas (α), means, standard deviations, and zero-order correlations of the study variables were computed. A path analysis with a maximum likelihood estimation was applied to test the overall fit of the hypothesized model and hypotheses in AMOS 21 (IBM, Armonk, NY, USA) [21]. Gender was entered as a co-variate since it was found to affect the strength of path estimates [9]. The current sample size ($n = 179$) is generally adequate for path analysis [20]. Model fit was evaluated through chi-square statistics to the degree of freedom ratio (χ^2/df), comparative fit index (CFI), Tucker-Lewis index (TLI), root mean square error of approximation (RMSEA), and standardized root mean square residual (SRMR) [22]. A value of χ^2/df smaller than 3.0, CFI/TLI values over 0.95, and RMSEA/SRMR values that are less than 0.06 represent a good fit [23]. To examine the mediation effects, mediation analyses using bootstrapping approach with 5000 replications were used to generate bias-corrected confidence intervals (CIs) of path estimate. A 95% CI that did not include zero indicates a significantly indirect effect [24].

3. Results

Table 1 presents the results of internal reliability, descriptive statistics, and zero-order correlations. The (sub) scales showed an adequate to excellent internal reliability (Cronbach's $\alpha = 0.71$ to 0.92). Participants reported moderate to high levels of autonomous/controlled motivation, attitude, subjective norm, PBC, behavioral intention, and fluid intake behavior. The zero-order correlations between the study variables yielded small to medium effect sizes.

Table 1. Descriptive statistics, internal reliability, and zero-order correlations among the study variables.

	1.	2.	3.	4.	5.	6.	7.	8.
1. T1 Autonomous motivation	1							
2. T1 Controlled motivation	0.45 **	1						
3. T1 Attitude	0.56 **	0.24 **	1					
4. T1 Subjective norm	0.47 **	0.40 **	0.49 **	1				
5. T1 Perceived behavior control	0.33 **	0.12	0.43 **	0.47 **	1			
6. T1 Intention	0.58 **	0.36 **	0.47 **	0.59 **	0.43 **	1		
7. T2 Behavior	0.25 **	0.22 **	0.16 *	0.26 **	0.17 *	0.20 **	1	
8. Age	0.10	0.00	0.11	0.05	−0.06	0.09	0.13	1
9. Gender	−0.02	−0.10	0.02	0.19 **	0.15 *	0.07	−0.09	0.03
Range	1–7	1–7	1–7	1–7	1–7	1–7	1–5	17–26
Mean	4.77	2.43	6.02	4.23	5.37	4.73	2.43	20.75
Standard deviation	1.17	1.12	1.15	1.34	1.17	1.49	0.77	2.24
Cronbach's α	0.78	0.77	0.92	0.75	0.82	0.85	0.71	—

T1 = baseline, T2 = one-month after the baseline, * $p < 0.05$, ** $p < 0.01$.

The results of the path analysis supported the proposed model: $\chi^2_{(5)} = 6.90$, $\chi^2/df = 1.38$, CFI = 0.995, TLI = 0.971, RMSEA = 0.046, SRMR = 0.030. Figure 1 presents the detailed path estimates. In line with H1 and H2, autonomous motivation positively predicted the three social cognitive variables ($\beta = 0.34$ to 0.56, $p < 0.01$), while controlled motivation exerted no effects on attitude/PBC ($\beta = 0.00/-0.02$, $p = 0.98/0.85$), but a significant effect on subjective norms ($\beta = 0.26$, $p < 0.01$). Autonomous motivation ($\beta = 0.33$, $p < 0.01$), subjective norm ($\beta = 0.35$, $p < 0.01$), and PBC ($\beta = 0.14$, $p = 0.03$) were positive predictors of intention, which subsequently predicted pre-exercise fluid intake behavior ($\beta = 0.23$, $p < 0.01$). Therefore, H3 was partially supported and H4 was confirmed. Autonomous/controlled motivation and the three social cognitive variables explained 48% of the total variance in intention. SDT- and TPB-based constructs only explained 6.5% of the total variance in behavior.

Table 2 shows the results of mediation analysis. In line with H5, the three social cognitive variables were found to mediate the relationships between autonomous/controlled motivation and intention ($\beta = 0.20/0.09$, $p = 0.00/0.02$). The direct link between PBC and pre-exercise fluid intake was not significant ($\beta = 0.07$, $p = 0.39$). Furthermore, the relationships between subjective norm/PBC and pre-exercise fluid intake behavior were fully mediated by intention ($\beta = 0.07/0.03$, $p = 0.01/0.03$), and intention was not a mediator in the path between attitude and behavior ($\beta = 0.01$, $p = 0.36$). Therefore, H6 was partially supported. H7 was partially confirmed given autonomous motivation ($\beta = 0.13$, $p = 0.003$), but not for controlled motivation ($\beta = 0.02$, $p = 0.23$) had an indirect effect on behavior via the three social cognitive variables and intention.

Table 2. Mediation analyses showing the standardized direct, indirect, and total effects of the model.

Effect (Corresponding Hypothesis If Applicable)	β	p	95% CI
Direct effects			
Autonomous motivation → Attitude (H1)	0.56	<0.001	[0.43, 0.69]
Autonomous motivation → Subjective norm (H1)	0.35	0.001	[0.20, 0.49]
Autonomous motivation → PBC (H1)	0.33	<0.001	[0.17, 0.49]
Controlled motivation → Attitude (H2)	0.00	0.99	[−0.13, 0.13]
Controlled motivation → Subjective norm (H2)	0.26	0.001	[0.11, 0.40]
Controlled motivation → PBC (H3)	−0.02	0.83	[−0.15, 0.12]
Autonomous motivation → Intention (H3)	0.33	<0.001	[0.18, 0.49]
Attitude → Intention (H3)	0.06	0.46	[−0.09, 0.19]
Subjective norm → Intention (H3)	0.35	0.001	[0.17, 0.51]
PBC → Intention (H3)	0.15	0.04	[0.01, 0.27]
Intention → FIB (H4)	0.20	0.01	[0.04, 0.35]
Indirect effects			
Autonomous motivation → TPB constructs → Intention (H5)	0.20	<0.001	[0.10, 0.32]
Controlled motivation → TPB constructs → Intention (H5)	0.09	0.02	[0.02, 0.18]
Attitude → Intention → FIB (H6)	0.01	0.36	[−0.02, 0.05]
Subjective norm → Intention → FIB (H6)	0.07	0.01	[0.01, 0.15]
PBC → Intention → FIB (H6)	0.03	0.03	[0.01, 0.08]
Autonomous motivation → TPB constructs → Intention → FIB (H7)	0.13	0.003	[0.04, 0.22]
Controlled motivation → TPB constructs → Intention → FIB (H7)	0.02	0.23	[−0.01, 0.05]
Total effects			
Autonomous motivation → Intention	0.54	<0.001	[0.42, 0.64]
Controlled motivation → Intention	0.09	0.02	[0.02, 0.12]
Attitude → FIB	0.01	0.36	[−0.02, 0.05]
Subjective norm → FIB	0.07	0.01	[0.01, 0.15]
PBC → FIB	0.10	0.20	[−0.05, 0.23]
Autonomous motivation → FIB	0.13	0.003	[0.04, 0.22]
Controlled motivation → FIB	0.02	0.23	[−0.01, 0.05]

β = standardized parameter estimate, 95% confidence interval (CI) = 95% confidence interval, PBC = perceived behavioral control, theory of planned behavior (TPB) constructs = attitude, subjective norm, and PBC, FIB = fluid intake behavior.

4. Discussion

The aim of the present prospective study was to use a multi-theory model that integrates SDT- and TPB-based constructs and hypotheses to understand athletes' pre-exercise fluid intake. Findings generally supported a number of effects found in early research that applied the integrated model to understand other health behaviors [9,14,15], including the effects of autonomous motivation and the three social cognitive variables on intention, which subsequently predicted pre-exercise fluid intake behavior. Overall, SDT- and TPB-based variables explained a small amount of the total variance in pre-exercise fluid intake behavior (6.5%).

Focusing first on the proposed prediction of the three social cognitive variables by autonomous motivation (H1), our results are parallel to earlier research that showed that autonomous motivation was a positive predictor of the three social cognitive variables [9,12,14]. This finding implies that the more the athletes were autonomously motivated to engage in taking fluid before exercise, the more likely they were to hold a positive evaluation of the behavior, regarding such behavior as socially appropriate, and perceive a strong sense of personal control over the action. H2 was also supported in that controlled motivation was a positive predictor of subjective norms, but not for attitude and PBC after controlling for autonomous motivation. Previous research has shown that controlled motivation relative to autonomous motivation has a limited role in predicting the three social cognitive variables [16,25]. In addition, since controlled motivation reflects externally referenced contingencies such as obtaining rewards and avoiding social pressure, it tends not to be aligned with attitude and PBC, but with subjective norm, which reflects one's beliefs about socially appropriate behaviors [25]. Hagger and Chatzisarantis [9] asserted that subjective norms may reflect both autonomous and controlled aspects of social cognitive belief on future health behavior engagement, which explains why both autonomous and controlled motivation were positively related to subjective norm in this research.

H3, being partially supported as the path from attitude to intention, was not significant. The finding seemed to contradict with the tenets of TPB [8]. However, there was a positive association between attitude and intention ($r = 0.47$, $p < 0.01$), based on the results of zero-order correlation. Therefore, it is highly possible that attitude had a limited effect on intention after controlling for the subjective norm and PBC. Furthermore, the subjective norm exerted a larger effect than PBC on intention (0.35 vs. 0.14). The context where a behavior is situated may affect the predictive ability of the three social cognitive variables [8]. As such, the subjective norm is likely the strongest predictor of intention in the context of pre-exercise fluid intake. There is a strong social component in pre-exercise fluid intake behavior, and university athletes' intention is mainly influenced by their beliefs about significant others' expectations (e.g., teammates). Observably, athletes have a lot of exposure to teammates' normative influences since they train together most of the time.

It is important to note that this is the first research to extend the TPB in understanding athletes' pre-exercise fluid intake behaviors. Their intention was found to positively predict pre-exercise fluid intake in our study. This finding is consistent with H4 and the TPB [8]. However, the effect size of the intention-behavior link is small ($\beta = 0.20$) and a similar effect was also found in early prospective research [9,26]. The small effect may be due to the intention-behavior gap [27]. To bridge the intention-behavior gap, theorists have suggested a number of solutions such as including implementation intention, planning, maintenance self-efficacy, action control, and self-control in the process of the intention-behavior relationship [6,26–28]. Another possible avenue is to use the dual-process approach [29–31]. Some health behaviors may be affected by the impulsive process, in which automaticity or habit implicitly governs the behavioral execution. Future research may incorporate automatic factors (e.g., implicit attitude or habit) into the integrated model that may provide additional avenues for the target behavior [5,25].

With regard to the mediation effects, the relationship between autonomous motivation and intention was partially mediated through the three social cognitive variables, while controlled motivation was fully mediated through them. This finding is consistent with H5 and early research [9,25], which suggests two possible routes by which superordinate motivational antecedents from SDT may predict intention. Namely, a mediated route that includes intention and its proximal predictors (i.e., the three social cognitive variables), and a direct route that directly affects intention independent of the belief-orientated decision-making process [26]. H6 was only partially supported, since intention was found to fully rather than partially mediate the relationship between PBC and fluid intake behavior. Lack of a direct effect from PBC to behavior is possible due to the measure of PBC. Our PBC measure reflects perceived rather than actual control beliefs. According to Ajzen [8], when the PBC measure reflects actual control over behavior, PBC will predict behavior directly. Although we found that autonomous motivation had an indirect effect on fluid intake behavior via the three social cognitive variables and intention, the finding is similar to the findings of meta-analytic studies of the integrated model [9,32]. Although motivation may also form a direct effect on health behavior [25], the mediation of social cognitive variables addresses the importance of understanding the proximal decision-making process to enhance the variance of intention and behavior.

Even though the present research has several strengths (e.g., the first research to test the integrated model in the area of pre-exercise fluid intake behavior), it is not without its limitations. First, the participants of this study were university athletes in China, which means the present findings may not be generalized into athletes in other age groups, educational levels, or cultures. Future research should examine whether the findings can be replicated across diverse populations. Second, the ongoing debate on the effectiveness of pre-exercise hydration status (e.g., [33]) could somewhat reduce the practical implications of the present study. However, the current guidelines are widely accepted, and the effective pre-exercise hydration status has not been proven to be deleterious on performance. Third, we relied entirely on self-reported measures that are subject to recall bias and response tendency [34]. Objective measures representing the effectiveness of behavioral adherence to pre-exercise fluid intake (e.g., urine specific gravity and body weight) should be used in future research. Lastly, even though a two-wave prospective survey design was used in this research, it is insufficient to conclude the temporal and causal nature of the relationships that are found in the integrated model. A panel design or intervention research is necessary to provide stronger evidence for the conclusions.

5. Conclusions

Our survey extended and tested the integrated model in the context of pre-exercise fluid intake among athletes. We generally found support for the model and its related hypotheses. Our findings suggest that there are multiple potential routes for pre-exercise fluid intake behavior, which provide preliminary evidence for the development of pre-exercise fluid intake interventions. Intervention programs should target all of the relevant routes to increase the intention and behavior of pre-exercise fluid intake. For example, since autonomous motivation has both substantially direct and indirect effects on intention, it would be useful to increase athletes' autonomous motivation. According to SDT [10], autonomy-supportive behaviors (e.g., providing choices in selecting different types of fluid and creating a caring climate during behavior changing processes) can be an effective way to enhance their autonomous motivation.

Supplementary Materials: The following is available online at http://www.mdpi.com/2072-6643/10/5/646/s1. Table S1: Scale items for constructs of the integrated model of pre-exercise fluid intake.

Author Contributions: C.L., F.-H.S., and D.K.C.C. conceived and designed the study. C.L. and L.Z. conducted the data collection. C.L. and D.K.C.C. analyzed the data. All the authors wrote the paper.

Acknowledgments: This research was supported by the Internal Research Grant of The Education University of Hong Kong [RG99/2015–2016]. The publication fee was supported by the Department of Health and Physical Education, The Education University of Hong Kong.

Conflicts of Interest: The authors declare no conflict of interest.

References

1. Caspersen, C.J.; Powell, K.E.; Christenson, G.M. Physical activity, exercise, and physical fitness: Definitions and distinctions for health-related research. *Public Health Rep.* **1985**, *100*, 126–131. [PubMed]
2. Institute of Medicine. *Dietary Reference in Takes for Water, Sodium, Chloride, Potassium and Sulfate*; National Academy Press: Washington, DC, USA, 2005.
3. Sawka, M.; Burke, L.; Eichner, E.; Maughan, R.; Montain, S.; Stachenfeld, N. American College of Sports Medicine position stand. Exercise and fluid replacement. *Med. Sci. Sports Exerc.* **2007**, *39*, 377–390. [PubMed]
4. Volpe, S.L.; Poule, K.A.; Bland, E.G. Estimation of prepractice hydration status of National Collegiate Athletic Association Division I athletes. *J. Athl. Train.* **2009**, *44*, 624–629. [CrossRef] [PubMed]

5. Hagger, M.S.; Chatzisarantis, N.L.D. An integrated behavior-change model for physical activity. *Exerc. Sport Sci. Rev.* **2014**, *42*, 62–69. [CrossRef] [PubMed]
6. Hagger, M.S.; Luszczynska, A.; de Wit, J.; Benyamini, Y.; Burkert, S.; Chamberland, P.E.; Chater, A.; Dombrowski, S.U.; van Dongen, A.; French, D.P. Implementation intention and planning interventions in health psychology: Recommendations from the Synergy Expert Group for research and practice. *Psychol. Health* **2016**, *31*, 814–839. [CrossRef] [PubMed]
7. Deci, E.L.; Ryan, R.M. *Intrinsic Motivation and Self-Determination in Human Behavior*; Plenum Press: New York, NY, USA, 1985.
8. Ajzen, I. The theory of planned behavior. *Organ. Behav. Hum. Decis. Process.* **1991**, *50*, 179–211. [CrossRef]
9. Hagger, M.S.; Chatzisarantis, N.L. Integrating the theory of planned behaviour and self-determination theory in health behaviour: A meta-analysis. *Br. J. Health Psychol.* **2009**, *14*, 275–302. [CrossRef] [PubMed]
10. Deci, E.L.; Ryan, R.M. The "what" and" why" of goal pursuits: Human needs and the self-determination of behavior. *Psychol. Inq.* **2000**, *11*, 227–268. [CrossRef]
11. Chan, D.; Dimmock, J.; Donovan, R.; Hardcastle, S.; Lentillon-Kaestner, V.; Hagger, M.S. Self-determined motivation in sport predicts anti-doping motivation and intention: A perspective from the trans-contextual model. *J. Sci. Med. Sport* **2015**, *18*, 315–322. [CrossRef] [PubMed]
12. Hamilton, K.; Cox, S.; White, K.M. Testing a model of physical activity among mothers and fathers of young children: Integrating self-determined motivation, planning, and the theory of planned behavior. *J. Sport Exerc. Psychol.* **2012**, *34*, 124–145. [CrossRef] [PubMed]
13. Chan, D.K.-C.; Hagger, M.S. Theoretical integration and the psychology of sport injury prevention. *Sports Med.* **2012**, *42*, 725–732. [PubMed]
14. Chan, D.K.-C.; Fung, Y.-K.; Xing, S.; Hagger, M.S. Myopia prevention, near work, and visual acuity of college students: Integrating the theory of planned behavior and self-determination theory. *J. Behav. Med.* **2014**, *37*, 369–380. [CrossRef] [PubMed]
15. Kor, K.; Mullan, B.A. Sleep hygiene behaviours: An application of the theory of planned behaviour and the investigation of perceived autonomy support, past behaviour and response inhibition. *Psychol. Health* **2011**, *26*, 1208–1224. [CrossRef] [PubMed]
16. Leblanc, V.; Bégin, C.; Corneau, L.; Dodin, S.; Lemieux, S. Gender differences in dietary intakes: What is the contribution of motivational variables? *J. Hum. Nutr. Diet.* **2015**, *28*, 37–46. [CrossRef] [PubMed]
17. Riebl, S.K.; Estabrooks, P.A.; Dunsmore, J.C.; Savla, J.; Frisard, M.I.; Dietrich, A.M.; Peng, Y.; Zhang, X.; Davy, B.M. A systematic literature review and meta-analysis: The Theory of Planned Behavior's application to understand and predict nutrition-related behaviors in youth. *Eat. Behav.* **2015**, *18*, 160–178. [CrossRef] [PubMed]
18. Pelletier, L.G.; Dion, S.C.; Slovinec-D'Angelo, M.; Reid, R. Why do you regulate what you eat? Relationships between forms of regulation, eating behaviors, sustained dietary behavior change, and psychological adjustment. *Motiv. Emot.* **2004**, *28*, 245–277. [CrossRef]
19. Hagger, M.S.; Lonsdale, A.J.; Hein, V.; Koka, A.; Lintunen, T.; Pasi, H.; Lindwall, M.; Rudolfsson, L.; Chatzisarantis, N.L. Predicting alcohol consumption and binge drinking in company employees: An application of planned behaviour and self-determination theories. *Br.J. Health Psychol.* **2012**, *17*, 379–407. [CrossRef] [PubMed]
20. Hair, J.; Anderson, R.; Babin, B.; Black, W. *Multivariate Data Analysi*, 7th ed.; Pearson: Upper Saddle River, NJ, USA, 2010.
21. Arbuckle, J.L. *IBM SPSS AMOS 20 User's Guide*; IBM Corporation: Armonk, NY, USA, 2011.
22. Kline, R.B. *Principles and Practice of Structural Equation Modeling*, 2nd ed.; The Guilford Press: New York, NY, USA, 2005.
23. Hu, L.; Bentler, P.M. Cutoff criteria for fit indexes in covariance structure analysis: Conventional criteria versus new alternatives. *Struct. Equ. Model.* **1999**, *6*, 1–55. [CrossRef]
24. Hayes, A.F. *Introduction to Mediation, Moderation, and Conditional Process Analysis: A Regression-Based Approach*; Guilford Publications: New York, NY, USA, 2013.
25. Hamilton, K.; Kirkpatrick, A.; Rebar, A.; Hagger, M.S. Child sun safety: Application of an Integrated Behavior Change model. *Health Psychol.* **2017**, *36*, 916–926. [CrossRef] [PubMed]
26. Caudwell, K.M.; Hagger, M.S. Predicting alcohol pre-drinking in Australian undergraduate students using an integrated theoretical model. *Appl. Psychol. Health Well-Being* **2015**, *7*, 188–213. [CrossRef] [PubMed]

27. Sniehotta, F.F.; Scholz, U.; Schwarzer, R. Bridging the intention-behaviour gap: Planning, self-efficacy, and action control in the adoption and maintenance of physical exercise. *Psychol. Health* **2005**, *20*, 143–160. [CrossRef]

28. Hagger, M.S.; Leaver, E.; Esser, K.; Leung, C.M.; Pas, N.T.; Keatley, D.A.; Chan, D.K.C.; Chatzisarantis, N.L.D. Cue-induced smoking urges deplete cigarette smokers' self-control resources. *Ann. Behav. Med.* **2013**, *46*, 394–400. [CrossRef] [PubMed]

29. Hagger, M.S.; Trost, N.; Keech, J.; Chan, D.K.C.; Hamilton, K. Predicting sugar consumption: Application of an integrated dual-process, dual-phase model. *Appetite* **2017**, *116*, 147–156. [CrossRef] [PubMed]

30. Keatley, D.A.; Chan, D.K.C.; Caudwell, K.; Chatzisarantis, N.L.D.; Hagger, M.S. A consideration of what is meant by automaticity and better ways to measure it. *Front. Psychol.* **2015**, *5*, 1537. [CrossRef] [PubMed]

31. Hollands, G.J.; Marteau, T.M.; Fletcher, P.C. Non-conscious processes in changing health-related behaviour: A conceptual analysis and framework. *Health Psychol. Rev.* **2016**, *10*, 381–394. [CrossRef] [PubMed]

32. Hagger, M.S.; Chatzisarantis, N.L. The trans-contextual model of autonomous motivation in education: Conceptual and empirical issues and meta-analysis. *Rev. Educ. Res.* **2016**, *86*, 360–407. [CrossRef] [PubMed]

33. Wall, B.A.; Watson, G.; Peiffer, J.J.; Abbiss, C.R.; Siegel, R.; Laursen, P.B. Current hydration guidelines are erroneous: Dehydration does not impair exercise performance in the heat. *Br. J. Sports Med.* **2015**, *49*, 1077–1083. [CrossRef] [PubMed]

34. Chan, D.K.C.; Ivarsson, A.; Stenling, A.; Yang, X.S.; Chatzisarantis, N.L.D.; Hagger, M.S. Response-order effects in survey methods: A randomized controlled crossover study in the context of sport injury prevention. *J. Sport Exerc. Psychol.* **2015**, *37*, 666–673. [CrossRef] [PubMed]

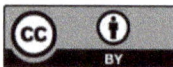

nutrients

MDPI

Article

Beverage Consumption among Adults in the Balearic Islands: Association with Total Water and Energy Intake

Asli Emine Özen [1], Maria del Mar Bibiloni [2], Cristina Bouzas [2], Antoni Pons [2] and Josep A. Tur [2,*]

[1] Department of Gastronomy and Culinary Arts, Reha Midilli Foça Faculty of Tourism, Dokuz Eylül University, Foça-Izmir 35680, Turkey; asli.ozen@deu.edu.tr

[2] Research Group on Community Nutrition and Oxidative Stress, University of the Balearic Islands & CIBEROBN, 07122 Palma de Mallorca, Spain; mar.bibiloni@uib.es (M.d.M.B.); cristinabouvel@gmail.com (C.B.); antonipons@uib.es (A.P.)

* Correspondence: pep.tur@uib.es; Tel.: +34-971-173146

Received: 7 July 2018; Accepted: 21 August 2018; Published: 23 August 2018

Abstract: The paper seeks to describe beverage consumption and examine the association between beverage consumption and total water intake and total energy intake of the adult population in the Balearic Islands. Beverage consumption, total water intake, and total energy intake were obtained by using two 24-h diet recalls from a cross-sectional nutritional survey carried out in the Balearic Islands (n = 1386). The contribution of beverages to total water intake and total energy intake were also assessed. Beverages accounted for 65–71% of total water intake and 29–35% of it provided by drinking water. Food moisture contributed 31–37% of total water intake. The mean daily total water intake from all sources was around 2.2 L for men and 1.9 L for women and slightly lower than the proposed adequate intake (AI) recommendations of the European Food Safety Authority (EFSA). The mean total energy intake was 2222 kcal/day and beverages contributed 10.3% of total energy intake for men and 9.5% for women. Energy intake from beverages varied with age. In both sexes, milk was the main beverage contributed to total energy intake. The energy contribution of caloric soft drinks was 1.8% for men and 1.2% for women and energy intake from these beverages was significantly higher among younger adults. Water was the main beverage in the diet, followed by milk and hot beverages. Beverages were mainly consumed in the main meal times (breakfast, lunch, and dinner) in both sexes. The main findings of this study indicate that consumption of sugar-sweetened beverages (caloric soft drinks and commercial fruit juice) is higher among young adults, consumption of alcoholic beverages is higher among males aged 26 and older, and TWI (total water intake) is lower than the EFSA recommendations. These findings may be used to develop effective, healthy eating and drinking policies and campaigns.

Keywords: beverage consumption; water consumption; total water intake; total energy intake; adults; Balearic Islands

1. Introduction

Water intake is very essential for human life because water accounts for 50–60% of adult body mass and we need water for the enzymatic and chemical reactions and excretion of metabolic waste from our body [1]. While in our early ancestors' diet consisted of only drinking water and breast milk [2,3], our beverage choices are vast.

The European Food Safety Authority (EFSA) estimates that 70–80% of total water intake (TWI) comes from drinking water and beverages, while the remaining 20–30% is obtained from food moisture [4]. However, estimates of the Spanish population fall slightly outside these estimations [5]. The contribution of foods and beverages to the TWI for the Spanish population are 32% and 68% [5], respectively. Still, drinking water is the main source of water in the diet of all age groups, and consumption of other beverages varies according to age [6–12].

Many beverages contribute to total energy intake (TEI). The average energy contribution of beverages to TEI among European countries varies from 7 to 16% (e.g., 7% in Italy [13], 8% in France [14], 12% in Spain [5], and 16% in the UK [15]). Alcoholic beverages are the main contributors to energy intake, followed by milk [14,15].

Recent studies of TWI and beverage consumption and the association between beverage consumption and energy intake among Spaniards have been published [5,12]. A recent study suggested that the population of the Balearic Islands is undergoing a nutrition transition [16]. We, therefore, investigated beverage consumption and TWI, with special attention to the types of beverages consumed and their calorie contribution to total energy intake in a nationally representative sample from the Balearic Islands.

2. Methods

2.1. Study Population

Subjects of this study were participants in the OBEX (Obesity and oxidative stress) project which is a population based cross-sectional nutritional survey. The data collection took place between 2009 and 2010. The sample population was derived from residents aged 16–65 years registered in the official population census of the Balearic Islands. The sampling technique included stratification according to municipality size, age, and sex of inhabitants, and the samples were randomization into subgroups, with the Balearic Islands municipalities being the primary sampling units, and individuals within these municipalities comprising the final sample units. The theoretical sample size was set at 1500 individuals and the one specific relative precision of 5% (type I error = 0.05; type II error = 0.10), and the final sample was 1386 (92.4% participation). Pregnant women were excluded from this study. This study was conducted according to the guidelines laid down in the Declaration of Helsinki, and all procedures involving human subjects were approved by the Balearic Islands' Ethics Committee (Palma de Mallorca, Spain) No. IB/1128/09/PI. Written informed consent was obtained from all subjects and, when they were under 18 years, also from their parents or legal tutors.

2.2. General Questionnaire and Anthropometrics

A questionnaire collected the following information: age, marital status, educational level (grouped according to years and type of education: low, <6 years at school; medium, 6–12 years of education; high, >12 years of education), and socioeconomic level (classified as low, medium, and high according to the methodology described by the Spanish Society of Epidemiology) [17].

Information about smoking habits and alcohol consumption was collected and grouped as non-smoker, ex-smoker, smoker, and non-drinker, occasional drinker, daily drinker (1–2 drinks/day), and heavy drinker (more than three drinks/day).

Anthropometric [18] and blood pressure (BP) [19] measurements have been described in full elsewhere. BMI was computed as weight/height^2 (kg/m^2) and study participants were categorized as healthy weight (BMI < 24.9 kg/m^2), overweight (25 kg/m^2 < BMI < 29.9 kg/m^2), and obese (BMI $\geq$ 30 kg/m^2) [20]. Hypertension was defined as either having a systolic blood pressure (SBP) of $\geq$140 mmHg or diastolic blood pressure (DBP) of $\geq$90 mmHg, currently under antihypertensive treatment, or previously diagnosed for hypertension.

2.3. Physical Activity Assessment

Physical activity (PA) was evaluated according to guidelines for data processing and analysis of the International Physical Activity Questionnaire [21] in the short form. The PA levels were estimated by using metabolic equivalents of task (MET). MET scores for different level activities were established based on the Compendium of Physical Activities [22]. On the basis of their total weekly MET scores, the subjects were divided into three groups: "low", "moderate", and "high" levels of PA.

2.4. Assessment of Beverage Consumption and Energy Intake

Beverage, food, and energy intakes were assessed by averaging two non-consecutive 24 h dietary recalls. To prevent seasonal variations, 24 h dietary recalls were administered in the warm season (May–September) and in the cold season (November–March). Furthermore, to account for day-to-day intake variability, the two 24-h recalls were administered from Monday to Sunday. Participants reported all foods and beverages consumed throughout the day: breakfast, second breakfast, lunch, afternoon snack, dinner, and outside of meal times. A manual of sets of photographs [23] was used for the estimation of portion size. Well-trained dieticians administered the recalls and verified and quantified the information obtained from the 24 h recalls.

Beverages were categorized into 11 groups; water (tap water and bottled water), full-fat milk, low/non-fat milk (semi-skimmed and skimmed milk), 100% fruit juice (all kinds of natural fruit juice), commercial fruit juice (all kinds of fruit juice sweetened with sugar), caloric soft drinks (all kinds of carbonated soft drinks, sugar added iced tea and energy beverages), diet soda (low calorie carbonated soft drinks), coffee, tea, alcoholic beverages (wine, beer, vodka, whisky, liquor), and other beverages (beer without alcohol, diet milkshake, soy milk, rice milk, oat milk, fermented milk drink with sugar, fermented milk drink, kefir, horchata, chocolate milkshake, isotonic drinks). Total milk included full-fat milk and low/non-fat milk, hot beverages included coffee and tea, and total fruit juice included all kinds of fruit juice were also calculated. TWI and TEI were calculated using a computer program (ALIMENTA®, NUCOX, Palma, Spain) based on Spanish [24,25] and European Food Composition Tables [26], and complemented with food composition data available for the Balearic food items [27]. Total water intake was calculated as drinking water plus water from all other beverages and moisture from all foods. Identification of underreporting participants was based on the Goldberg cut-off [28]. Adults whose reported energy intake (EI)/basal metabolic rate (BMR) was <0.9585 were classified as under-reporters (n = 328), and they were excluded from the current study.

2.5. Statistics

Statistical analyses were performed using SPSS for Windows, version 24.0 (SPSS Inc., Chicago, IL, USA). For descriptive purposes, absolute numbers and percentages of participants were calculated for demographic and lifestyle characteristics and differences tested by χ^2. Average daily beverage consumption, TWI (g/day) and TEI (kcal/day) were calculated and differences across means were evaluated by using analysis of variance. Differences in mean daily water, beverage and energy intake across age groups within sex were assessed by using student t-tests with Bonferroni correction for multiple testing. Partial correlations between the consumption of different types of beverages and TWI, water intake from beverages and foods, TEI, energy intake from beverages and foods were adjusted for gender, age, and BMI. For all statistical tests, $p < 0.05$ was taken as the significant level.

3. Results

3.1. Description of the Survey Sample

Survey respondents ranged from 16 to 65 years (mean 32 years) (Table 1). Overweight prevalence was higher among men (41%) than women (32%). Men were likely to be single heavy drinker and have hypertension; women reported engaging in less physical activity.

Table 1. Socio-demographic and lifestyle characteristics of study population.

Characteristics	Male (*n* = 410)		Female (*n* = 654)		
	n	%	*n*	%	χ^2
Age (years)					<0.001
16–25	201	49	228	36	
26–45	150	37	290	45	
46–65	57	14	122	19	
BMI					<0.001
Healthy weight	232	57	445	68	
Overweight	143	35	159	24	
Obese	35	9	49	8	
Marital Status					0.003
Not married	304	75	426	67	
Married	103	25	213	33	
Education Level					ns
Low	136	34	185	29	
Medium	144	36	224	35	
High	124	31	228	36	
Employment Status					ns
Low	174	43	240	37	
Medium	40	10	81	13	
High	195	48	324	50	
Smoking status					ns
Non smoker	241	61	374	59	
Ex-smoker	48	12	82	13	
Smoker	108	27	174	28	
Alcohol consumption					<0.001
Non drinkers	91	23	207	32	
Very occasional drinkers	151	37	263	41	
Daily drinkers	125	31	140	22	
Heavy drinkers	37	9	29	5	
Hypertension					0.038
No hypertension	288	71	483	76	
Have hypertension	116	29	149	24	
Physical Activity					<0.001
Low	164	41	431	67	
Moderate	132	33	174	30	
High	102	26	43	7	

BMI: Body Mass Index; Not married includes: single, divorced, widowed, and separated. ns: Not statistically significant.

3.2. Contribution of Beverages and Food Moisture to Daily Diet

Daily mean beverage consumption was stratified by gender and age as presented in Table 2. Consumption of full-fat milk, fruit juice, and caloric soft drinks tended to decrease with age in both sexes. Men consumed two times more caloric soft drinks (*p* < 0.001) and alcoholic beverage (*p* < 0.001) than women, while tea (*p* < 0.001) consumption was much higher in women.

The contribution of foods and beverages to daily TWI (g/day) and TEI (kcal/day), by gender and age group, are presented in Table 3. In total, beverages accounted for 71.1% and 65.4% of TWI for men and women, respectively, while the contribution of all foods to TWI was 28.9% for men and 34.6% for women. The mean daily TWI from all sources was around 2.2 L for men and 1.9 L for women. Energy intake from beverages was higher in men than in women and slightly increased with age. The mean TEI of the study population was 2222 (±19) kcal/day, and beverages contributed 9.5% of TEI for females and 10.3% for males.

3.3. Contribution of Beverage Type to Diet

The contribution of beverages to daily water and energy intake by gender and age is presented in Table 4. Water was the most consumed beverage for both sexes and drinking water alone accounted for 31.7% of the TWI for men and 29.2% of the TWI for women. Among other beverages, hot beverages (mainly coffee) and milk were the main sources of TWI for both sexes.

Table 2. Mean daily beverage consumption (g/day) by gender and age group.

Beverages	Male					Female				
	16-25 Mean (SE)[1]	26-45 Mean (SE)[1]	46-65 Mean (SE)[1]	Total Mean (SE)[1]	p Value	16-25 Mean (SE)[1]	26-45 Mean (SE)[1]	46-65 Mean (SE)[1]	Total Mean (SE)[1]	p Value
Water	839.5 (57.3)	817.7 (69.2)	845.3 (110.7)	831.4 (40.7)	ns	709.8 (47.5)	636.0 (38.7)	748.8 (79.3)	688.5 (28.5)	ns
Milk total	228.8 (15.3) [a]	194.8 (14.6) [ab]	150.6 (20.1) [b]	205.6 (9.7) *	0.021	176.4 (9.4)	165.4 (8.2)	181.1 (11.6)	173.4 (5.4)	ns
Full-fat milk	111.8 (11.8) [a]	85.9 (9.9) [ab]	59.4 (12.5) [b]	95.2 (7.1) ***	0.032	94.0 (8.8) [a]	61.0 (6.1) [b]	47.7 (9.4) [b]	70.0 (4.5)	<0.001
Low/non-fat milk	117.0 (13.1)	108.9 (14.0)	91.2 (17.0)	110.4 (8.6)	ns	82.5 (7.9) [a]	104.4 (7.5) [ab]	133.4 (10.8) [b]	103.4 (5.0)	0.001
Fruit juice total	111.4 (14.6) [a]	83.0 (12.9) [ab]	49.1 (13.5) [b]	92.3 (8.8) ***	0.049	96.5 (9.3) [a]	63.8 (7.0) [b]	36.0 (8.7) [b]	70.4 (4.9)	<0.001
100% fruit juice	22.7 (7.3)	28.9 (6.2)	21.1 (8.2)	24.8 (4.4)	ns	20.3 (4.0)	23.7 (3.9)	26.9 (2.7)	23.1 (2.7)	ns
Commercial fruit juice	88.7 (13.2) [a]	54.1 (11.8) [ab]	28.1 (9.3) [b]	67.5 (8.0) *	0.019	76.3 (8.9) [a]	40.1 (6.1) [b]	11.1 (4.1) [c]	47.5 (4.4)	<0.001
Caloric soft drinks	219.5 (24.7) [a]	84.9 (9.3) [b]	48.1 (17.4) [b]	145.4 (14.0) ***	<0.001	129.4 (17.8) [a]	68.6 (9.7) [b]	19.6 (6.9) [c]	79.7 (7.8)	<0.001
Light soft drinks	11.8 (5.5) [a]	38.9 (9.3) [b]	10.5 (7.4) [a]	21.5 (4.5) *	0.014	19.3 (10.6)	36.6 (7.5)	14.4 (6.4)	25.7 (5.1)	ns
Hot beverages total	207.7 (21.8)	181.0 (20.4)	174.2 (26.8)	194.7 (13.6)	ns	219.0 (17.8)	190.1 (11.2)	202.5 (17.7)	202.1 (8.7)	ns
Coffee	194.7 (20.8)	152.3 (19.3)	142.6 (25.8)	173.0 (13.0) ***	ns	193.5 (17.5) [a]	128.2 (8.7) [b]	121.6 (13.1) [b]	150.4 (7.8)	<0.001
Tea	12.9 (5.7)	28.7 (7.1)	31.6 (10.7)	21.7 (4.1) ***	ns	25.4 (5.6) [a]	61.96 (8.3) [b]	80.9 (14.4) [b]	51.7 (5.0)	<0.001
Alcoholic beverages	46.3 (15.8) [a]	161.0 (37.0) [b]	179.2 (36.8) [b]	107.0 (16.7) **	0.001	25.0 (11.0)	51.1 (7.2)	52.4 (10.3)	41.9 (5.4)	ns
Other beverages	3.6 (2.2) [a]	45.0 (9.5) [b]	33.4 (13.7) [b]	22.9 (4.2) ***	<0.001	13.9 (4.5) [a]	28.72 (4.6) [ab]	34.2 (8.4) [b]	24.3 (3.0)	0.031
Total beverage	1668.6 (57.8)	1606.3 (86.5)	1490.4 (115.2)	1620.7 (45.4) *	ns	1390.2 (52.8)	1242.7 (42.0)	1290.9 (79.3)	1307.3 (30.4)	ns

* $p < 0.05$, ** $p < 0.01$, *** $p < 0.001$ (Significantly different from females). Superscript lowercase letters denote significant differences across age group within sex (analysis of variance with Bonferroni correction). ns: not statistically significant. [1] Standard Error Means.

Table 3. Contribution of food and beverages to total water (g/day) and energy (kcal/day) intake by gender and age group.

	Age Group	Water from Beverages[1]		Water from Foods[1]		Total Water Intake (TWI)[1]	Energy from Beverages[1]		Energy from Foods[1]		Total Energy Intake (TEI)[1]
		Mean (SE)[1]	%	Mean (SE)[1]	%	Mean (SE)[1]	Mean (SE)[1]	%	Mean (SE)[1]	%	Mean (SE)[1]
Male	16–25 years	1604.7 (57.1)[a]	78.4	544.8 (39.3)[a]	21.6	2149.6 (62.5)	262.7 (13.1)	10.1	2359.1 (48.4)[a]	89.9	2621.8 (51.0)[a]
	26–45 years	1542.7 (84.2)	66.8	749.2 (37.9)[b]	33.2	2291.9 (84.9)	258.3 (15.0)	10.6	2192.6 (51.9)[b]	89.6	2450.9 (54.6)[a]
	46–65 years	1438.6 (114.8)	63.1	824.8 (50.8)[b]	36.9	2263.4 (125.8)	233.8 (18.6)	10.5	1976.8 (59.6)[c]	89.5	2210.6 (64.1)[b]
	Total	1558.7 (44.6) ***	71.1	658.4 (44.6)	28.9	2217.1 (47.0) ***	257.1 (8.9) ***	10.3	2244.5 (32.6) ***	89.7	2499.5 (33.9) ***
Female	16–25 years	1343.6 (52.2)	73.5	530.0 (28.7)[a]	26.5	1873.6 (54.9)	205.7 (9.7)	9.6	1931.6 (33.1)[a]	90.4	2137.3 (35.0)[a]
	26–45 years	1202.6 (41.8)	62.1	724.9 (22.8)[b]	37.9	1925.7 (44.6)	190.2 (7.4)	9.4	1863.1 (28.5)[a]	90.6	2050.5 (29.3)[a]
	46–65 years	1249.3 (78.9)	58.8	825.7 (33.1)[c]	41.2	2074.9 (87.2)	172.6 (10.4)	9.3	1704.4 (34.4)[b]	90.4	1877.0 (35.4)[b]
	Total	1264.8 (30.2)	65.4	673.4 (16.2)	34.6	1937.4 (32.4)	192.4 (5.2)	9.5	1857.2 (18.9)	90.5	2048.1 (19.4)
Total		1380.4 (25.7)	68.1	667.5 (14.0)	31.9	2047.4 (27.3)	217.6 (4.8)	9.8	2008.1 (18.0)	90.2	2222.0 (18.9)

*** $p < 0.001$ (Significantly different from females). Superscript lowercase letters denote significant differences across age group within sex (analysis of variance with Bonferroni correction). [1] Standard Error Means.

Table 4. Contribution of beverages to total water and energy intake by gender and age group.

	Contribution to Water Intake								Contribution to Energy Intake							
	Male				Female				Male				Female			
	Age Group				Age Group				Age Group				Age Group			
	16-25	26-45	46-65	Total	16-25	26-45	46-65	Total	16-25	26-45	46-65	Total	16-25	26-45	46-65	Total
Total intake, Mean(SE)[1]	2149.6	2291.9	2263.4	2217.1	1873.6	1925.7	2074.9	1937.4	2621.8	2450.9	2210.6	2499.5	2137.3	2050.5	1877.0	2048.1
	(62.5)	(84.9)	(125.8)	(47.0)***	(54.9)	(44.6)	(87.2)	(32.4)	(51.0)[a]	(54.6)[a]	(64.1)[b]	(33.9)***	(35.0)[a]	(29.3)[a]	(35.4)[b]	(19.4)
From Beverages (%)	78.4	66.8	63.1	71.1	73.5	62.1	58.8	65.4	10.1	10.6	10.5	10.3	9.6	9.4	9.3	9.5
Water (%)	33.3	29.6	32.1	31.7	31.5	27.3	28.5	29.2	0.0	0.0	0.0	0.0	0.0	0.0	0.0	0.0
Milk total (%)	11.1	8.3	6.4	9.4	10	8.5	9.5	9.3	4.7	4.3	3.8	4.5	4.6	4.1	4.4	4.4
Full-fat milk (%)	5.5	3.6	2.6	2.5	5.5	3.2	2.5	2.2	2.7	2.4	1.8	2.5	2.8	1.9	1.8	2.2
Low/non-fat milk (%)	5.6	4.8	3.8	2	4.5	5.3	7.0	2.2	2.0	1.9	2.0	2.0	1.9	2.2	2.6	2.2
Fruit juice total (%)	5.2	3.5	2.2	4.1	5.3	3.1	1.5	3.6	2.0	1.5	1.3	1.7	2.1	1.4	1.0	1.6
100% fruit juice (%)	0.9	1.4	0.8	1.1	1.2	1.2	1.1	1.1	0.4	0.6	0.4	0.5	0.5	0.6	0.7	0.6
Commercial fruit juice (%)	4.3	2.0	2.0	1.3	4.1	1.9	0.4	2.4	1.6	1.0	0.7	1.3	1.8	0.9	0.3	1.1
Caloric soft drinks (%)	10.9	3.6	1.9	6.9	7.1	3.7	0.8	4.3	2.7	1.0	0.8	1.8	1.7	1.0	0.8	1.2
Light soft drinks (%)	0.8	1.8	0.6	1.1	1.0	2.0	1.0	1.4	0.0	0.0	0.0	0.0	0.0	0.0	0.0	0.0
Hot beverages total (%)	11.7	8.8	7.8	10.2	14.2	11.2	10.9	12.2	0.1	0.2	0.3	0.2	0.2	0.4	0.6	0.4
Coffee (%)	11.2	7.4	6.6	9.2	12.8	7.9	6.7	9.4	0.1	0.1	0.2	0.1	0.1	0.2	0.2	0.1
Tea (%)	0.5	1.4	1.3	0.9	1.4	3.3	4.2	2.7	0.1	0.1	0.1	0.1	0.1	0.3	0.4	0.3
Alcoholic beverages (%)	1.8	6.9	8.4	4.6	0.9	2.6	3.1	2.1	0.4	2.6	3.7	1.7	0.5	1.5	1.6	1.2
Other beverages (%)	0.2	1.4	1.1	0.8	0.8	1.5	1.4	1.2	0.2	0.9	0.7	0.5	0.5	1.0	0.9	0.8

*** $p < 0.001$ (Significantly different from females). Superscript lowercase letters denote significant differences across age group within sex (analysis of variance with Bonferroni correction). [1] Standard Error Means.

In both males and females, milk was the principal beverage contributor of TEI. Among younger adults, the contribution of commercial fruit juice and caloric soft drinks to TEI was higher, while the energy contribution of alcoholic beverages was higher in middle-aged men.

3.4. Distribution of Beverages during Day

Figure 1 shows the mean daily consumption of beverages during each meal time for males and females. Milk, fruit juices, and hot beverages (coffee and tea) were mainly consumed for breakfast in both sexes. Alcoholic beverages were mainly consumed during lunch and dinner. Other beverages were more evenly spread throughout the day, with slightly higher consumption during lunch and dinner. The main part of the water consumption was concentrated in the afternoon, and the highest water intake was observed outside of the meal times.

Percentage of total beverage consumption during each meal time is presented in Figure 2. Beverage consumption during dinner was significantly higher in middle-aged men than others, while a higher proportion of older women preferred to consume their beverages during dinner.

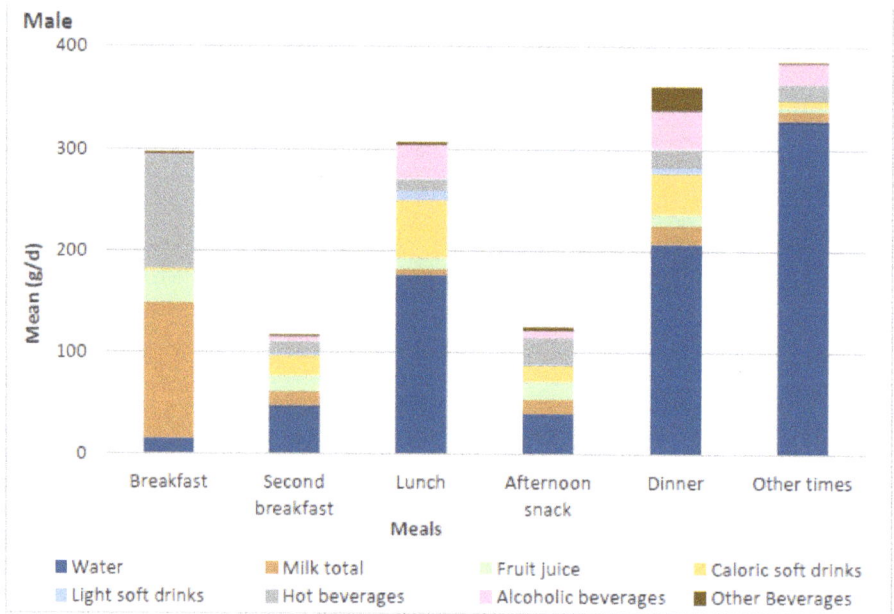

Figure 1. *Cont.*

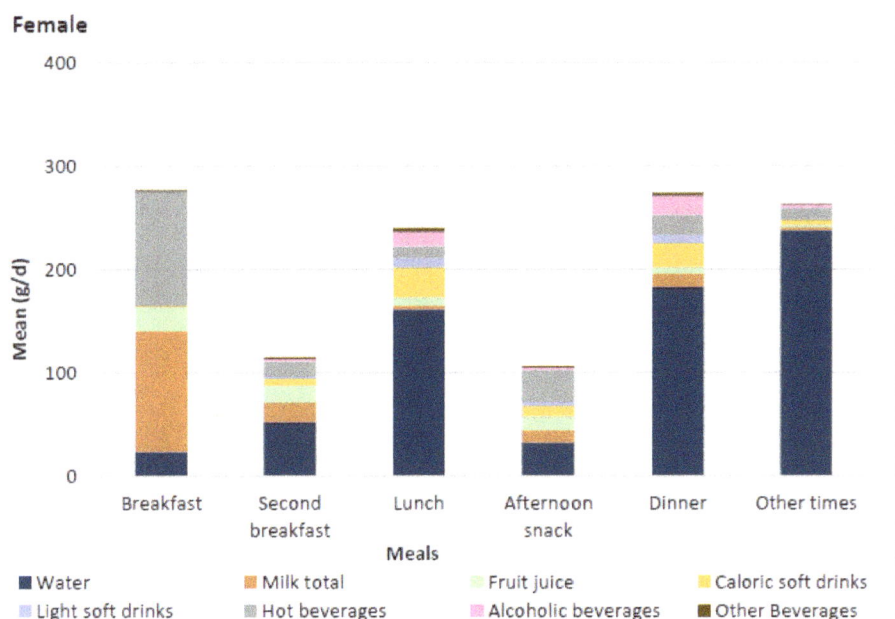

Figure 1. Daily mean beverage consumption during different meals by gender.

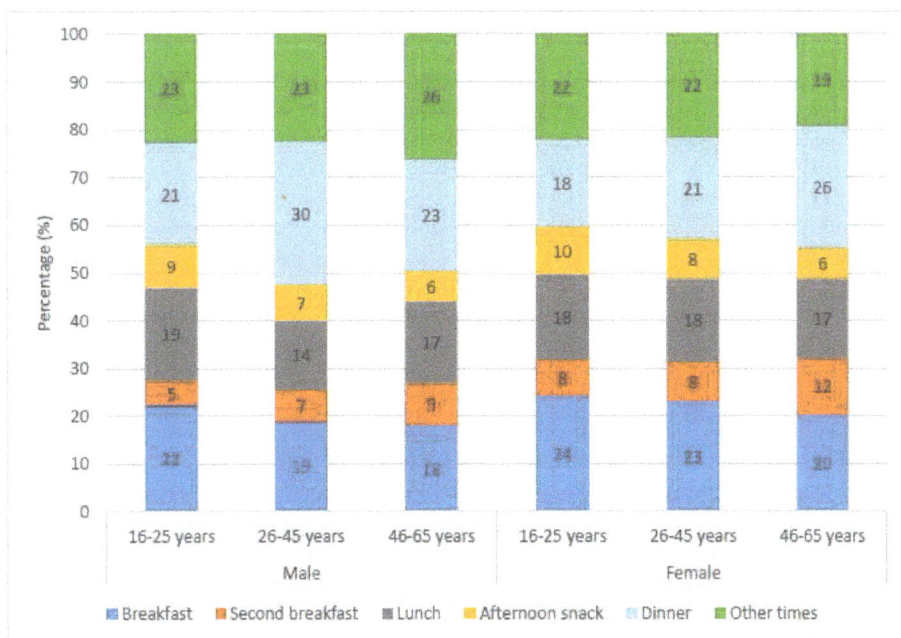

Figure 2. Percentage of total beverage consumption during different meals by gender and age group.

In Table 5, we assessed the correlation between the consumption of different types of beverages and TWI, water from beverages and foods, TEI, energy intake from beverages and foods. Water consumption was highly correlated with the total beverage consumption, water intake from beverages and TWI. Consumption of caloric soft drinks was associated with energy intake from foods and beverages and also TEI. In other cases, correlation coefficients were generally unremarkable.

Table 5. Partial correlation between the consumption of different types of beverages and TWI, water from beverages and foods, TEI, energy intake from beverages and foods (adjusted for gender, age, BMI, and PA).

Beverages	Total Beverage	Water from Beverages	Water from Foods	TWI	Energy from Beverages	Energy from Foods	TEI
Water	0.837 *	0.853 *	0.107 *	0.851 *	−0.163 *	0.051 *	−0.016
Full-fat milk	0.142 *	0.130 *	−0.166 *	0.047 *	0.374 *	0.092 *	0.186 *
Low/non-fat milk	0.140 *	0.135 *	−0.087 *	0.083 *	0.079 *	0.021	0.033
100% fruit juice	−0.052	−0.057	0.003	−0.055	0.050	−0.070 *	−0.052
Commercial fruit juice	−0.074 *	−0.086 *	−0.014	−0.088 *	0.165 *	0.020	0.070 *
Caloric soft drinks	0.107 *	0.082 *	−0.189 *	−0.019	0.340 *	0.178 *	0.275 *
Light soft drinks	0.070 *	0.076 *	−0.068 *	0.037	−0.077 *	0.009	−0.016
Coffee	0.296 *	0.291 *	−0.567 *	−0.012	0.181 *	0.080 *	0.134 *
Tea	0.059	0.062 *	0.079 *	0.098 *	−0.033	0.031	0.021
Alcoholic beverages	0.191 *	0.179 *	−0.101 *	0.117 *	0.141 *	0.108 *	0.153 *
Other beverages	0.047	0.025	−0.111 *	0.079 *	0.068 *	−0.042	−0.019

* $p < 0.05$ (statistically significant); TWI: Total Water Intake; TEI: Total Energy Intake; BMI: Body Mass Index; PA: Physical Activity.

4. Discussion

The present study investigated the beverage consumption and TWI and TEI from beverages among Balearic adults. The results show that mean TWI was 2.2 L for men and 1.9 L for women in the study population and slightly lower than the proposed AIs of water, which are 2.5 L for males and 2 L for females by the EFSA [4]. Water recommendations of EFSA are applied only to conditions of moderate environmental temperature and moderate physical activity levels [4]. TWI below the recommended values might be related with the low physical activity level of the study population. We observed that more than half of the study population had a low physical activity level.

According to the estimation of EFSA, beverages contribute 70–80% of TWI and foods contribute 20–30% of TWI [4]. While men met these estimations, among women water intake from foods was higher, 35%. This difference can be explained with the high vegetable consumption of women as these contain a high amount of food moisture. We observe that women consumed more vegetables (172 g/day) than men did (142 g/day) (data not shown), and this finding is in line with a previous study [29].

In this study, water was the principal beverage, and water accounted for 31% of TWI. In parallel to our findings, drinking water was the main beverage among the entire Spanish population [12,30]. Within other beverages, hot beverages were the main contributor to TWI, followed by milk and caloric soft drinks.

Energy intake from beverages varied within sex and age-specific groups and mean energy intake of the whole population is 9.8% which was lower than those of the entire Spanish population [12]. Overall, milk is the main beverage, accounting for energy intake, followed by alcoholic beverages and caloric soft drinks. In general, energy contribution of caloric soft drinks was 1.8% for men and 1.2% for women in our study population, but energy intake from these beverages was significantly higher among younger adults, especially in men (2.7% of TEI). In addition to caloric soft drinks, energy intake from commercial fruit juice was higher among younger adults. In comparison with the US population (5.7%) [31], energy intake from caloric soft drinks is lower in the Balearic population, but in view of the adverse health effect of caloric soft drinks [32–34], high consumption of these beverages among younger people should be discouraged by health authorities.

Another issue to be raised is the higher energy intake from alcoholic beverages of adults aged 26 and older, particularly men. Many older adults have chronic health conditions, and therefore, they take numerous medications; alcohol intake may interact with these medications [35]. Mean daily alcoholic beverage intake of the study population was below the recommended limits of alcohol and low to moderate alcohol consumption has some health benefits [36,37]. However the body composition changes with age and the amount of total body water decreases, which results in higher blood alcohol concentration in older than younger adults for the same amount of alcohol intake [38]. Close attention needs to be paid by health authorities for identifying high alcohol consumption of older adults since they are at a greater risk of alcohol-related harm than younger drinkers.

Adults in the Balearic Islands consumed more beverages during main meal times. Type of beverages varied between different meal times. Hot beverages, milk, and fruit juices were mainly consumed at breakfast, while water consumption was the lowest during breakfast. Fruit juice and milk have more effects on hunger and satiety than water, and these beverages satisfy thirst like water [39]. This might explain the beverage preferences of the study population and low water consumption during breakfast. Similar to our findings, milk and fruit juices were commonly consumed beverages for breakfast in Norway [40].

Earlier studies have suggested that consumption of sugar-sweetened beverages was related to high levels of energy intake [41,42]. In line with this, consumption of caloric soft drinks was positively correlated with TEI and also energy intake from food. Consumption of caloric soft drinks not only adds empty calories to the diet, but also regular consumption of these energy-dense beverages may affect the food choices and total caloric intake [43].

Some of the strengths of the present study consist of the use of a large and representative sample of Balearic adults. Misreporting of energy intake is an acknowledged problem in all dietary assessment methods [44,45]; Goldberg cut-off methods [28] were applied to exclude under-reporters. Several limitations of the present study need to be mentioned. First, the food and beverage intake and physical activity (IPAQ questionnaire) data are gathered using self-reported questionnaires and might be influenced by recording errors. Estimation of portion size is a usual weakness of self-reported dietary assessment methods; however, we used a manual of sets of photographs to avoid this weakness. Another limitation of the study is its cross-sectional design, which limits conclusions regarding causality. We used two 24 h dietary recalls. Dietary intakes estimated by means of two 24 h dietary recalls are not suitable for determining the usual intake distributions [46]; therefore, we do not attempt to describe the usual intake distributions of daily water intake. We present population means and standard errors for the beverage consumption, TWI, and TEI.

5. Conclusions

Although the energy contribution of beverages is low among the Balearic Islands population, there are some issues requiring the attention of health authorities for promoting healthy drinking. The main findings of this study indicate that consumption of sugar-sweetened beverages (caloric soft drinks and commercial fruit juice) is higher among young adults, consumption of alcoholic beverages is higher among males aged 26 and older, and TWI is lower than the EFSA recommendations. These findings may be used to develop effective, healthy eating and drinking policies and campaigns.

Author Contributions: A.E.O. and J.A.T. conceived, designed and devised the study; M.d.M.B. collected and supervised the samples; A.E.O., M.d.M.B., C.B., and J.A.T. analyzed the data and wrote the manuscript; all read and approved the final manuscript; A.P. and J.A.T. obtained funding.

Funding: The study was supported by the Instituto de Salud Carlos III (Program for the Promotion of Biomedical Research and Health Sciences, projects 05/1276, 08/1259, 11/01791, 14/00636 and 17/01827, Red Predimed RETIC RD06/0045/1004, and CIBEROBN CB12/03/30038), grant to research group No. 35/2011 (Balearic Islands Government), COST Action CA16112, and UE-FEDER funds. The funders had no role in the design or conduct of the study; collection, management, analysis and interpretation of the data; or preparation, review and approval of the manuscript.

Conflicts of Interest: None of the authors have any financial or non-financial competing interests to disclose.

Abbreviations

AI	adequate intake
BMR	basal metabolic rate
DBP	diastolic blood pressure
EFSA	European Food Safety Authority
EI	energy intake
FFQ	food frequency questionnaire
IPAQ	International Physical Activity Questionnaire
MD	Mediterranean diet
MET	metabolic equivalent
PA	physical activity
BP	systolic blood pressure
SPSS	Statistical Package for the Social Sciences
TEI	total energy intake;
TWI	total water intake

References

1. World Health Organisation. *Nutrients in Drinking Water*; World Health Organisation: Geneva, Switzerland, 2005.
2. Wolf, A.; Bray, G.A.; Popkin, B.M. A short history of beverages and how our body treats them. *Obes. Rev.* **2008**, *9*, 151–164. [CrossRef] [PubMed]
3. Popkin, B.M. Patterns of beverage use across the lifecycle. *Physiol. Behav.* **2010**, *100*, 4–9. [CrossRef] [PubMed]
4. Agostoni, C.; Bresson, J.-L.; Fairweather-Tait, S.; Flynn, A.; Golly, I.; Korhonen, H.; Lagiou, P.; Løvik, M.; Marchelli, R.; Martin, A.; et al. Scientific Opinion on Dietary reference values for water. *EFSA J.* **2010**, *8*. [CrossRef]
5. Nissensohn, M.; Sánchez-Villegas, A.; Galan, P.; Turrini, A.; Arnault, N.; Mistura, L.; Ortiz-Andrellucchi, A.; Edelenyi, F.S.; D'Addezio, L.; Serra-Majem, L. Beverage Consumption Habits among the European Population: Association with Total Water and Energy Intakes. *Nutrients* **2017**, *9*, 383. [CrossRef] [PubMed]
6. Storey, M.L.; Forshee, R.A.; Anderson, P.A. Beverage consumption in the US population. *J. Am. Diet. Assoc.* **2006**, *106*, 1992–2000. [CrossRef] [PubMed]
7. Garriguet, D. Beverage consumption of children and teens. *Health Rep.* **2008**, *19*, 17–22. [PubMed]
8. Garriguet, D. Beverage consumption of Canadian adults. *Health Rep.* **2008**, *9*, 23–29.
9. Barquera, S.; Hernandez-Barrera, L.; Tolentino, M.L.; Espinosa, J.; Ng, S.W.; Rivera, J.A.; Popkin, B.M. Energy intake from beverages is increasing among Mexican adolescents and adults. *J. Nutr.* **2008**, *138*, 2454–2461. [CrossRef] [PubMed]
10. Barquera, S.; Campirano, F.; Bonvecchio, A.; Hernández-Barrera, L.; Rivera, J.A.; Popkin, B.M. Caloric beverage consumption patterns in Mexican children. *Nutr. J.* **2010**, *21*. [CrossRef] [PubMed]
11. Bellisle, F.; Thornton, S.N.; Hebel, P.; Denizeau, M.; Tahiri, M. A study of fluid intake from beverages in a sample of healthy French children, adolescents and adults. *Eur. J. Clin. Nutr.* **2010**, *84*, 350–355. [CrossRef] [PubMed]
12. Nissensohn, M.; Sánchez-Villegas, A.; Ortega, R.M.; Aranceta-Bartrina, J.; Gil, Á.; González-Gross, M.; Varela-Moreiras, G.; Serra-Majem, L. Beverage Consumption Habits and Association with Total Water and Energy Intakes in the Spanish Population: Findings of the ANIBES Study. *Nutrients* **2016**, *8*, 232. [CrossRef] [PubMed]
13. Mistura, L.; D'Addezio, L.; Turrini, A. Beverage Consumption Habits in Italian Population: Association with Total Water Intake and Energy Intake. *Nutrients* **2016**, *8*, 674. [CrossRef] [PubMed]
14. de Edelenyi, F.S.; Druesne-Pecollo, N.; Arnault, N.; González, R.; Buscail, C.; Galan, P. Characteristics of Beverage Consumption Habits among a Large Sample of French Adults: Associations with Total Water and Energy Intakes. *Nutrients* **2016**, *8*, 627. [CrossRef] [PubMed]
15. Gibson, S.; Shirreffs, S.M. Beverage consumption habits "24/7" among British adults: Association with total water intake and energy intake. *Nutr. J.* **2013**, *12*. [CrossRef] [PubMed]

16. Tur, J.A.; Serra-Majem, L.; Romaguera, D.; Pons, A. Does the diet of the Balearic population, a Mediterranean type diet, still provide adequate antioxidant nutrient intakes? *Eur. J. Nutr.* **2005**, *44*, 204–213. [CrossRef] [PubMed]

17. La Medición de la Clase Social en Ciencias de la Salud. Available online: https://www.seepidemiologia.es/documents/dummy/LA%20MEDICION%20DE%20LA%20CLASE%20SOCIAL-4.pdf (accessed on 10 March 2012).

18. Ozen, A.E.; BibiloniMdel, M.; Pons, A.; Tur, J.A. Sociodemographic and lifestyle determinants of functional food consumption in an adult population of the Balearic Islands. *Ann. Nutr. Metab.* **2013**, *63*, 200–207. [CrossRef] [PubMed]

19. González, M.; del Mar Bibiloni, M.; Pons, A.; Llompart, I.; Tur, J.A. Inflammatory markers and metabolic syndrome among adolescents. *Eur. J. Clin. Nutr.* **2012**, *66*, 1141–1145. [CrossRef] [PubMed]

20. Body Mass Index-BMI. Available online: http://www.euro.who.int/en/health-topics/disease-prevention/nutrition/a-healthy-lifestyle/body-mass-index-bmi (accessed on 28 July 2018).

21. IPAQ International Physical Activity Questionnaire. Guide-Lines for Data Processing and Analysis of the International Physical Activity Questionnaire (IPAQ). Available online: https://sites.google.com/site/theipaq (accessed on 20 July 2012).

22. The Compendium of Physical Activities Tracking Guide. Available online: http://prevention.sph.sc.edu/tools/docs/documents_compendium.pdf (accessed on 20 July 2012).

23. Gómez, C.; Kohen, V.L.; Nogueira, T.L. *GuíaVisual de Alimentos y Raciones*; EDIMSA: Madrid, Spain, 2007.

24. Moreiras, O.; Carbajal, A.; Cabrera, L.; Cuadrado, C. *Tablas de Composicion de Alimentos*, 7th ed.; Piramide: Madrid, Spain, 2003.

25. Mataix, V.J.; Manas, A.M. *Tabla de Composicion de AlimentosEspañoles*, 4th ed.; Editorial Universidad de Granada: Granada, Spain, 2003.

26. Feinberg, M.; Favier, J.C.; Ireland-Ripert, J. *Repertoire General des Aliments (Food Composition Tables)*; Tec & Doc Lavoisier: Paris, France, 1995.

27. Ripoll, L. *Cocina de las Islas Baleares*, 5th ed.; L. Ripoll Pub. Co.: Palma de Mallorca, Spain, 1992.

28. Black, A.E. Critical evaluation of energy intake using the goldberg cut-off for energy intake: Basal metabolic rate. A practical guide to its calculation, use and limitations. *Int. J. Obes.* **2000**, *24*, 1119–1130. [CrossRef]

29. Salas, R.; del Mar Bibiloni, M.; Zapata, M.E.; Coll, J.L.; Pons, A.; Tur, J.A. Balearic adults have low intakes of fruits and vegetables compared with the dietary guidelines for adults in Spain. *Nutr. Res.* **2013**, *33*, 204–210. [CrossRef] [PubMed]

30. Ferreira-Pêgo, C.; Babio, N.; Fenández-Alvira, J.M.; Iglesia, I.; Moreno, L.A.; Salas-Salvadó, J. Fluid intake from beverages in Spanish adults; cross-sectional study. *Nutr. Hosp.* **2014**, *29*, 1171–1178. [CrossRef] [PubMed]

31. Drewnowski, A.; Rehm, C.D.; Constant, F. Water and beverage consumption among adults in the United States: Cross-sectional study using data from NHANES 2005–2010. *BMC Public Health* **2013**, *13*. [CrossRef] [PubMed]

32. Vartanian, L.R.; Schwartz, M.B.; Brownell, K.D. Effects of soft drink consumption on nutrition and health: A systematic review and meta-analysis. *Am. J. Public Health* **2007**, *97*, 667–675. [CrossRef] [PubMed]

33. Malik, V.S.; Popkin, B.M.; Bray, G.A.; Despres, J.P.; Willett, W.C.; Hu, F.B. Sugar-sweetened beverages and risk of metabolic syndrome and type 2 diabetes: A meta-analysis. *Diabetes Care* **2010**, *33*, 2477–2483. [CrossRef] [PubMed]

34. Hu, B.F. Resolved: There is sufficient scientific evidence that decreasing sugar-sweetened beverage consumption will reduce the prevalence of obesity and obesity-related diseases. *Obes. Rev.* **2013**, *14*, 606–619. [CrossRef] [PubMed]

35. Denton, F.T.; Spencer, B.G. Chronic health conditions: Changing prevalence in an aging population and some implications for the delivery of health care services. *Can. J. Aging* **2010**, *29*, 11–21. [CrossRef] [PubMed]

36. Krenz, M.; Korthuis, R.J. Moderate ethanol ingestion and cardiovascular protection: From epidemiologic associations to cellular mechanisms. *J. Mol. Cell. Cardiol.* **2012**, *52*, 93–104. [CrossRef] [PubMed]

37. Arranz, S.; Chiva-Blanch, G.; Valderas-Martínez, P.; Medina-Remón, A.; Lamuela-Raventós, R.M.; Estruch, R. Wine, beer, alcohol and polyphenols on cardiovascular disease and cancer. *Nutrients* **2012**, *4*, 759–781. [CrossRef] [PubMed]

38. Dufour, M.C.; Archer, L.; Gordis, E. Alcohol and the elderly. *Clin. Geriatr. Med.* **1992**, *8*, 127–141. [CrossRef]

39. Almiron-Roig, E.; Drewnowski, A. Hunger, thirst, and energy intakes following consumption of caloric beverages. *Physiol. Behav.* **2003**, *79*, 767–773. [CrossRef]
40. Paulsen, M.M.; Myhre, J.B.; Andersen, L.F. Beverage Consumption Patterns among Norwegian Adults. *Nutrients* **2016**, *8*, 561. [CrossRef] [PubMed]
41. Mathias, K.C.; Slining, M.M.; Popkin, B.M. Foods and beverages associated with higher intake of sugar-sweetened beverages. *Am. J. Prev. Med.* **2013**, *44*, 351–357. [CrossRef] [PubMed]
42. An, R. Beverage consumption in relation to discretionary food intake and diet quality among US adults, 2003 to 2012. *J. Acad. Nutr. Diet.* **2016**, *116*, 28–37. [CrossRef] [PubMed]
43. Bell, E.A.; Castellanos, V.H.; Pelkman, C.L.; Thorwart, M.L.; Rolls, B.J. Energy density of foods affects energy intake in normal-weight women. *Am. J. Clin. Nutr.* **1998**, *67*, 412–420. [CrossRef] [PubMed]
44. Macdiarmid, J.; Blundell, J. Assessing dietary intake: Who, what and why of under-reporting. *Nutr. Res. Rev.* **1998**, *11*, 231–253. [CrossRef] [PubMed]
45. Livingstone, M.B.; Black, A.E. Markers of the validity of reported energy intake. *J. Nutr.* **2003**, *133*, 895S–920S. [CrossRef]
46. National Cancer Institute (NIH). Usual Dietary Intakes. Available online: https://epi.grants.cancer.gov/diet/usualintakes/ (accessed on 29 July 2018).

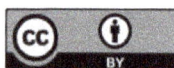

nutrients

MDPI

Article

"Your Body Feels Better When You Drink Water": Parent and School-Age Children's Sugar-Sweetened Beverage Cognitions

Kaitlyn M. Eck [1,*], Aleksandr Dinesen [1], Elder Garcia [2], Colleen L. Delaney [1],
Oluremi A. Famodu [2], Melissa D. Olfert [3], Carol Byrd-Bredbenner [1] and Karla P. Shelnutt [2]

[1] Department of Nutritional Sciences, Rutgers University, 26 Nichol Avenue, New Brunswick, NJ 08901, USA;
     ard180@sebs.rutgers.edu (A.D.); colleenldelaney90@gmail.com (C.L.D.);
     bredbenner@sebs.rutgers.edu (C.B.-B.)
[2] Department of Family, Youth, and Community Sciences, University of Florida, Gainesville, FL 32611, USA;
     elder89@ufl.edu (E.G.); oluremifamodu@tcomn.com (O.A.F.); kpagan@ufl.edu (K.P.S.)
[3] Division of Animal and Nutritional Sciences, West Virginia University, 1194 Evansdale Dr. G28,
     West Virginia University, Morgantown, WV 26506, USA; Melissa.Olfert@mail.wvu.edu
*   Correspondence: kmd260@scarletmail.rutgers.edu; Tel.: +1-732-932-9827

Received: 15 August 2018; Accepted: 2 September 2018; Published: 5 September 2018

Abstract: Sugar-sweetened beverages (SSBs) are a leading source of added sugar in the American diet. Further, ingestion of added sugars from SSBs exceeds recommendations. Thus, interventions that effectively reduce SSB consumption are needed. Focus group discussions with parents ($n = 37$) and school-aged children between the ages of 6 and 11 years ($n = 41$) from Florida, New Jersey, and West Virginia were led by trained moderators using Social Cognitive Theory as a guide. Trends and themes that emerged from the content analysis of the focus group data indicated that both parents and children felt that limiting SSBs was important to health and weight control. However, parents and children reported consuming an average of 1.85 ± 2.38 SD and 2.13 ± 2.52 SD SSB servings/week, respectively. Parents and children were aware that parent behaviors influenced kids, but parents reported modeling healthy SSB behaviors was difficult. Busy schedules, including more frequent parties and events as children get older, were another barrier to limiting SSBs. Parents were most successful at limiting SSBs when they were not in the house. This qualitative research provides novel insights into parents' and children's cognitions (e.g., beliefs, attitudes), barriers, and facilitators related to SSB ingestion. Consideration of these insights during nutrition intervention development has the potential to improve intervention effectiveness in reducing SSB intake.

Keywords: sugar-sweetened beverages; children; parents; social cognitive theory; nutrition education; health promotion

1. Introduction

Sugar sweetened beverages (SSBs) are a leading source of added sugars in the American diet [1]. Ingestion of these beverages is positively associated with excess body weight [2–4] as well as an increased risk of metabolic syndrome and its associated conditions, including cardiovascular disease and type 2 diabetes [5–8]. Currently, 20% of school-aged children (6 to 11 years) in the United States are classified as obese [9]. The Academy of Nutrition and Dietetics has identified SSBs as a contributor to childhood overweight and obesity; hence, this organization's Pediatric Weight Management Guidelines recommend limited intake of these beverages by children [10].

The Dietary Guidelines for Americans recommend keeping added sugar intake to less than 10% of an individual's daily calorie intake [11]; however, many Americans exceed this advice [1,12–14].

For instance, nearly 66% of school-aged children are consuming at least one SSB each day and as a result they are consuming over 7% of their total daily calories from these beverages [14]. Sugary drinks provide 60% of the total calories from added sugar in the diets of children in the U.S. [15].

In addition to its links to obesity and related physical and mental health effects [16–18], sugary beverages have negative consequences on oral health in children [19,20]. SSBs also displace nutrient-dense beverages, especially dairy milk [21,22], a key source of calcium, potassium, and vitamin D in the diets of American children [23]. Additionally, there is a positive relationship between SSB intake and weakened bones and increased risk of fractures [24].

Several studies have attempted to elucidate factors influencing SSB consumption. One factor is family behaviors, with a positive correlation between parent and child SSB intake [25–27], which is indicative of the observational learning construct of the Social Cognitive Theory [28,29]. Another factor affecting SSB intake is behavioral facilitators [28–30], also a Social Cognitive Theory construct. Environmental conditions [28–30] where there is greater SSB availability in the home, appear to facilitate SSB drinking [25,26,31]. Another environmental condition promoting consumption of sugary drinks is location of eating—as the frequency of eating away from home rises, so does SSB intake [32].

In recent years, consumption of sugary drinks has declined [33]. However, there is considerable opportunity to further reduce intake of these calorie-dense, nutrient-bare beverages. A greater understanding of factors supporting SSB consumption as well as those that help reduce it could lead to more effective behavior change and obesity prevention programs. Thus, this study aimed to qualitatively explore factors affecting SSB intake with the goal of creating recommendations that inform the development of health promotion and obesity prevention materials predicated on the Social Cognitive Theory that aim to reduce sugary drink intake of parents and school-aged children (6 to 11 years).

2. Materials and Methods

The Institutional Review Boards at the authors' universities approved the procedures for this investigation. All parents gave informed consent for their children as well as themselves. Prior to data collection, children gave verbal assent.

2.1. Sample

Parents who resided in Florida, New Jersey, or West Virginia and had one or more children aged 6 to 11 years were recruited to enroll in focus groups discussing home and lifestyles changes to promote child health and development. Electronic (website, emails) and paper recruitment announcements were distributed at workplaces, schools, community centers, and other locations frequented by parents. Recruitment announcements were in English and Spanish and specified that focus groups would take about 60 min and that participants would receive $25. The announcements also invited parents to sign up their school-age children for a 30-min focus group discussion and indicated child participants would receive $15. Parents and children participating in the focus groups were not necessarily related. Focus group size was intentionally kept small to permit everyone to fully participate.

2.2. Instruments

Before focus groups began, parents completed a brief survey to report demographic characteristics (e.g., age, highest education level) and frequency of SSB intake. Children completed a similar form.

A semi-structured questionnaire based on key Social Cognitive Theory (SCT) constructs (i.e., attitudes toward SSB, barriers to reducing SSB intake, and facilitators for reducing SSB intake) was developed. SCT considers both inter- and intra-personal factors influencing behavior performance including self-efficacy, collective efficacy (belief that a group is able to perform a behavior change), and observational learning (learning by watching others perform a behavior) [28–30], which makes it suitable to employ in family-based interventions. Furthermore, SCT addresses the interaction between people and their environment—a bidirectional influence between these that is referred to as reciprocal determinism [28–30]. The notion of reciprocal determinism also makes SCT a good fit for home-based interventions where family members' behaviors affect and are affected by their home environment.

Prior to commencing the study, all data collectors were trained to conduct the focus groups in a uniform manner using standard procedures [34]. English and Spanish focus groups were conducted separately to accommodate the parents' language preference. All child focus groups were in English because all were fluent in this language. Younger children (ages 6 to 9) participated in focus groups separate from those comprised of older, more mature children (ages 9 to 11). At each focus group, a second trained researcher took comprehensive notes of the discussion and transcribed the notes within 48 h of the focus group, including translating Spanish language focus group notes. The researcher moderating the focus group reviewed the notes and discussed them with the note-taker to ensure they were a clear, complete, and correct record.

2.3. Data Analysis

Descriptive statistics summarizing data collected in the survey administered before the focus group were conducted were calculated using SPSS version 21.0 (Chicago, IL, USA). Three researchers trained in standard content analysis procedures independently categorized focus group data into themes (Miles and Huberman 1994 [35], Harris, Gleason et al. 2009 [36]). Content analysis generates objective, systematic descriptions [37] that permit drawing "replicable and valid inferences from the data to their context" [38]. The independent content analysis findings were compared and researchers discussed them to reach consensus. Focus group data were continually analyzed during the data collection period to determine when no new information was being revealed (i.e., data saturation was reached) and data collection could end [39].

3. Results

A total of 37 parents (97% female) participated in 1 of 13 focus group discussions about beverages. Three of these focus groups were performed in Florida (*n* = 13 parents), 5 in New Jersey (*n* = 12 parents), and 4 in West Virginia (*n* = 12 parents). Parents were 36.3 ± 5.13 SD years old and had 2.42 ± 0.91 SD children under 18 living at home. The group was well educated, with 57% having obtained a baccalaureate degree or higher. Two-thirds of the parents completed the focus groups in English, with the remainder in Spanish.

A total of 41 school-aged children (ages 6 to 11 years) participated in 1 of 15 focus group discussions about beverages. Five of these focus groups were performed in Florida (*n* = 12 children), 5 in New Jersey (*n* = 13 children), and 5 in West Virginia (*n* = 16 children). The average age of the children was 8.46 ± 1.85 SD years. Participants had 1.17 ± 2.645 SD older siblings and 1.50 ± 1.57 SD younger siblings.

3.1. Parent Focus Groups

Survey results illustrated that parents consumed an average of 1.85 ± 2.38 SD SSBs per week. A comparison of SSB intake by language spoken and state of residence indicated intake was similar. Additionally, no differences were discerned in focus group data by language or state of residence, so data are presented in aggregate.

3.1.1. Parents' Attitudes toward SSB Consumption

The majority of parents felt that limiting sugary beverages like soft drinks is "very important" for their children's overall health and wellbeing commenting, "young kids can have health problems from the sugar". Parents recognized the value of reducing SSB consumption, indicating that "sugary drinks have empty calories, no vitamins, and lack the ability to keep you full" and these drinks "can affect kids so much that children become overweight". One noted, "I feel like, if I knew what I know now at their age, I wouldn't have had to get a gastric sleeve". On the other hand, another commented "I don't try to tell them (kids) about gaining weight because I don't want them to think about body images at their age".

Another common concern was oral health, with parents commenting on the "effect [SSBs have on] their teeth", with others extending the effects to complexion and other physical aspects—"it's really a whole body thing". Other health conditions, such as kidney stones and diabetes, were mentioned by parents who had a family history of these conditions.

Behavior and adequate sleep were common themes in focus groups, with parents observing that "I see a palpable change in my kids when they are sugared up" and "it disrupts sleeping habits". Numerous respondents indicated that SSBs made their children "hyperactive", "bounce off the walls", and "rowdier".

Some participants alluded to "addictive" qualities of these drinks. "The more sugar they start to take in, the more sugar they want". Caffeine also was of concern to some parents who indicated that they "try to limit their caffeine intake so they (kids) don't get addicted to it" and "kids don't need the caffeine".

A few commented on environmental/geographical influences on beverage intake. One parent said, "in southern West Virginia, soda is normal, and it was difficult to change when I realized that it wasn't normal and healthy".

3.1.2. Parents' Perceived Barriers to Limiting SSB Consumption

A common barrier to limiting children's SSB intake was parental role modeling. Most parents reported that their children commonly want to partake in whatever their mother or father do: "they see an example and they imitate it" and "if I consume it, they are going to consume it". Some acknowledged that being a role model was challenging because "I really like soda, so it can be hard to limit them" and "if they (children) see you drinking it (SSB), they want it". Some parents also did not realize that some beverages were sweetened, "I used to give Gatorade, but the dentist said no".

Busy schedules were another barrier that parents faced in curtailing SSB intake in that time scarcity enabled decisions that limited access to healthier alternatives. For example, parents reported feeling like they were "living at Wawa and Wendy's during the sports season and school year" where sugary drink options were common and healthy alternatives were limited. Fast food restaurants, gas stations, and convenience "stores have such a small selection of water and then huge selections of sugary drinks; so every time we are in the gas station or something, he asks for a pop". Parents also raised the concern of limited availability of healthy alternatives at after school events, remarking "school-related activities don't always have a lot of water and you can only find pop and sweetened tea at sporting events".

Parents felt that SSB intake had increased as children got older. One parent stated, "his consumption has increased exponentially" and another reported "now they drink them (SSB) more; when they were younger, they didn't drink them. I even find bottles of soda hidden under their beds now". Children's growing maturity and independence was seen as an obstacle to limiting SSB intake. As kids got older, they were purchasing lunch more often and parents were "unsure of how much sugary beverages they drink when they buy lunches at school". And, "it is more difficult to control the consumption of juices and sugar (when kids are at school)". Parents felt kids' beverage choices at home were influenced by school experiences, noting that "the school gives the option for flavored milk", so now they have "had to switch to chocolate or strawberry milk (at home)". Another parent reported that when "other parents give sugary drinks for school lunches . . . my kid says, 'why can't I bring that, too?'".

Another aspect of children's increasing age that got in the way of keeping SSB intake in check was that, as they got older, they "have more involvements, which often mean more celebrations and sugar intake". They attend more "school activities, friends' birthday parties, and get togethers" where soda was readily available. One parent commented, "I blame little league baseball—he used to get a hotdog and a soda after a game; he had never had it (SSB) until he was 8 years old".

SSB purchases of other family members also presented roadblocks to limiting intake of these beverages. "In my house the only problem is that my sister lives with us and she will buy soda and then they (kids) will drink it. I can't stop her from buying soda because she is an adult, since they see her drinking it they will ask her for soda and drink it". Responsibilities outside the home presented another obstacle because parents were not able to supervise children's consumption of sugary beverages during these times: "It's difficult to limit their drink consumption when I'm not home because they will get what they want". Another obstacle, television, made it "more complicated" for parents to control children's SSB intake because it provided frequent exposure to advertisements for these drinks.

3.1.3. Parents' Strategies for Overcoming Barriers to Limiting SSB Consumption

The number one strategy for limiting sugary beverage intake was environmental control: "keeping them (SSB) out of the house" and "don't buy them". Another common approach to regulating SSB consumption was to "set boundaries" and reserve sugary drinks for "special occasions". For instance, "Friday night is pizza night and my children get a soda beverage, but it's not (a) regular (occurrence)". Occasional intake of SSBs was recognized by some parents as being important for teaching self-control, because "you cannot forbid her to do it or else she will go crazy later when it's available". "My basic rule is water or milk, but exceptions at parties or events with other kids. They probably have it like 3 times a month—so not often, but they have learned what they should have". However, other parents were more rigid in their approach (e.g., "I force them to drink water; if they don't want water, then they don't get anything" and "I distribute (SSB0, and I use child-locks for all of my pantries").

Making "milk and water the drinks of choice" in their homes and being sure "kids grew up with the mind set to enjoy and prefer water" were other methods parents used to limit SSB intake. To boost children's preference for water, parents tried "cutting up lemons and limes in the water to give it a little punch", serving "agua fresca" (water infused with fruit), and making "it more interesting . . . have fruit and ice in it" or add "sugar-free flavored water packets". To encourage healthier drink options, parents also proposed environmental solutions. For example, "having an accessible fridge where they can reach for water", "keeping a large Brita filter in the refrigerator" and having "an array of water bottles" and "fun cups for the kids to drink out of" were identified as useful tools for encouraging water intake over SSB.

Another approach was to lower sugar intake from beverages. Parents "cut juice with water". They also reduced the sugar content of flavored milk by "putting in mostly white milk with just a little chocolate (drink mix)". Parents also touted the benefits of diet soft drinks to children, describing them as "sugar-free flavored water" and seltzer water as healthy alternatives to sugary drinks. One parent used portion control as a means to control SSB intake: "get them a little glass if they ask".

Promoting various qualities of beverages was another tactic parents employed to limit SSB intake. For instance, the health benefits of alternative beverage options were conveyed when parents reminded children that "milk helps bones", "milk will make their teeth white", and will help you "get stronger and taller". Parents also promoted the benefits of water. "When you do drink water, when your kids are well hydrated, it shows in everything—your eyes aren't as puffy, your skin feels clearer—(this) translates over to kids. When your kids are hydrated, they aren't as sluggish and it keeps your body at its best. Sharing that with the kids keeps them at their best". Some parents helped children think about calories from SSB by telling them if they "do not have soda, they can use those calories to have something more enjoyable". Thirst quenching abilities also were invoked ("juice and soda are going to make you thirstier"). Others pointed out that "it's helpful to have the orthodontist and dentist" endorse milk and water and the importance of limiting SSBs.

Many parents recognized that "setting a good example" was an effective way to help kids keep SSB intake under control. One mother observed, "seeing me drink water helps them. The mirrored behavior is important". Parents also were motivated to drink more water themselves and encourage their children to do the same because, "your body feels better when you drink water and you feel better about yourself".

3.2. Children's Focus Groups

Survey results indicated that children had an average intake of 2.13 ± 2.52 SD servings weekly of SSBs. A review of children's responses indicated that SSB intake was similar across age and state of residence. Focus group data were similar across age groups and state, so data were combined.

3.2.1. Children's Attitudes toward SSB Consumption

Kids reported drinking a wide array of SSBs, with intake ranging from infrequent ("we don't have them often, maybe once a month") to often ("I have them once a day or I have a little more than that"). These beverages were consumed at meals or alone. Several kids reported having SSBs more frequently on the weekend and at events like birthday parties and when going out to eat. Some participants indicated "you can only drink it sometimes, but not a lot".

Reasons many children gave for limiting consumption of SSBs were "it's very important because if you drink too much, it is not good for you" and "sugar is kind of bad for you" "because might have too much energy, get sugar rushes" and makes them "hyper" and "hard to go to sleep". Health effects were common explanations children gave for limiting SSBs; these ranged from general (they could "get a stomachache" or "get sick") to more specific health effects (sugary drinks are "bad for your teeth", "not good for your skin", "not good for your kidneys", or "are not good for your health because they can cause diabetes"). Some commented that SSBs are "bad for your bodies because of the calories, I think" and "you can also start getting fat".

A few children linked calories in SSB with energy expenditure and discounted the importance of limiting SSBs if balanced with exercise, "I ran yesterday, so I don't need to limit it (SSB)". One commented, "it is less important for us (to limit SSBs) than for them (parents) because they don't burn a lot of calories like we do".

Some children commented on hydrating qualities of drinks. "When I play outside, I drink water instead of sugary drinks because you cramp if you don't have water and have too much sugary drinks" and understood that "it is important to drink a lot of water or you will get dehydrated". Kids also connected SSB consumption to decreased athletic performance and energy levels saying, "when I go to recess, I will run slower".

Although most children felt keeping SSB intake under control was important, some did not. "I don't think it's important because I love sugar, and it tastes good".

3.2.2. Children's Perception of Their Parents' Attitudes toward SSB Consumption

Most children thought parents felt it was important to limit SSB intake because parents tell them, "if you drink a lot of it (SSB), you can get sick" and that parents "get happy if you don't drink a lot of sugary drinks" but "get mad if I drink too much". Other ways parents conveyed to children that it was important to control sugary beverages was that parents told kids "not to drink a lot of them", set limits on the number of SSBs kids can drink ("My mom says to only have one can of soda a day"), controlled access ("my parents only buy 1 or 2 (boxes of pop), but they put it somewhere where I can't reach or see it"), set "rules requiring us to drink water or milk", and rewarded kids for drinking water.

Others concluded that parents believed it was important to limit SSB because parents promoted healthier beverages "she (mom) fills up big pitchers with water and we have to drink that", or "mom and dad set goals not to buy them". Conversely, parental behaviors led one child to surmise, "dad doesn't care, he drinks soda".

3.2.3. Children's Perceived Barriers to Limiting SSB Consumption

Although most kids understood the importance of limiting SSB intake, they noted many barriers hindered their efforts. A commonly mentioned theme was parental influence. Many children indicated that they want to do what their parents do—"I want what my parents have. When my parents drink pop, I want it, too". Another child remarked, "I have iced tea that my dad drinks a lot and sometimes I steal it and drink it". Another participant indicated, "every time my mom drinks soda, we see it and then we get jealous". Parental behaviors were not limited to sugary drinks: "it (soda) does make me want to have what they have. But if they have milk or water, I'll drink it, too".

Another common barrier to limiting sugary drinks was the taste. "I drink soda because it tastes good. I'm not judging water because it has no taste, it's just clear". There also was a social aspect that made limiting SSBs difficult as well. Many children reported that "I usually have them (SSB) at parties" or on "special occasions, like birthdays and holidays". Having their own money to buy sugary drinks presented a roadblock to curbing SSB intake for some. The home environment presented another obstacle: "we keep around 100 cans (of soda) at home in our basement". Another barrier was wanting to be like siblings or friends, "my friend is allowed to drink whatever she wants" and using these beverages as a reward (we get) a little everyday if we have good behavior").

3.2.4. Children's Strategies for Overcoming Barriers to SSB Consumption

Children indicated that parents play the largest role in helping them limit SSBs and gave various strategies parents could use. One common suggestion was for parents to not drink sugary beverages themselves—"tell parents not to drink a lot of soda" because "it makes me want it when they drink sugary drinks". Role modeling healthy behavior was another strategy: "my mom drinks a lot of water so it makes me want to drink water."

Teaching kids about sugary drinks was another approach children recommended parents try: "show your kids a video to educate them and tell them what these drinks are made of and why they are not healthy" or "have them (kids) write paragraphs of why they are drinking so much sugar". Explaining the disadvantages of SSBs was another idea children had: "you still feel thirsty after drinking a sugary drink, but not if you drink water", "if you drink it [after sports practice], then its wasting what you just worked off", and "tell kids they could get sick" and "it's not good for the kidneys". On the other hand, some thought parents could explain the advantages of healthier drinks, and they could "explain it's good for sports" and that "water is healthy".

Children also proposed that parents impose limits on SSBs, such as "2 sugary drinks a day" or "only let children drink juice if they drink a lot of water" and "give us certain drink choices and we can only choose from those". Another method kids thought parents should try was to promote milk and water, offer kids incentives (e.g., "if you drink water or milk, then you get a reward"), or when kids refuse water or milk, punish them (e.g., "put children in timeout because they will learn their lesson").

To lower intake of sugary beverages, kids proposed making "it more difficult to get pop", drinking more water ("water helps me drink less sugary drinks"), buying "soda without sugar in it" and "healthy drinks", diluting juice with water, and making healthier options more appealing ("flavor the drinks or make something creative like smoothies", "drink out of straws with loops", "put raspberries in the drink"). Other strategies children thought parents could use were "have them [children] drink 3 bottles of water before they can drink sugary drinks" and "trick them–dye water to make it look like juice".

Children also suggested environmental controls that restrict access to SSBs: "I've been to friends' houses and they will have 5 to 8 boxes (of soda) at a time, but we don't have a lot of boxes at a time–it's easier when you don't have as much around". Other environmental controls were to hide sugary drinks, "just don't buy it", have healthy options available ("have lots of milk, instead"), and "get the good drinks for them and bring it to them".

They also thought that small serving sizes ("don't give them a lot"), limiting access to certain times or events (e.g., after practice, weekends), and setting goals for healthier beverages ("I aim for 8 bottles of water every day") would be helpful ways to control SSB intake. Finally, kids recommended being role models themselves ("don't drink sugary drinks around siblings ... they are likely to see what you are drinking and would like that drink").

4. Discussion

This study aimed to explore the cognitions, barriers, and facilitators related to SSB intake of school-age children and parents of school-age children. A second aim was to use the finding to create recommendations for future nutrition education programs targeting limited SSB consumption based on constructs from the Social Cognitive Theory (Table 1). Social Cognitive Theory [28–30] provides a useful framework for categorizing factors known to promote behavior change and thus was used to organize future programming recommendations.

Table 1. Recommendations for Interventions Targeting Limiting Sugar-Sweetened Beverage Intake in Families with School-Age Children.

Social Cognitive Theory Recommendations for Future Interventions Promoting Reduced Sugar Sweetened Beverage (SSB) Intake	
Outcome Expectations	Expand SSB outcome expectations to include weight management and oral health.
Outcome Expectations	Expand SSB outcome expectations to include the negative effect of caffeine in coffee and energy drinks.
Reciprocal Determinism	Teach parents and children about actual SSB behaviors to improve their perceived norms of this behavior.
Outcome Expectations	Expand SSB outcome expectations to include the positive effects of choosing flavored milk in moderation over other SSBs.
Facilitation	Provide oral health professionals with nutrition education materials and training to enable them to help families decrease SSB intake.
Facilitation	Provide parents with strategies to break from geographic and/or cultural norms that encourage SSB consumption.
Facilitation	Provide opportunities for parents to develop strategies that control SSB availability in the home environment, such as limiting amount of SSB on hand and purchasing them only at the time of consumption.
Facilitation	Provide parents with opportunities to develop more authoritative parental feeding skills and an understanding of how this type of parenting can facilitate child development.
Facilitation	Inform parents about school meal program guidelines and policies and encourage them to visit children's school cafeteria.
Facilitation	Provide tips for identifying healthier, on-the-go beverage options, including planning ahead for busy days.
Facilitation	Share quick and easy ways to incorporate healthy beverages in meals and snacks.
Facilitation	Provide parents with time management strategies.
Observational Learning	Explain the importance of healthy role modeling to parents and encourage parents to make better beverage choices to demonstrate healthier beverage choices to children.
Self-efficacy	Build parents' confidence in their ability to provide healthier alternatives to SSBs and enjoy more nutrient-dense beverage.

The findings from this study reveal that most parents and children accurately perceive the negative health effects of excessive SSB intake. For instance, both parents and children knew that sugary beverages lacked important nutrients [40]. In addition, they accurately reported that SSBs can promote weight gain and contribute to health problems [41]. However, not all participants were fully cognizant of these negative health benefits, thereby highlighting an opportunity to expand their knowledge as well as reinforce the knowledge of those who are more informed.

Some parents and children were aware of the effect of SSB on oral health and mentioned dental health professionals as sources of SSB-related information. According to the American Academy of Pediatric Dentistry, frequent consumption of SSBs increases the risk of dental caries [42]. Helping parents and children fully realize the potential outcomes of SSB on oral health could be an important component of future nutrition education programming to elicit reductions in sugary beverage intake. Furthermore, the American Dental Association recognizes the role of dental professionals in promoting healthy lifestyles and behavior change to reduce the incidence of obesity by collaborating with other health care professionals and organizations [43]. General oral health recommendations include visiting the dentist twice a year, which provides an opportunity for nutrition education professionals to develop theory-based training programs to train oral health professionals to discuss limiting SSBs with families and provide educational materials and training that oral health professionals can provide to families to help them limit SSB consumption in children [43].

A negative outcome expectation of SSB consumption shared by some parents and children was hyperactivity. Although this belief is commonly held by many consumers, the effect of sugar on behavior in children remains unclear. Although a landmark 1995 meta-analysis published in the Journal of the American Medical Association concluded that sugar did not have an effect on behavior [44], more recent cross-sectional data suggest that risk for hyperactivity/inattention does rise as SSB consumption increases [44]. Helping parents and kids understand that SSB increase may affect behavior in some people could help them implement behaviors to curb intake of these drinks.

Participants' observation that SSB consumption affects sleep patterns is supported by research reporting links between dietary sugar and sleep duration [45]. The 2014 Sleep in America® Poll revealed that nearly one in three children age 6 to 11 years in the Unites States gets 8 h or less of sleep each night [46], falling short of the National Sleep Foundation's recommended 9 to 11 h per night [47]. The link between short sleep duration and increased BMI is well established [48]. Decreased sleep duration associated with SSB consumption may further exacerbate the association between SSB consumption and BMI.

Parents were also correct to express concern about the effect of caffeine in SSBs on children's behavior. Three-quarters of the young children in a study evaluating caffeine consumption were caffeine consumers, and caffeine consumption was negatively correlated with average number of sleep hours [49]. In addition, caffeine can have negative cardiovascular effects in children [50]. While caffeinated soda consumption in children has declined over the years, more children are consuming trendy coffee and energy drinks high in sugar and caffeine [51]. Future nutrition education programs should build knowledge of the negative effects of caffeine from SSB and offer strategies for limiting caffeine consumption.

Although SSB consumption reported by participants did not differ by geographic location, parents in West Virginia commented that SSB consumption was a normal part of their lifestyle and culture, which they felt made it especially difficult to decrease consumption. The Theory of Reasoned Action postulates that an individual's behaviors are influenced by perceived social norms, or the extent to which they believe others support engaging in a particular behavior [52]. Similarly, the construct of reciprocal determinism from SCT suggests that individuals' behaviors are influenced by their environment, including cultural influences [29]. The potential effect of geography and culture on SSB intake is important to consider in nutrition education programs. Cultural norms can both precipitate and reinforce positive, as well as negative behaviors. For example, a study aiming to improve adolescent normative beliefs related to smoking found that students' perceived prevalence of smoking was linked to their risk of smoking, as was their beliefs that smoking was popular among "successful/elite elements of society" [53]. The study also found that disapproval of smoking by friends and family was significantly negatively associated with adolescent smoking behaviors [53]. Future interventions may promote behavior change by aiming to alter normative beliefs related to SSB consumption.

A common barrier to limiting children's SSB intake was parental role modeling. Children tend to model their parents' eating behaviors, lifestyle, eating-related attitudes, and body image satisfaction [54]. In the current study, both parents and kids recognized that children were affected by parent actions. In fact, children suggested parents not drink as much SSB as a strategy to help kids decrease their own intake, however some parents indicated that it was a struggle to not consume SSBs. Several studies have demonstrated a positive association between parent knowledge about diet and health and positive parental influence on children's beverage intake [31,55–57], thereby highlighting the importance of building parent knowledge of the importance of limiting SSBs to motivate them to limit child SSB intake. Often parents reported turning to quick, sugary beverage options due to the time constraints and limited healthy options at convenience stores. Providing strategies for healthy beverage options on-the-go as part of nutrition education interventions could enable families to reduce SSB intake, as would building parents' time management skills.

Another barrier noted was parents' lack of knowledge of the school food environment and policies that promote healthy eating in this setting. It was evident from the focus groups that many parents were not aware of federal guidelines designed to ensure school beverage options are nutrient dense [58]. Instead, parents felt that their children's beverage choices at home were negatively influenced by school experiences. Studies consistently show that students who participate in the National School Lunch Program (NSLP) consume more fruits, vegetables, and milk and less SSBs and low-nutrient, energy-dense items than non-participants [59,60]. A cross-sectional study exploring the relationship between school lunch participation and dietary patterns also indicated that children who participated in NSLP consumed less than one-third the average amount of energy from SSBs as non-participants [59].

Findings from the current study suggest parental disapproval of flavored milk in the school setting. Federal guidelines allow non-fat flavored milk as part of the NSLP, which has been endorsed by the American Academy of Pediatrics [61] and the Academy of Nutrition and Dietetics [62,63] as part of an overall healthy diet. Additionally, a recent systematic review reported that flavored milk increases overall milk intake by 28% [64]. Most other SSBs contain more added sugar than flavored milks, which provides an opportunity to teach parents and children to make better SSB choices, such as flavored milk in moderation when away from home.

Both children and parents recognized the importance of the home food environment in promoting healthy beverage choices and suggested not purchasing SSBs as a key strategy to limiting consumption [25,62,65]. Similarly, in a qualitative study with Latino adolescents and their parents, youth cited home availability as a key factor driving their SSB consumption [66]. Research supports the effectiveness of this strategy in that the availability of soft drinks in the home is strongly associated with soft drink consumption. Future nutrition interventions should promote SSBs as a beverage to consume on occasion rather than every day and should suggest that SSBs be purchased at the time of consumption rather than kept on-hand in the house.

Both parents and children in the study reported here indicated the importance of setting boundaries for SSB intake. Recommendations by children that parents incentivize or punish children as a means for promoting healthier beverage intake suggests kids have experienced non-recommended authoritarian parental feeding practices. In general, an authoritative feeding style, where parents use supportive and responsive feeding practices to encourage heathy eating, is associated with healthier dietary behaviors and BMI [67,68], although a more restrictive parental feeding style was associated with less soft drink consumption in teenagers [69]. Helping parents and children recognize the benefits of authoritative feeding styles could help families now, as well as future families of the current generation of children, form healthier dietary habits, including limited SSB intake.

Previous research has shown that interventions that focus on environmental changes are most successful at reducing SSB consumption in school-age children [70]. This is particularly true for interventions that target the home rather than school environment [71]. Interventions aimed at teaching parents of school-aged children to set goals for making health-related behavior changes for their families can be effective at reducing children's SSB consumption [72]. The success of these interventions is congruent with some recommendations in Table 1, including facilitating behavior change by adjusting the home environment and building parent self-efficacy for making behavior changes.

5. Conclusions

This qualitative research provides important information regarding parents' and children's cognitions (e.g., beliefs, attitudes), barriers, and facilitators related to children's SSB consumption. To the authors' knowledge, this study is the first to qualitatively explore SSB cognitions and use them to generate recommendations for future nutrition programming aiming to lower SSB intake. However, the small sample size limits the ability to detect ethnic differences in study participants. Furthermore, self-selection bias may have resulted in a sample that is not representative of the general population.

Achieving the goal of limited SSB consumption is important given that SSBs are a significant source of added sugars in the diets of children and are considered an important contributor to the obesity epidemic [73]. Educating both parents and children is important because parents serve as household food gatekeepers and children's role models and, as children age, they have more opportunities to make their own beverage choices. Future research should aim to implement the recommendations generated by this study in interventions and assess their effectiveness in helping families reach the goal of reduced SSB intake and associated health outcomes.

Author Contributions: Data curation, K.M.E., E.G., C.L.D. and O.A.F.; Formal analysis, K.M.E., A.D., E.G., C.L.D., O.A.F. and C.B.-B.; Funding acquisition, M.D.O., C.B.-B. and K.P.S.; Methodology, K.M.E., M.D.O., C.B.-B., K.P.S.; Writing–original draft, K.M.E., S.D., E.G., C.B.-B.; Writing-Review & Editing, All authors.; Funding Acquisition, C.B.-B., M.D.O. and K.P.S.

Funding: This research was funded by United States Department of Agriculture, National Institute of Food and Agriculture, grant number 2017-680001-26351

Conflicts of Interest: The authors declare no conflict of interest.

References

1. Drewnowski, A.; Rehm, C.D. Consumption of added sugars among us children and adults by food purchase location and food source. *Am. J. Clin. Nutr.* **2014**, *100*, 901–907. [CrossRef] [PubMed]

2. Ochoa, M.C.; Moreno-Aliaga, M.J.; Martínez-González, M.A.; Martínez, J.A.; Marti, A. Predictor factors for childhood obesity in a Spanish case-control study. *Nutrition* **2007**, *23*, 379–384. [CrossRef] [PubMed]

3. Athanasopoulos, D.; Garopoulou, A.; Dragoumanos, V. Childhood obesity and associated factors in a rural Greek Island. *Rural Remote Health* **2011**, *11*, 1–9.

4. Malik, V.S.; Pan, A.; Willett, W.C.; Hu, F.B. Sugar-sweetened beverages and weight gain in children and adults: A systematic review and meta-analysis. *Am. J. Clin. Nutr.* **2013**, *98*, 1084–1102. [CrossRef] [PubMed]

5. Malik, V.S.; Popkin, B.M.; Bray, G.A.; Després, J.-P.; Willett, W.C.; Hu, F.B. Sugar-sweetened beverages and risk of metabolic syndrome and type 2 diabetes: A meta-analysis. *Diabetes Care* **2010**, *33*, 2477–2483. [CrossRef] [PubMed]

6. Imamura, F.; O'Connor, L.; Ye, Z.; Mursu, J.; Hayashino, Y.; Bhupathiraju, S.N.; Forouhi, N.G. Consumption of sugar sweetened beverages, artificially sweetened beverages, and fruit juice and incidence of type 2 diabetes: Systematic review, meta-analysis, and estimation of population attributable fraction. *BMJ* **2015**, *351*. [CrossRef] [PubMed]

7. Rodríguez, L.A.; Madsen, K.A.; Cotterman, C.; Lustig, R.H. Added sugar intake and metabolic syndrome in us adolescents: Cross-sectional analysis of the national health and nutrition examination survey 2005–2012. *Public Health Nutr.* **2016**, *19*, 2424–2434. [CrossRef] [PubMed]

8. Stanhope, K.L. Sugar consumption, metabolic disease and obesity: The state of the controversy. *Crit. Rev. Clin. Lab. Sci.* **2016**, *53*, 52–67. [CrossRef] [PubMed]

9. Hales, C.M.; Carroll, M.D.; Fryar, C.D.; Ogden, C.L. Prevalence of obesity among adults and youth: United States. *NCHS Data Brief* **2017**, *288*, 1–8.

10. Hoelscher, D.M.; Kirk, S.; Ritchie, L.; Cunningham-Sabo, L. Position of the academy of nutrition and dietetics: Interventions for the prevention and treatment of pediatric overweight and obesity. *J. Acad. Nutr. Diet.* **2013**, *113*, 1375–1394. [CrossRef] [PubMed]

11. Health, U.D.O.; Services, H. *Dietary Guidelines for Americans 2015–2020*; Skyhorse Publishing Inc.: New York, NY, USA, 2017.

12. Ervin, R.; Kit, B.; Carroll, M.; Ogden, C. Consumption of added sugar among U.S. Children and adolescents, 2005–2008. *NCHS Data Brief* **2012**, *87*, 1–8.

13. Ervin, R.B.; Ogden, C.L. Consumption of added sugars among us adults, 2005–2010. *NCHS Data Brief* **2013**, 1–8.

14. Rosinger, A.; Herrick, K.; Gahche, J.; Park, S. Sugar-sweetened beverage consumption among U.S.; Adults, 2011–2014. *NCHS Data Brief* **2017**, *270*, 1–8.

15. Watowicz, R.; Anderson, S.; Kaye, G.; Taylor, C. Energy contribution of beverages in us children by age, weight, and consumer status. *Child. Obes.* **2015**, *11*, 475–483. [CrossRef] [PubMed]

16. Gishti, O.; Gaillard, R.; Durmus, B.; Abrahamse, M.; van der Beek, E.M.; Hofman, A.; Franco, O.H.; de Jonge, L.L.; Jaddoe, V.W. BMI, total and abdominal fat distribution, and cardiovascular risk factors in school-age children. *Pediatr. Res.* **2015**, *77*, 710–718. [CrossRef] [PubMed]

17. Kumar, S.; Kelly, A.S. Review of childhood obesity: From epidemiology, etiology, and comorbidities to clinical assessment and treatment. *Mayo Clin. Proc.* **2017**, *92*, 251–265. [CrossRef] [PubMed]

18. Zuba, A.; Warschburger, P. The role of weight teasing and weight bias internalization in psychological functioning: A prospective study among school-aged children. *Eur. Child Adolesc. Psychiatry* **2017**, *26*, 1245–1255. [CrossRef] [PubMed]

19. Armfield, J.M.; Spencer, A.J.; Roberts-Thomson, K.F.; Plastow, K. Water fluoridation and the association of sugar-sweetened beverage consumption and dental caries in Australian children. *Am. J. Public Health* **2013**, *103*, 494–500. [CrossRef] [PubMed]

20. Wilder, J.; Kaste, L.; Handler, A.; Chapple-McGruder, T.; Rankin, K. The association between sugar-sweetened beverages and dental caries among third-grade students in Georgia. *J. Public Health Dent.* **2016**, *76*, 76–84. [CrossRef] [PubMed]

21. Keller, K.; Kirzner, J.; Pietrobelli, A.; St-Onge, M.; Faith, M. Increased sweetened beverage intake is associated with reduced milk and calcium intake in 3- to 7-year-old children at multi-item laboratory lunches. *J. Am. Diet. Assoc.* **2009**, *109*, 497–501. [CrossRef] [PubMed]

22. Leung, C.; DiMatteo, S.; Gosliner, W.; Ritchie, L. Sugar-sweetened beverage and water intake in relation to diet quality in U.S. Children. *Am. J. Prev. Med.* **2018**, *54*, 394–402. [CrossRef] [PubMed]

23. Keast, D.; Fulgoni, V.; Nicklas, T.; O'Neil, C. Food sources of energy and nutrients among children in the united states: National health and nutrition examination survey 2003–2006. *Nutrients* **2013**, *5*, 283–301. [CrossRef] [PubMed]

24. Handel, M.; Heitmann, B.; Abrahamsen, B. Nutrient and food intakes in early life and risk of childhood fractures: A systematic review and meta-analysis. *Am. J. Clin. Nutr.* **2015**, *102*, 1182–1195. [CrossRef] [PubMed]

25. Grimm, G.C.; Harnack, L.; Story, M. Factors associated with soft drink consumption in school-aged children. *J. Am. Diet. Assoc.* **2004**, *104*, 1244–1249. [CrossRef] [PubMed]

26. Verloigne, M.; Van Lippevelde, W.; Maes, L.; Brug, J.; De Bourdeaudhuij, I. Family-and school-based correlates of energy balance-related behaviours in 10–12-year-old children: A systematic review within the energy (European energy balance research to prevent excessive weight gain among youth) project. *Public Health Nutr.* **2012**, *15*, 1380–1395. [CrossRef] [PubMed]

27. Mazarello Paes, V.; Hesketh, K.; O'Malley, C.; Moore, H.; Summerbell, C.; Griffin, S.; van Sluijs, E.; Ong, K.; Lakshman, R. Determinants of sugar-sweetened beverage consumption in young children: A systematic review. *Obes. Rev.* **2015**, *16*, 903–913. [CrossRef] [PubMed]

28. Bandura, A. Health promotion by social cognitive means. *Health Educ. Behav.* **2004**, *31*, 143–164. [CrossRef] [PubMed]

29. Kelder, S.; Hoelscher, D.; Perry, C. How individuals, enviornments, and health behavior interact. In *Health Behavior, Theory, Research, and Practice*, 5th ed.; Glanz, K., Rimer, B., Viswanath, K., Eds.; Jossey-Bass: San Francisco, CA, USA, 2015; pp. 165–184.

30. Bandura, A. *A Social Learning Theory*; Prentice-Hall: Englewood Cliffs, NJ, USA, 1977.

31. Zahid, A.; Davey, C.; Reicks, M. Beverage intake among children: Associations with parent and home-related factors. *Int. J. Environ. Res. Public Health* **2017**, *14*. [CrossRef] [PubMed]

32. Van Ansem, W.J.; van Lenthe, F.J.; Schrijvers, C.T.; Rodenburg, G.; van de Mheen, D. Socio-economic inequalities in children's snack consumption and sugar-sweetened beverage consumption: The contribution of home environmental factors. *Br. J. Nutr.* **2014**, *112*, 467–476. [CrossRef] [PubMed]

33. Rehm, C.; Drewnowski, A. Trends in consumption of solid fats, added sugars, sodium, sugar-sweetened beverages, and fruit from fast food restaurants and by fast food restaurant type among us children, 2003–2010. *Nutrients* **2016**, *8*. [CrossRef] [PubMed]

34. Then, K.; Rankin, J.; Ali, E. Focus group research: What is it and how can it be used? *Can. J. Cardiovasc. Nurs.* **2014**, *24*, 16–22. [PubMed]

35. Miles, M.B.; Huberman, A.M. *Qualitative Data Analysis*; Sage Publications: Thousand Oaks, CA, USA, 1994.

36. Harris, J.E.; Gleason, P.M.; Sheean, P.M.; Boushey, C.; Beto, J.A.; Brummer, B. An introduction to qualitative research for food and nutrition professionals. *J. Am. Diet. Assoc.* **2009**, *109*, 80–90. [CrossRef] [PubMed]

37. Elo, S.; Kyngas, H. The qualitative content analysis process. *J. Adv. Nurs.* **2008**, *62*, 107–115. [CrossRef] [PubMed]

38. Kirppendorff, K. Content Analysis: An Introduction to Its Methodology. Available online: file:///C: /Users/carolbb225-2/Downloads/intro_to_content_analysis%20(1).pdf (accessed on 25 August 2018).

39. Fusch, P.I.; Ness, L.R. Are we there yet? Data saturation in qualitative research. *Qual. Rep.* **2015**, *20*, 1408–1416.

40. Mrdjenovic, G.; Levitsky, D.A. Nutritional and energetic consequences of sweetened drink consumption in 6-to 13-year-old children. *Pediatrics* **2003**, *142*, 604–610. [CrossRef] [PubMed]

41. Basu, S.; McKee, M.; Galea, G.; Stuckler, D. Relationship of soft drink consumption to global overweight, obesity, and diabetes: A cross-national analysis of 75 countries. *Am. J. Public Health* **2013**, *103*, 2071–2077. [CrossRef] [PubMed]

42. American Academy of Pediatric Dentistry. Policy on dietary recommendations for infants, children, and adolescents. *Policy Man.* **2012**, *37*, 2015–2016.

43. Mallonee, L.F.; Boyd, L.D.; Stegeman, C. A scoping review of skills and tools oral health professionals need to engage children and parents in dietary changes to prevent childhood obesity and consumption of sugar sweetened beverages. *J. Public Health Dent.* **2017**, *77*, S128–S135. [CrossRef] [PubMed]

44. Schwartz, D.L.; Gilstad-Hayden, K.; Carroll-Scott, A.; Grilo, S.A.; McCaslin, C.; Schwartz, M.; Ickovics, J.R. Energy drinks and youth self-reported hyperactivity/inattention symptoms. *Acad. Pediatr.* **2015**, *15*, 297–304. [CrossRef] [PubMed]

45. Franckle, R.L.; Falbe, J.; Gortmaker, S.; Ganter, C.; Taveras, E.M.; Land, T.; Davison, K.K. Insufficient sleep among elementary and middle school students is linked with elevated soda consumption and other unhealthy dietary behaviors. *Am. J. Prev. Med.* **2015**, *74*, 36–41. [CrossRef] [PubMed]

46. National Sleep Foundation. *Sleep in America Poll: Sleep in the Modern Family*; National Sleep Foundation: Arlington, VA, USA, 2014.

47. Hirshkowitz, M.; Whiton, K.; Albert, S.M.; Alessi, C.; Bruni, O.; DonCarlos, L.; Hazen, N.; Herman, J.; Katz, E.S.; Kheirandish-Gozal, L. National sleep foundation's sleep time duration recommendations: Methodology and results summary. *Sleep Health* **2015**, *1*, 40–43. [CrossRef] [PubMed]

48. Zhang, J.; Zhang, Y.; Jiang, Y.; Sun, W.; Zhu, Q.; Ip, P.; Zhang, D.; Liu, S.; Chen, C.; Chen, J. Effect of sleep duration, diet, and physical activity on obesity and overweight elementary school students in Shanghai. *J. Sch. Health* **2018**, *88*, 112–121. [CrossRef] [PubMed]

49. Warzak, W.J.; Evans, S.; Floress, M.T.; Gross, A.C.; Stoolman, S. Caffeine consumption in young children. *Peadiatrics* **2011**, *158*, 508–509. [CrossRef] [PubMed]

50. Temple, J.L.; Ziegler, A.M.; Graczyk, A.; Bendlin, A.; Sion, T.; Vattana, K. Cardiovascular responses to caffeine by gender and pubertal stage. *Pediatrics* **2014**. [CrossRef] [PubMed]

51. Branum, A.M.; Rossen, L.M.; Schoendorf, K.C. Trends in caffeine intake among us children and adolescents. *Pediatrics* **2014**, *134*, e112–e119. [CrossRef] [PubMed]

52. Montano, D.E.; Kasprzyk, D. Theory of reasoned action, theory of planned behavior, and the integrated behavioral model. In *Health Behavior: Theory, Research and Practice*; Jossey Bass Publishers: San Francisco, CA, USA, 2015; pp. 95–124.

53. Primack, B.A.; Switzer, G.E.; Dalton, M.A. Improving measurement of normative beliefs involving smoking among adolescents. *Arch. Pediatr. Adolesc. Med.* **2007**, *161*, 434–439. [CrossRef] [PubMed]

54. Scaglioni, S.; De Cosmi, V.; Ciappolino, V.; Parazzini, F.; Brambilla, P.; Agostoni, C. Factors influencing children's eating behaviours. *Nutrients* **2018**, *10*. [CrossRef] [PubMed]

55. Harris, T.S.; Ramsey, M. Paternal modeling, household availability, and paternal intake as predictors of fruit, vegetable, and sweetened beverage consumption among African American children. *Appetite* **2015**, *85*, 171–177. [CrossRef] [PubMed]

56. Hart, L.M.; Damiano, S.R.; Cornell, C.; Paxton, S.J. What parents know and want to learn about healthy eating and body image in preschool children: A triangulated qualitative study with parents and early childhood professionals. *BMC Public Health* **2015**, *15*. [CrossRef] [PubMed]

57. Hennessy, M.; Bleakley, A.; Piotrowski, J.T.; Mallya, G.; Jordan, A. Sugar-sweetened beverage consumption by adult caregivers and their children: The role of drink features and advertising exposure. *Health Educ. Behav.* **2015**, *42*, 677–686. [CrossRef] [PubMed]

58. Food and Nutrition Service. National school lunch program and school breakfast program: Nutrition standards for all foods sold in schools as required by the healthy, hunger-free kids act of 2010. *Fed. Regist.* **2016**, *78*, 50131–50151.

59. Briefel, R.R.; Wilson, A.; Gleason, P.M. Consumption of low-nutrient, energy-dense foods and beverages at school, home, and other locations among school lunch participants and nonparticipants. *J. Acad. Nutr. Diet.* **2009**, *109*, S79–S90. [CrossRef] [PubMed]

60. Ohri-Vachaspati, P. Parental perception of the nutritional quality of school meals and its association with students' school lunch participation. *Appetite* **2014**, *74*, 44–47. [CrossRef] [PubMed]

61. Murray, R.; Bhatia, J.; Okamoto, J.; Allison, M.; Ancona, R.; Attisha, E.; De Pinto, C.; Holmes, B.; Kjolhede, C.; Lerner, M. Snacks, sweetened beverages, added sugars, and schools. *Pediatrics* **2015**, *135*, 575–583.

62. Marion, J.; Franz, M. Use of nutritive and non-nutritive sweetener. *J. Am. Diet. Assoc.* **1993**, *93*, 816–821.

63. Patel, A.I.; Moghadam, S.D.; Freedman, M.; Hazari, A.; Fang, M.-L.; Allen, I. The association of flavored milk consumption with milk and energy intake, and obesity: A systematic review. *Am. J. Prev. Med.* **2018**, *111*, 151–162. [CrossRef] [PubMed]

64. Fayet-Moore, F. Effect of flavored milk vs plain milk on total milk intake and nutrient provision in children. *Nutr. Rev.* **2016**, *74*, 1–17. [CrossRef] [PubMed]

65. Campbell, K.J.; Crawford, D.A.; Salmon, J.; Carver, A.; Garnett, S.P.; Baur, L.A. Associations between the home food environment and obesity-promoting eating behaviors in adolescence. *Obesity* **2007**, *15*, 719–730. [CrossRef] [PubMed]

66. Bogart, L.M.; Elliott, M.N.; Ober, A.J.; Klein, D.J.; Hawes-Dawson, J.; Cowgill, B.O.; Uyeda, K.; Schuster, M.A. Home sweet home: Parent and home environmental factors in adolescent consumption of sugar-sweetened beverages. *Pediatrics* **2017**, *17*, 529–536. [CrossRef] [PubMed]

67. Sleddens, E.F.; Gerards, S.M.; Thijs, C.; De Vries, N.K.; Kremers, S.P. General parenting, childhood overweight and obesity-inducing behaviors: A review. *Pediatr. Obes.* **2011**, *6*, e12–e27. [CrossRef] [PubMed]

68. Shloim, N.; Edelson, L.R.; Martin, N.; Hetherington, M.M. Parenting styles, feeding styles, feeding practices, and weight status in 4–12 year-old children: A systematic review of the literature. *Front. Psychol.* **2015**, *6*. [CrossRef] [PubMed]

69. Van der Horst, K.; Kremers, S.; Ferreira, I.; Singh, A.; Oenema, A.; Brug, J. Perceived parenting style and practices and the consumption of sugar-sweetened beverages by adolescents. *Health Educ. Res.* **2007**, *22*, 295–304. [CrossRef] [PubMed]

70. Avery, A.; Bostock, L.; McCullough, F. A systematic review investigating interventions that can help reduce consumption of sugar-sweetened beverages in children leading to changes in body fatness. *J. Hum. Nutr. Diet.* **2016**, *28*, 52–64. [CrossRef] [PubMed]

71. Vargas-Garcia, E.; Evans, C.; Perstwich, A.; Sykes-Muskett, B.; Hooson, J.; Cade, J. Interventions to reduce consumption of sugar-sweetened beverages or increase water intake: Evidence from a systematic review and meta-analysis. *Obes. Rev.* **2017**, *18*, 1350–1363. [CrossRef] [PubMed]

72. Fulkerson, J.A.; Friend, S.; Horning, M.; Flattum, C.; Draxten, M.; Neumark-Sztainer, D.; Gurvich, O.; Garwick, A.; Story, M.; Kubik, M.Y. Family home food environment and nutrition-related parent and child personal and behavioral outcomes of the healthy home offerings via the mealtime environment (home) plus program: A randomized controlled trial. *J. Acad. Nutr. Diet.* **2018**, *118*, 240–251. [CrossRef] [PubMed]

73. Tucker, L.A.; Tucker, J.M.; Bailey, B.W.; LeCheminant, J.D. A 4-year prospective study of soft drink consumption and weight gain: The role of calorie intake and physical activity. *Am. J. Health Promot.* **2015**, *29*, 262–265. [CrossRef] [PubMed]

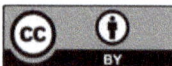

nutrients

MDPI

Article

Moderate Beer Intake and Cardiovascular Health in Overweight Individuals

Teresa Padro [1,2], Natàlia Muñoz-García [1], Gemma Vilahur [1,2], Patricia Chagas [1,3], Alba Deyà [1], Rosa Maria Antonijoan [4] and Lina Badimon [1,2,5,*]

[1] Cardiovascular ICCC-Program, Research Institute Hospital de la Santa Creu i Sant Pau, IIB-Sant Pau, 08025 Barcelona, Spain; tpadro@santpau.cat (T.P.); nmunoz@santpau.cat (N.M.-G.); gvilahur@santpau.cat (G.V.); patriciachagas.ufsm@hotmail.com (P.C.); albadeya4@gmail.com (A.D.)
[2] CIBERCV Instituto de Salud Carlos III, 28029 Madrid, Spain
[3] Department of Food and Nutrition, Universidade Federal de Santa Maria, Palmeira das Missões RS 98300000, Brasil
[4] Medicament Research Center (CIM), Research Institute Hospital de la Santa Creu i Sant Pau, IIB-Sant Pau, 08025 Barcelona, Spain; rantonijoana@santpau.cat
[5] Cardiovascular Research Chair, UAB, 08025 Barcelona, Spain
* Correspondence: lbadimon@santpau.cat; Tel.: +34-935-565-880; Fax: +34-935-565-559

Received: 8 August 2018; Accepted: 28 August 2018; Published: 5 September 2018

Abstract: Consistent epidemiological evidence indicates that low-to-moderate alcohol consumption is inversely associated with cardiovascular event presentation, while high levels of alcohol intake are associated to increased cardiovascular risk. Little is known on the effects of moderate beer intake in the metabolic syndrome. The aim of this study is to investigate the effects of moderate and regular daily intake of beer with meals in overweight (body mass index (BMI) of 28–29.9 kg/m^2) or obese class 1 (BMI of 30–35 kg/m^2) individuals without other cardiovascular risk factors (dyslipidemia, type 2-diabetes, hypertension) focusing on the effects related to changes in weight, in lipoproteins and vascular endothelial function. We have performed an open, prospective two-arms longitudinal crossover study to investigate the effects associated with regular consumption (four week) of alcohol-free-beer (0 g alcohol/day) or traditional-beer (30 g alcohol/day in men and 15 g alcohol/day in women) on anthropometrical and biochemical parameters, liver and kidney function biomarkers, and vascular endothelial function. After four-week intervention with traditional and/or alcohol-free beer, BMI did not show any significant change and values for liver and kidney functions were within the normal levels. Moderate traditional beer intake did not affect lipid levels—however it significantly increased the antioxidant capacity of high density lipoprotein (HDL). In addition, apoB-depleted serum (after the four-week intervention period) showed a higher potential to promote cholesterol efflux from macrophages. Beer consumption did not induce vascular endothelial dysfunction or stiffness. In summary, our results based on a 12-week prospective study provide evidence that moderate intake of beer (traditional and alcohol-free) does not exert vascular detrimental effects nor increases body weight in obese healthy individuals. In contrast, moderate intake of beer increases the anti-oxidative properties of HDL and facilitates cholesterol efflux, which may prevent lipid deposition in the vessel wall.

Keywords: cardiovascular-risk-factors; overweight; obesity; fermented-beverage; lipoprotein-oxidation; HDL-antioxidant-capacity; cholesterol-efflux; endothelial-function

1. Introduction

Epidemiological studies have reported a J-shaped relationship between alcohol intake and cardiovascular disease (CVD). Therefore, low-to-moderate drinkers have a lower risk of developing coronary heart disease and less mortality compared to both heavy drinkers and abstainers, being the heavy drinkers the ones with the highest risk [1–3]. However, the benefits of alcohol consumption are widely discussed and remain controversial regarding the type of beverage [4–6] and drinking pattern [7,8]. Mukamal et al. reported that alcohol intake distributed over the week inversely associates with the risk of myocardial infarction, independently of the type of beverage or the proportion consumed with meals [7]. In contrast, results of the INTERHART Study, a case-control study examining the relationship between alcohol consumption and the long- and short-term risk of myocardial infarction (MI) in all inhabited continents of the world, highlights the importance of the type of alcohol consumed and the pattern of alcohol use as modifiers of the relationship between alcohol and myocardial infarction [8]. In agreement, some studies indicate that low-to-moderate alcohol consumption does not have a net mortality benefit compared to abstainers because the rates of mortality and cardiovascular disease (CVD) risk from alcohol are significantly altered by study design and characteristics as well as confounding factors [9–12]. Regarding the type of beverage, early studies supported the benefits of wine on cardiovascular outcomes and mortality and depicted that a J-shaped relationship was found in wine, but neither in beer nor spirits [13,14]. However, more recently, an updated meta-analysis study reported by Costanzo et al. [15] provided evidence that the J-shaped association is found in both wine and beer, but not in spirits. Fermented beverages, both wine and beer, are rich in antioxidants, mainly polyphenolic compounds [5,16,17], that are missing in spirit beverages.

Beer is one of the most consumed alcoholic beverages in the world; in America it is the most popular alcoholic beverage, contributing up to 55.3% of the alcohol consumed [18]. Studies on traditional- and non-alcoholic beer consumption are needed to evidence their effects in different factors contributing to cardiovascular health and their benefit/risk ratios. Here, we are reporting a clinical study aimed to investigate beneficial and detrimental effects of moderate and regular intake of beer in overweight or obese class-1 individuals without other cardiovascular risk factors (CVRF) such as dyslipidemia, type 2-diabetes or hypertension, focusing on the effects related to changes in weight, on lipoprotein atheroprotective effects and vascular endothelial function.

2. Materials and Methods

2.1. Subjects

Healthy adult men and women between ages of 40–60 years ($N = 36$), non-smokers, regular but moderate beer consumers (self-reported alcohol consumption), and with overweight (body mass index (BMI) of 28–29.9 kg/m^2) or obesity class 1 (BMI of 30–35 kg/m^2) were invited to participate in the study through word of mouth and a newspaper advertisement. Moderate beer drinking was defined according to the "Dietary Guidelines for Americans 2015–2020," U.S. Department of Health and Human Services and U.S. Department of Agriculture, (https://www.niaaa.nih.gov/alcohol-health/overview-alcohol-consumption/moderate-binge-drinking) and refers up to 1 drink per day for women, and up to 2 drinks per day for men. Subjects were excluded if they reported extensive consumption of beer (>60 g day of ethanol), existing chronic illnesses including cancer, overt hyperlipidemia, diabetes mellitus, hypertension, heart, liver or kidney disease. Other exclusion criteria included the use of lipid-lowering drugs, beta-blockers or diuretics, history of CVD, psychiatric illness or treatment of psychotropic drugs, intolerance to alcoholic beverages or being in a weight-loss program. To confirm health status, all subjects underwent a complete physical examination conducted by the study physician before entry into the study. The study complies with the Declaration of Helsinki and was approved by the Human Ethical Review Committee of the Hospital "Santa Creu i Sant Pau" of Barcelona (Ref 14/186; 12 November 2014). Informed written consent was obtained from all participants before entering the study.

2.2. Study Design and Dietary Monitoring

The study was an open, randomized two-arm longitudinal cross-over trial with a 4 week intervention period (Figure 1). All subjects were subjected to two 4-week treatment sequences, separated by a 4-week wash-out period. Before the initiation of the intervention, individuals were subjected to a 4-week run-in period. At the end of the run-in period, subjects were randomly allocated to receive one of the two treatment sequences (study arm-1: traditional beer in the first intervention period and alcohol-free beer in the second intervention period; study-arm-2: non-alcoholic beer in the first intervention period and traditional beer in the second intervention period). During the intervention periods, men and women were instructed to drink two cans (660 mL beer) and one can (330 mL beer), respectively, of traditional beer (15 g of ethanol and 604 mg polyphenols/can) or alcohol-free beer (0.0 g alcohol and 414 mg polyphenols/can) per day. During the run-in and wash-out periods and throughout the intervention phases the participants were asked to maintain their physical activity level and usual dietary habits, abstaining from drinking alcoholic beverages and alcohol-free beer out of those provided as part of the study. Dietary habits, determined by using food frequency questionnaires, were recorded prior to each visit, and rare changes in diet habits were reported.

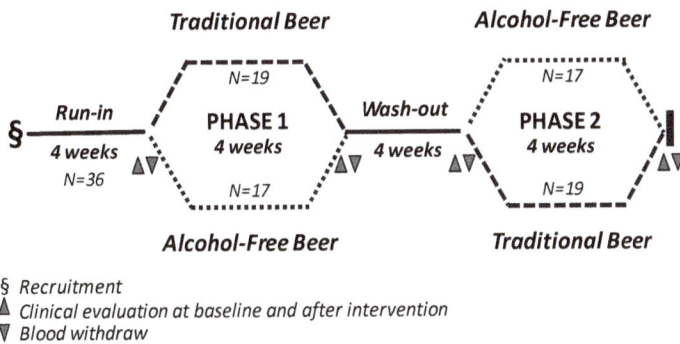

§ Recruitment
▲ Clinical evaluation at baseline and after intervention
▼ Blood withdraw

Figure 1. Flow diagram describing the study design.

Compliance was monitored by regular telephone contact with participants and interviewing them at the end of each intervention period. Participants also recorded whether they had consumed beer on a diary card each day. Moreover, at the end of each intervention period, a clinician assessed any side effects or symptoms such as flushing, bloating, dizziness, vomiting, diarrhea, with possible association with the study interventions.

Traditional and alcohol-free beers were of the lager type from the same Spanish commercial brand. The phenolic composition derived from the traditional and alcohol-free beer interventions and the daily intake according to the gender is provided in Supplementary Table S1.

2.3. Blood Samples

Twelve hour fasting blood samples were collected on days 1 and 28 (baseline and endpoint of the first treatment period) and on days 56 and 84 (baseline and endpoint of the second treatment period). Blood samples were collected without anticoagulant or in ethylenediamine tetraacetic acid (EDTA)-containing Vacutainer tubes for serum and plasma preparation, respectively. Serum and plasma fractions were separated by centrifugation at $1800 \times g$ for 20 min and stored at -80 °C until used.

2.4. Anthropometric Data, Blood Pressure, Serum Lipid Profile and Other Biochemical Measurements

Anthropometric measurements were determined at baseline, before starting the intervention, and at the end of the intervention periods (see Figure 1). The BMI was calculated using the formula body weight (Kg)/height (m^2) [19]. Waist circumference (WC) was measured between the lowest rib and the iliac crest with the participant standing.

Serum biochemical measurements were performed using routine commercially available assays for glucose levels, hepatic and renal markers, hemogram and standard serum lipid profile including triglycerides, total cholesterol (TC) and HDL (high density lipoprotein) cholesterol (Roche Diagnostics, Basel, Switzerland). As there were no cases of hypertriglyceridemia, LDL (low density lipoprotein) cholesterol was calculated using the Friedewald equation. Glomerular filtration rate was obtained according to the CKD-EPI Levey equation [20].

2.5. LDL and HDL Sample Preparation, Purity Control and Oxidation Assays

2.5.1. Lipoprotein Preparation

LDL (density range 1.019–1.063 g/mL) and HDL (density range 1.063–1.210 g/mL) were obtained from plasma-EDTA from individual samples by sequential ultracentrifugation, according to the method originally described by Havel et al. [21] and modified by De Juan-Franco et al. [22]. Briefly, plasma was adjusted to a density of 1.019 g/mL with a concentrated salt solution (potassium bromide) and centrifuged at $225,000 \times g$ (18 h) in a Beckman L-60 ultracentrifuge with a fixed-angle type 50.4 Ti rotor (Beckman, Brea, CA, USA). After removal of the top layer, containing very low and intermediate density lipoproteins (VLDL and IDL), the density of the infranatant was adjusted to 1.063 g/mL, followed by centrifugation for 20 h at $225,000 \times g$ and LDL were collected from the top of the tube. Lastly, the process was repeated adjusting plasma density to 1.210 g/mL and samples ultracentrifuges at $225,000 \times g$ for 24 h, at 4 °C, to allow HDL to float and separate from lipoprotein deficient serum.

In addition, LDLs to be used in the TRAP assay were isolated from a pool of plasma obtained from normolipemic subjects and obtained as described above in a Beckman Optima L-100 XP with a fixed- angle type 50.2 Ti (Beckman, Brea, CA, USA).

LDL and HDL fractions were dialyzed against phosphate buffer saline 1X (PBS 1X) for 24 h. LDL- and HDL-protein content was determined by the colorimetric assay BCA (Pierce, Thermo Fischer Scientific, Waltham, MA, USA), and adjusted to 100 µg/mL. Samples were left protected of light at 4 °C until analysis. LDL and HDL purity was routinely analyzed by electrophoresis in agarose gels (SAS-MX Lipo 10 kit, Helena Biosciences, Gateshead, UK).

2.5.2. Conjugated Dienes Assay

Susceptibility of LDL to copper-induced oxidation was assessed by determining the formation of conjugated dienes. Briefly, freshly prepared LDL samples adjusted to 100 µg/mL with PBS 1X were analyzed by incubation with a copper (II) sulfate ($CuSO_4 \cdot 5H_2O$) solution at a final concentration of 5 µM. The change of absorbance was determined during 2.5 h at 37 °C using a SpectraMax 190 Microplate reader (Molecular Devices, Philadelphia, PA, USA) by continuously monitoring the formation of conjugated dienes, a product of lipid peroxidation with absorbance peak at 234 nm. The total amount of conjugated dienes was calculated as previously described [23].

2.5.3. HDL Antioxidant Potential

The antioxidant potential of HDL was assessed by performing the total radical-trapping antioxidative potential (TRAP) test [24], a method based on the capability of HDL to prevent LDL oxidation. Briefly, HDL and LDL lipoproteins were diluted in PBS 1X to a final concentration of 100 µg protein/mL. LDL derived from the control plasma pool were incubated with $CuSO_4 \cdot 5H_2O$ (final concentration of 20 µM) in the absence/presence of HDL from each individual subject for 4 h (37 °C). Afterward, oxidation was stopped with 1 mM EDTA and samples incubated with 10 µM DCFH-DA (2′,7′-dichlorodihydrofluorescein diacetate) for detection of the oxidation level [25]. Intensity of fluorescence was determined with a Typhoon FLA9500 (GE Healthcare, Chicago, IL, USA) set at $\lambda ex = 500$ nm and $\lambda em = 520$ nm. Final fluorescence measurements were expressed as the percentage of oxidized LDL generated in the presence of HDL relative to the oxidation level when LDLs were incubated in the absence of HDL.

2.6. HDL Cholesterol Efflux Capacity Assay

The cholesterol efflux capacity of HDL was determined in cholesterol-loaded murine macrophages as previously reported [26,27]. To this end, J774A.1 mouse macrophages were cultured in RPMI 1640 (Roswell Park Memorial Institute medium) containing 10% of heat-inactivated FBS (Fetal bovine serum), 2 mM glutamine, 100 U/mL penicillin, 100 U/mL streptomycin and 10 µg/mL gentamicin at 37 °C in a humidified atmosphere of 5% CO_2.

For the experiments, macrophages (1.5×10^5 cells/well seeded in 6-well culture plates) were labeled for 48 h with [$1\alpha, 2\alpha$ (n)$^{-3}$H cholesterol] (GE Healthcare, Chicago, IL, USA) at 1 µCi per well. Cells were equilibrated overnight in 0.2% bovine serum albumin (BSA) and thereafter incubated with RPMI media containing 5% apoB-depleted serum (4 h, 37 °C) to promote cholesterol efflux from the [^{3}H] cholesterol-labeled cells. Radioactivity signal was quantified in both media and cells and the percentages of cholesterol efflux calculated by expressing the radioactive cholesterol released to the medium as the fraction (%) of the total radioactive cholesterol present in the well (radioactivity in the cell + radioactivity in medium).

2.7. Vascular Endothelial Function and Arterial Stiffness

Endothelial function and arterial stiffness were assessed by digital plethysmography using the EndoPAT2000-device (Itamar Medical Ltd., Caesarea, Israel). Measurements were performed according to the manufacturer's instructions in subjects resting in supine position and both hands on the same level in a comfortable, thermoneutral environment, with a temperature of 21–24 °C. Arterial systolic and diastolic blood pressure and heart rate frequency were measured before starting the test. Pneumatic probes were placed on each index finger and a blood pressure cuff on one arm (study arm), while the contralateral arm served as a control (control arm). After a 10-min equilibration period, the blood pressure cuff on the study arm was inflated to 60 mmHg above systolic pressure for 5 min. The cuff was then deflated to induce reactive hyperemia (RH), whereas the signals from both PAT channels (Probe 1 and Probe 2) were recorded by a computer.

The recording was initiated after 25 min of rest. After 5 min baseline recording, the blood pressure cuff was inflated to 60 mmHg above systolic blood pressure and no less than 200 mmHg. Occlusion was confirmed by visual confirmation of complete attenuation of the PAT signal from the test arm. After 5 min occlusion, the cuff was deflated, and the recording continued for 5 min during the reactive hyperemia phase. Recordings from the non-occluded arm served as an internal control correcting for systemic changes in vascular tone. Endothelial function and arterial stiffness were calculated using the EndoPAT software package version 3.4.4. Endothelial function was given as the reactive hyperemia index (RHI) and the arterial stiffness as the augmentation index (AI) and AI standardized to a pulse of 75/min (AI@75) [28].

2.8. Inflammatory Markers

Plasma levels of CRP (C-reactive protein), TNF-α (Tumour Necrosis Factor-alpha), and IL-6 (Interleukin-6) were measured by an Enzyme-Linked ImmunoSorbent Assay (ELISA): High sensitivity CRP and TNF-α (Quantikine HS ELISA, R&D Systems, Minneapolis, MN, USA), IL-6: (AssayMax, AssaPro, St. Lake Charles, LA, USA). All assays were performed according to the manufacturer instructions.

2.9. Statistical Analysis

Statistical analyses were conducted using StatView 5.0.1 software (SAS Institute, Cary, NC, USA) and SPSS software (IBM SPSS Statistics 25.0.0, New York, NY, USA) except when indicated. Data are expressed by the number of cases (qualitative variable) and as mean ± SEM or median [IQR] for the quantitative variable. For all analyzed variables, values at the end of the run-in and the wash-out period were considered as the baseline value for the following intervention period. Differences in the baseline characteristics of the groups and in the percentage of change between intervention-diets were analyzed by unpaired Student's *t*-test for parametric variables and chi-square test for non-parametric variables. Effects of the 4-week interventions were evaluated using a paired Student's *t*-test (baseline and post-intervention values) or an analysis of variance (ANOVA) test introducing the different obesity and lipid-related variables as co-variable when required. All reported *p*-values are two-sided, and a *p*-value of 0.05 or less was considered to indicate statistical significance.

3. Results

3.1. Baseline Characteristics of the Study Population and Side Effects of Beer Consumption

Thirty-six subjects (21 men, 15 women) with an average age of 48.3 ± 5.4 years who were initially recruited for the study completed both intervention phases and were included in the final analysis. Table 1 shows the characteristics of study population at baseline, after the run-in period (Phase 1) and after the wash-out period (Phase 2), at the time of starting each intervention period. All subjects included in the study had overweight (BMI values in the range 28.0–29.9 kg/m^2, $N = 18$) or obesity class-1 (BMI values in the range 30.0–35.0 kg/m^2, $N = 18$). BMI was similar between men and women, being mean BMI 30.2 ± 0.4 kg/m^2 in men and 30.6 ± 0.7 kg/m^2 in women (Student's *t*-test, $p = 0.554$).

Table 1. Subject characteristics at baseline for phase 1 and for phase 2, at the time of starting each intervention period ($N = 36$).

	After Run-In Period	After Wash-Out Period	*p*-Value
Anthropometric parameters			
Sex (Men/Women)	21/15	21/15	
Weight (kg)	87.9 ± 2.3	88.2 ± 2.0	0.92
BMI (kg/m^2)	30.5 ± 0.5	30.6 ± 0.5	0.88
Waist circumference (cm)	100.4 ± 1.7	101.5 ± 1.5	0.63
Hemodynamic control			
Systolic blood pressure (mmHg)	127.1 ± 1.8	125.6 ± 1.8	0.57
Diastolic blood pressure (mmHg)	75.8 ± 1.5	75.1 ± 1.3	0.71
Cardiac Frequency (beats/min)	65.3 ± 1.6	64.9 ± 1.4	0.85
Biochemical parameters			
Glucose (mg/dL)	88.5 ± 1.6	89.2 ± 1.7	0.77
Creatinine (mg/dL)	0.77 ± 0.02	0.77 ± 0.02	0.75
Urea (mg/dL)	14.0 ± 0.6	14.8 ± 0.5	0.28
AST (U/L)	16.8 ± 0.7	16.9 ± 0.7	0.85
GGT (U/L)	20.5 ± 1.8	22.5 ± 1.9	0.46
Lipid parameters			
TC (mg/dL)	188.9 ± 4.5	191.4 ± 4.5	0.67
HDLc (mg/dL)	48.3 ± 1.7	48.8 ± 1.6	0.82
Non-HDLc (mg/dL)	140.5 ± 4.1	142.6 ± 4.3	0.71
LDLc (mg/dL)	124.1 ± 3.8	125.4 ± 3.9	0.80
VLDLc (mg/dL	16.4 ± 1.0	16.9 ± 1.0	0.58
TGL (mg/dL)	81.5 ± 4.8	85.6 ± 5.0	0.58

Baseline values after the four-week run-in and the four-week wash-out periods are expressed as mean $\pm$ SEM. Statistical analysis was performed with a Student's *t*-test for paired samples. Statistical significance: $p < 0.05$. BMI, body mass index; AST, aspartate transaminase; GGT, gamma-glutamyltransferase; TC, total cholesterol; HDLc, high density lipoprotein cholesterol; LDLc, low density lipoprotein cholesterol; VLDLc, very low density lipoprotein cholesterol; TGL, triglycerides.

As shown in Table 2, after a four-week intervention with traditional or alcohol-free beer, anthropometric variables such as body-weight, BMI, and waist circumference, the hemodynamic parameters, plasma levels of hepatic and kidney function, and hemogram profile remain within the normal physiological range. A modest increase (within the normal-range) in glucose and GGT levels was found after four-week intervention with traditional beer ($p < 0.05$).

Table 2. Anthropometric and hemodynamic variables, biochemical parameter and hemogram profile before and after four-week dietary intervention with alcohol-free and traditional and beer.

	Alcohol-Free Beer			Traditional Beer		
	Before Intervention	After Intervention	p-Value	Before Intervention	After Intervention	p-Value
Anthropometric parameters						
Weight (kg)	87.7 ± 2.3	88.1 ± 2.3	0.02	87.7 ± 2.3	88.1 ± 2.3	0.08
BMI (kg/m^2)	30.4 ± 0.5	30.5 ± 0.5	0.01	30.4 ± 0.5	30.4 ± 0.5	0.11
Waist circumference (cm)	99.7 ± 1.9	101.1 ± 1.5	0.11	100.5 ± 1.4	102.1 ± 1.3	0.06
Hemodynamic control						
Systolic blood pressure (mmHg)	125.4 ± 1.9	125.8 ± 1.8	0.76	125.3 ± 2.0	125.7 ± 2.0	0.82
Diastolic blood pressure (mmHg)	75.1 ± 1.6	75.2 ± 1.5	0.93	75.9 ± 1.5	74.9 ± 1.4	0.36
Cardiac Frequency (beats/min)	65.4 ± 1.7	63.9 ± 1.7	0.25	64.8 ± 1.5	66.0 ± 1.8	0.25
Biochemical parameters						
Glucose (mg/dL)	88.0 ± 1.6	88.8 ± 1.7	0.43	88.2 ± 2.0	90.1 ± 1.7	0.04
Creatinine (mg/dL)	0.76 ± 0.02	0.78 ± 0.13	0.03	0.78 ± 0.02	0.78 ± 0.02	0.84
Urea (mg/dL)	14.9 ± 0.6	15.0 ± 0.5	0.75	14.9 ± 0.6	15.6 ± 0.6	0.21
AST (U/L)	16.6 ± 0.7	16.3 ± 0.6	0.49	16.6 ± 0.6	17.2 ± 0.7	0.14
GGT (U/L)	21.5 ± 2.0	21.7 ± 1.9	0.82	20.6 ± 1.9	23.8 ± 2.0	0.00
Hemogram						
RBC (10^6 mm)	4.3 ± 0.1	4.3 ± 0.1	0.09	4.4 ± 0.1	4.3 ± 0.1	0.14
HCT (%)	36.7 ± 0.6	36.2 ± 0.6	0.14	37.2 ± 0.7	36.5 ± 0.5	0.21
PLT (10^3 mm^3)	198.9 ± 5.5	204.1 ± 6.7	0.17	200.9 ± 6.4	205.4 ± 6.2	0.26
MPV (Um^3)	8.4 ± 0.1	8.4 ± 0.1	0.74	8.4 ± 0.1	8.4 ± 0.1	0.41
WBC (10^3 mm^3)	5.8 ± 0.2	5.9 ± 0.2	0.27	5.9 ± 0.2	6.1 ± 0.2	0.36

Values before and after the four-week intervention period with alcohol-free and traditional beer expressed as mean ± SEM. Statistical analysis was performed with the Student's t-test for paired samples. Statistical significance: $p < 0.05$. RBC, red blood cells; HCT, hematocrit; PLT, platelet; MPV, mean platelet volume; WBC, white blood cells.

Similar results were found when women and men (42% and 58% respectively of the study population) were analyzed separately. Therefore, despite small differences were detected relative to baseline for cardiac frequency, aspartate transaminase (AST) levels, creatinine levels and estimated glomerular filtration, all changes remained within the normal physiological range in the men-subgroup (Supplementary Table S2). Changes relative to baseline induced by intervention with traditional or alcohol-free beer did not differ in the woman-subgroup (Supplementary Table S3). The fact that the changes were within normal range indicate that there was no toxicity associated to beer uptake in a highly compliant group.

3.2. Effects of Beer Consumption on Weight Indexes

Neither traditional nor alcohol-free beer induced any weight gain in the study population.

Table 3 shows evolution of weight, BMI, and waist circumference for men and women during the study period (12-week).

Table 3. Evolution of weight, BMI and waist circumference for men and women during the study period.

	Beer Intervention				*p*-Value
	Week-0	Week-4	Week-8	Week-12	
Men (N = 21)					
Weight (kg)	94.6 ± 2.5 [89.4–99.8]	94.9 ± 2.6 [89.6–100.3]	94.3 ± 2.4 [89.2–99.4]	94.8 ± 2.5 [89.6–100.1]	0.99
BMI (kg/m^2)	30.2 ± 0.5 [29.1–31.3]	30.4 ± 0.5 [29.3–31.5]	30.5 ± 0.5 [29.3–31.6]	30.4 ± 0.5 [29.3–31.5]	0.99
Waist-circumference (cm)	103.3 ± 2.2 [98.7–108.0]	103.7 ± 1.9 [99.8–107.6]	102.4 ± 1.6 [99.2–105.7]	103.9 ± 1.5 [100.8–107.1]	0.88
Women (N = 15)					
Weight (kg)	78.6 ± 2.2 [72.5–84.6]	78.8 ± 3.0 [72.5–85.1]	77.9 ± 3.1 [71.3–84.5]	78.4 ± 3.0 [71.9–84.9]	0.99
BMI (kg/m^2)	30.8 ± 0.9 [28.8–32.7]	30.8 ± 0.9 [28.8–32.8]	30.5 ± 1.0 [28.4–32.6]	30.6 ± 1.0 [28.6–32.7]	0.44
Waist-circumference (cm)	96.3 ± 2.5 [91.0–101.7]	98.4 ± 2.3 [93.5–103.3]	97.4 ± 2.5 [92.1–102.7]	98.3 ± 1.9 [94.2–102.4]	0.94

Values are given as mean ± SEM [95% confidence interval]; *p*-values obtained by analysis of variance (ANOVA) for 1 factor. Statistical significance: $p < 0.05$. The time-interval between week-4 and week-8 refers to the wash-out period. Beer intervention includes traditional and alcohol-free beer intake. BMI, body mass index.

3.3. Effect of Beer Consumption on Lipid Profile and Lipoprotein Functionality

3.3.1. Lipid Profile

Mean serum lipid concentration at baseline and after of each intervention period are presented in Table 4. Mean serum concentrations of TC, non-HDLc, LDLc, HDLc, VLDLc and TG did not show any significant change after intervention with traditional beer or alcohol-free beer, when the total population was considered. Interestingly, levels of HDLc and TC were significantly increased after intervention with traditional beer in the subgroup of subjects with LDLc levels < 130 mg/dL (moderate CVD risk), whereas this effect was not found in subjects with LDLc > 130 mg/dL (Table 5).

Table 4. Serum lipid levels before and after four-week dietary intervention with alcohol-free and traditional beer.

	Alcohol-Free Beer			Traditional Beer		
	Before Intervention	After Intervention	*p*-Value	Before Intervention	After Intervention	*p*-Value
TC (mg/dL)	189.3 ± 4.5	191.0 ± 4.7	0.63	189.9 ± 5.0	193.1 ± 4.5	0.33
HDLc (mg/dL)	47.7 ± 1.6	48.0 ± 1.7	0.69	48.2 ± 1.6	48.8 ± 1.5	0.41
Non-HDLc (mg/dL)	141.6 ± 4.0	143.0 ± 4.4	0.65	141.7 ± 4.5	144.2 ± 4.4	0.39
LDLc (mg/dL)	124.8 ± 3.8	125.6 ± 4.0	0.78	125.7 ± 4.3	126.1 ± 3.9	0.88
VLDLc (mg/dL)	16.8 ± 1.1	17.4 ± 1.2	0.43	16.0 ± 0.9	18.1 ± 1.4	0.06
TG (mg/dL)	83.5 ± 5.5	86.4 ± 6.0	0.43	79.5 ± 4.4	90.1 ± 6.9	0.06

Lipid data (mg/dL) are given as mean ± SEM. Differences for values before and after four-week intervention with alcohol-free and traditional beer were analyzed by paired Student's *t*-test. Statistical significance: $p < 0.05$. TC, total cholesterol; HDL, high density lipoproteins; LDL, low density lipoproteins; TG, triglycerides; VLDL, very-low density lipoproteins.

Table 5. Serum lipid levels before and after four-week dietary intervention with alcohol-free and traditional beer in subjects with LDLc at baseline below and above 130 mg/dL.

	Alcohol-Free Beer Intervention				Traditional Beer Intervention			
	Before	After	Δ	p-Value	Before	After	Δ	p-Value
Serum lipids-subjects with LDL < 130 mg/dL								
CT (mg/dL)	170.5 ± 3.5	176.5 ± 4.0	+6.0	0.14	170.6 ± 2.5	179.1 ± 3.8	+8.6	**0.04**
HDLc (mg/dL)	46.3 ± 2.2	47.0 ± 2.2	+0.7	0.34	46.6 ± 1.7	48.8 ± 1.7	+2.2	**0.01**
Non-HDLc (mg/dL)	124.2 ± 3.1	129.5 ± 4.3	+5.2	0.17	124.9 ± 2.6	130.5 ± 3.7	+5.6	0.12
LDLc (mg/dL)	108.8 ± 2.9	112.4 ± 3.5	+3.6	0.35	109.9 ± 2.2	114.2 ± 3.4	+4.3	0.18
VLDLc (mg/dL)	15.4 ± 1.4	17.1 ± 1.6	+1.6	0.08	15.0 ± 1.1	16.3 ± 1.3	+1.3	0.13
TG (mg/dL)	76.8 ± 6.8	84.9 ± 8.1	+8.2	0.08	74.7 ± 5.3	81.2 ± 6.7	+6.6	0.13
Serum lipids-subjects with LDL > 130 mg/dL								
CT (mg/dL)	215.6 ± 3.7	211.3 ± 6.9	-4.3	0.49	226.1 ± 5.5	221.4 ± 4.6	-4.7	0.22
HDLc (mg/dL)	49.7 ± 2.5	49.3 ± 2.6	-0.3	0.82	50.9 ± 3.5	49.7 ± 3.0	-1.1	0.46
Non-HDLc (mg/dL)	165.9 ± 2.6	161.9 ± 5.7	-4.0	0.43	175.2 ± 3.9	171.6 ± 4.8	-3.5	0.52
LDLc (mg/dL)	147.2 ± 2.5	144.1 ± 5.3	-3.1	0.51	157.2 ± 4.8	149.9 ± 4.7	-7.3	0.16
VLDLc (mg/dL)	18.7 ± 1.7	17.8 ± 1.9	-0.9	0.45	17.9 ± 1.5	21.7 ± 3.0	+3.7	0.22
TG (mg/dL)	92.9 ± 8.7	88.4 ± 9.3	-4.5	0.45	89.2 ± 7.6	107.8 ± 14.9	+18.6	0.22

Serum lipid values for subjects with moderate CVD risk (LDL < 130 mg/dL) and high (LDL > 130 mg/dL) are given as mean ± SEM. Differences for values before and after four-week intervention with alcohol-free and traditional beer were analyzed by paired Student's t-test. Δ Percentage of change in plasma lipids levels after four-week intervention with alcohol-free and traditional beer. $p \leq 0.05$ indicates statistical significance. TC, total cholesterol; HDL, high density lipoproteins; LDL, low density lipoproteins; TG, triglycerides; VLDL, very-low density lipoproteins.

3.3.2. LDL Susceptibility to Oxidation

The susceptibility of LDL to oxidation was assessed by the maximal amount of generated conjugated dienes (Dmax) and the maximum velocity of dienes production (Vmax), during in vitro incubation of purified LDL with cupric ions. Susceptibility of LDL to oxidation (Dmax and Vmax) did not relate to the baseline BMI, and did not differ significantly between men and women (data not shown).

Sixty-one percent of the participants (52% of men and 73% of women) showed lower susceptibility of LDLs to oxidation after four-week intervention with traditional beer as compared to control baseline LDLs, while around 42% of participants (43% of men and 40% of women) showed less susceptibility of LDLs to oxidation after alcohol-free beer intake ($p = 0.007$ for the difference in the response to both interventions by the X^2-test). Compared to baseline, mean level of Dmax was slightly lower (-8.0 ± 4.8 Dmax/mg LDL-protein) after intervention with traditional beer ($p = 0.052$; Figure 2A) and a similar trend was found for the kinetic of conjugated dienes (CD) generation (Decrease in Vmax: $p = 0.075$; Figure 2B), but changes were non-significant.

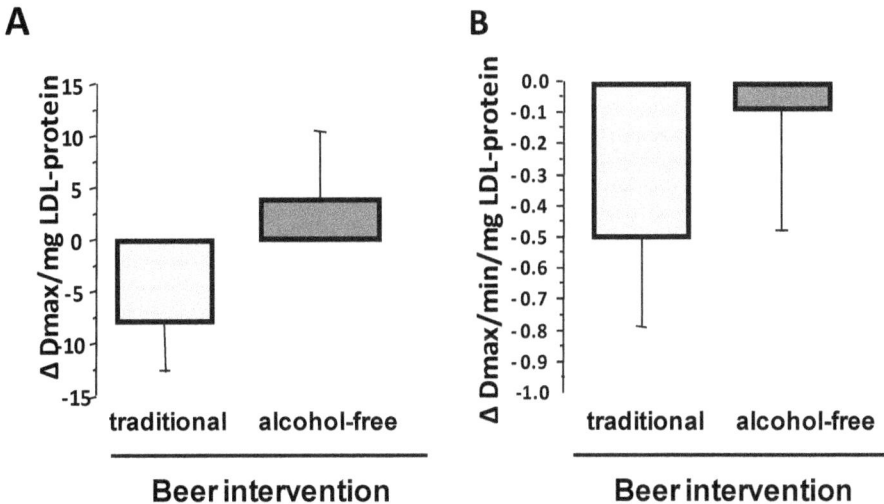

Figure 2. Effect of four-week intervention with alcohol-free and traditional beer on the susceptibility of plasma LDL to be oxidized. Values are given as change verses baseline for (**A**) maximal value for generated conjugate dienes, and (**B**) Vmax that conjugate dienes are generated. Bars refer to mean values and lines to standard error of the mean (SEM).

3.3.3. HDL Antioxidant Capacity

Susceptibility of LDL to oxidation (Dmax) in the presence of HDL was decreased to $47.3 \pm 1.8\%$ of the value obtained in the absence of high-density lipoproteins ($p < 0.001$). This value was unrelated to sex (men: $47.4 \pm 2.1\%$; women $47.3 \pm 3.51\%$). After four-week intake of both types of beer, HDL exhibited higher antioxidant effects than control baseline HDL ($p < 0.001$, Figure 3A). These beneficial effects on HDL of beer (5–40% decrease in LDL oxidation compared to the effect induced by HDL obtained at baseline) was found in 87% of the subjects after intervention with traditional beer and 80% after intake of alcohol-free beer (Figure 3B). This effect did not relate to sex (men: Traditional-beer, $-17.2 \pm 2.2\%$; alcohol-free beer: $-15.7 \pm 1.8\%$); women: Traditional-beer: $-13.8 \pm 3.0\%$; alcohol-free beer: $-11.3 \pm 4.2\%$).

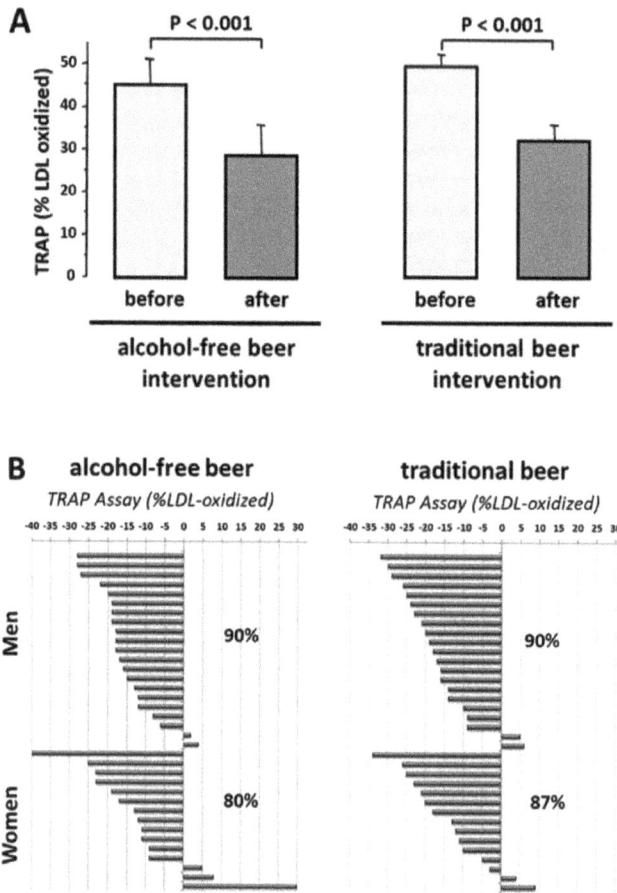

Figure 3. Effect of moderate beer consumption on HDL antioxidant capacity in subjects with overweight or obesity class-1. (**A**) Results are expressed as % of oxidized LDL referred to the value obtained in the absence of HDL. (**B**) Functional response of HDL to oxidative stress at individual level.

3.3.4. Effect of Beer Intake on HDL Cholesterol Efflux Capacity

After intervention with traditional beer, there was a statistically significant increase in the capacity of apoB-depleted serum to induce cholesterol efflux from macrophages in vitro ($p = 0.002$; Table 6). Intervention with alcohol-free beer did not induce any statistically significant change on cholesterol efflux mediated by the apoB-depleted serum.

Table 6. Effect of the intervention with alcohol-free and traditional beer on the cholesterol efflux induced by apoB-depleted serum in macrophages.

Cholesterol Efflux (%)	Alcohol-Free Beer			Traditional Beer		
	Before Intervention	After Intervention	*p*-Value	Before Intervention	After Intervention	*p*-Value
Total population (N = 36)	16.4 ± 0.4	16.6 ± 0.4	0.16	16.6 ± 0.4	17.2 ± 0.4	**0.02**
Men (N = 21)	16.9 ± 0.4	17.1 ± 0.5	0.47	16.9 ± 0.5	17.6 ± 0.5	0.09
Women (N = 15)	15.6 ± 0.7	16.0 ± 0.6	0.21	16.4 ± 0.7	16.8 ± 0.7	0.45

Cholesterol efflux values expressed as percentage and given as the mean ± SEM; *p*-values were analyzed by a Student's *t*-test for paired samples.

3.4. Plasma Inflammatory Markers and Beer Intervention

Regular intake of traditional or alcohol-free beer did not induce any increase in systemic inflammatory markers such as CRP, IL6, TNF alpha (Table 7).

Table 7. Effect of the intervention with alcohol-free and traditional beer on inflammatory markers.

Inflammatory Markers	Alcohol-Free Beer			Traditional Beer		
	Before Intervention	After Intervention	*p*-Value	Before Intervention	After Intervention	*p*-Value
PCR (ng/mL)	3.4 ± 0.6	4.1 ± 0.8	0.06	4.8 ± 1.2	4.4 ± 0.7	0.63
TNFα (ng/mL)	83.1 ± 0.96	2.0 ± 0.1	0.25	1.8 ± 0.1	2.0 ± 0.2	0.06
IL-6 (ng/mL)	0.03 ± 0.00	0.03 ± 0.01	0.20	0.03 ± 0.01	0.04 ± 0.01	0.58

Values of the inflammatory markers expressed in ng/mL and given as the mean ± SEM; *p*-values were obtained by Student's *t*-test for paired samples. CRP, C-reactive protein; TNF-α, tumor necrosis factor alpha; IL-6, interleukin-6.

3.5. Vascular Endothelial Function and Arterial Stiffness before and after Intervention

Mean value of vascular reactivity measured by the pulse amplitude response to hyperemia (response hyperemia index; RHI), in subjects with overweight or obesity was 1.69 ± 0.43. This value indicates normal endothelial function, because RHI values below 1.67 are categorized as endothelial dysfunction, whereas higher RHI values are considered normal function.

Four-week intervention with traditional or alcohol-free beer did not induce any statistically significant effect on the RHI level compared with baseline when the total study population was considered (before vs. after intervention: 1.71 ± 0.05 vs. 1.75 ± 0.07 and 1.67 ± 0.05 vs. 1.64 ± 0.05, for traditional and alcohol–free beer, respectively). Interestingly, 24 subjects that showed endothelial dysfunction at entry (baseline RHI values: 1.38 ± 0.03) had a statistically significant improvement in endothelial function after non-alcoholic beer intake, while those with values within the normal RHI range at entry (2.02 ± 0.11, N = 12) did not (RHI change: +0.092 ± 0.04 vs. −0.381 ± 0.11, *p* = 0.001). Similar trend was found after intervention with traditional beer, although differences did not achieve statistical significance (change in RHI group < 1.67 vs. RHI-group > 1.67: +0.137 ± 0.07 vs. −0.075 ± 0.13, *p* = 0.113). Indeed, changes in RHI value after beer intervention negatively correlated with RHI values at baseline (*r* = −0.567, *p* < 0.001). Therefore, beer intake did not induce any impairment in endothelial vascular reactivity and function.

The augmentation index (AI) was calculated based on the EndoPAT data and is considered a marker for the arterial stiffness. AI standardized to a pulse of 75/min (AI@75) gave baseline values of −5.61 ± 1.81 in men and +13.46 ± 3.62 in women (*p* < 0.001). Four-week intervention with traditional beer or with non-alcoholic beer did not lead to impairment in AI@75 values (traditional beer: +2.26 ± 1.43 verses baseline, *p* = 0.229; non-alcoholic beer: −1.23 ± 1.00 verses baseline, *p* = 0.123). Beer intake did not induce arterial stiffness.

3.6. Beer Consumption and Cardiovascular Risk Score

The risk of CVD in the study population was calculated on basis to the Framingham risk score (FRS), which gave a mean value of 7.8 ± 0.5, being the risk 8.7 ± 1.1 in women and 7.3 ± 0.5 in men. As shown in Table 8, the FRS was not increased after daily intake of alcohol-free or traditional beer during a total eight-week period. These values refer to a 10-year CV-risk of 3% in men and <1% in women at baseline. These percentages did not change after regular consumption of alcohol-free or traditional beer during four-week periods.

Table 8. Effect of beer consumption on the Framingham Risk Score (FRS).

	Alcohol-Free Beer				Traditional Beer			
	Before	After	10-Year Risk	*p*-Value	Before	After	10-Year Risk	*p*-Value
Total population (*N* = 36)	7.9 ± 0.5	7.8 ± 0.5	<1%	0.50	7.9 ± 0.5	7.8 ± 0.5	<1%	0.50
Men (N = 21)	7.3 ± 0.5	7.2 ± 0.5	3%	0.54	7.3 ± 0.5	7.2 ± 0.5	3%	0.54
Women (N = 15)	8.7 ± 1.1	8.7 ± 1.1	<1%	0.75	8.7 ± 1.1	8.7 ± 1.1	<1%	0.75

The Framingham score was calculated according to the guidelines provided in the Framingham Heart Study of NHLBI (National Heart, Lung & Blood Institute & Boston University) [29]. Values are expressed as mean ± SEM was analyzed by Student's *t*-test for paired samples.

4. Discussion

Although excessive alcohol consumption is unquestionably a health hazard, there is substantial evidence based on epidemiological and observational studies suggesting that a light-to-moderate regular alcohol intake has a protective effect in overall mortality, mainly from coronary artery disease [30]. This evidence is supported by data derived from experimental animal studies and prospective clinical trials suggesting that alcoholic beverages may exert different protective effects against atherosclerosis development either by modulating lipid metabolism, platelet activity, inflammation, and thrombogenic factors [31,32]. Despite the results of these studies, findings up to now are inconclusive. The balance between risks and benefits of moderate alcohol consumption in health is still under discussion [33,34]. Alcohol is the main active component in alcoholic beverages and as such considered as the causal factor in both beneficial and toxic effects. However, nowadays particular interest focuses on fermented alcoholic beverages such as wine or beer. In this respect, epidemiological evidence [17] and results from prospective clinical trials [5] suggests that these beverages with heterogenous content of non-alcoholic components might confer better cardiovascular protection than spirits.

In this study we performed a randomized, cross-over, prospective study to investigate benefits and risks of moderate intake of beer in low cardiovascular risk individuals with overweight or obesity class1 (BMI 27–35 kg/m^2). More specifically, effects related to changes in weight, on lipoprotein atheroprotective effects, and vascular endothelial function, were investigated. Our results provide consistent evidence that regular consumption of alcohol-free beer or traditional beer in moderate quantities (two cans a day for men and one can a day for women) over two periods of four weeks did not modify or only induced minimal changes within clinical normality range in plasma biomarkers of liver and kidney function, whereas significantly promoted atheroprotective properties of HDL, such as prevention of LDL oxidation and induction of cholesterol efflux from macrophages, considered a first step in the reverse cholesterol transport [35]. Supporting the findings of our study, Romeo et al. did not report any change regarding hepatic enzymes in younger healthy men and women of lesser BMI (24–25 kg/m^2) after a four-week alcohol abstinence and a four-week moderate consumption of a Pils-style beer [36].

One of the most important questions regarding moderate beer consumption is whether it induces an increase in body weight and waist circumference, since these anthropometric parameters are associated to the increase in cardiovascular risk [37] atherosclerosis [38] and also mortality [39,40].

Here, the moderate consumption of traditional or non-alcoholic beer for a total of eight weeks did not induce significant changes in body weight, BMI or waist circumference in our study population of overweight/obese, but otherwise healthy subjects. Interestingly, Chiva-Blanch et al. reported that regular intake of traditional or non-alcoholic beer did not alter the weight, BMI, or waist-hip ratio in men at high cardiovascular risk, because of previous clinical evidence of disease or presence of CVD risk factors [5].

Excessive alcohol intake has been associated with hypertension and atrial fibrillation [41]. In our study, moderate beer intake during 4 + 4 week-periods did not affect blood pressure or heart-rate. Moreover, moderate intake of regular beer did not modify glucose levels after a four week intervention in our adult population with baseline values below 90 mg/dL, neither affected plasma levels of liver enzymes nor biomarkers for kidney dysfunction beyond the normal range. It is to notice that four-week regular beer intake increased in 15% the plasma GGT levels, although the increase was within the standards considered normal. This finding can be justified due the fact that the alcohol is primordially metabolized by the enzyme alcohol dehydrogenase (ADH) in the hepatocytes [42] and therefore liver is a highly sensitive organ for detecting alcohol-induced changes [43–45].

Thus, the above results provided evidence that regular (daily) but moderate intake of beer during an eight-week intervention study does not induce harmful effects on the hepatic or renal function, neither affects body weight, plasma glucose or blood pressure pattern beyond the normal range in healthy subjects in spite of presenting with overweight or obesity. According to these findings, light-to-moderate beer consumption (women $\approx$ 15 g/day alcohol, men $\approx$ 30 g/day alcohol) does not show any detrimental effects and in contrast it might improve the atheroprotective profile of their HDL. However, further studies in larger and more heterogeneous populations with longer duration of beer consumption periods may be necessary to prove the effects of moderate beer intake on HDL function and their effect on the vessel wall and on CVD prevention.

A key element during atherosclerosis progression is the accumulation of cholesterol within macrophages in the arterial wall and their transformation in foam cells with a more atherogenic phenotype. In this respect, HDL have a relevant atheroprotective role by promoting the reverse cholesterol transport (RCT) from peripheral tissue (i.e., macrophages on the arterial intima) with the subsequent excretion of cholesterol out of the body after transport to the liver [46,47]. HDL has the capacity to remove cholesterol from cells acting as acceptor during the cholesterol efflux, which is the first step of the RCT [35,48]. By using apoB-depleted serum to measure of HDL function [49], we provided evidence that moderate but regular intake of traditional beer favors HDL-induced cholesterol efflux. It had previously been reported that alcohol consumption at the dose of 40 g alcohol/day for 17 to 23 days increased ABCA1-mediated cholesterol efflux [48]. Here, we have seen that the beneficial effect of beer intake on HDL efflux capacity is already evident after a low-moderate alcohol intake (15 g alcohol/day in women and 30 g alcohol/day in men) [50].

Using a preclinical swine model of dyslipidemia, we had shown that the intake of both alcohol and non-alcohol beer reduces the systemic oxidative stress triggered by hypercholesterolemia through a process mediated by HDL [51]. The current study in humans further supports the concept of a functional effect of beer intake, indistinctly of its alcohol content, enhancing the antioxidant capacity of HDL. Epidemiological and observational studies have associated the beneficial effects of alcohol in cardiovascular protection to their effect on plasma HDL cholesterol levels [52,53]. In this regard, results of a recently reported community-based study with more than 70.000 subjects over six years suggest that moderate alcohol consumption associates with less HDL-cholesterol decrease over time [6]. In our study, four-week regular intake of moderate amount of traditional beer only raised HDL levels in subjects with a low LDL-lipid profile (<130 mg/dL). However, the four-week term was already able to improve circulating HDL quality by rendering HDL particles functionally active to prevent LDL from oxidation and facilitate cell-cholesterol efflux.

Impaired endothelial function is the first step in the process of atherosclerosis, usually induced by dyslipidemia, even before the development of the fatty streak [54,55]. In our study there was no impairment in endothelial function due to beer intake in overweight/obese individuals with normal LDL levels. Previous studies have shown that regular beer-intake protects against hypercholesterolemia-induced coronary endothelial dysfunction as we have demonstrated in the hypercholesterolemic swine model [51]. Moreover, a beneficial effect on vascular endothelial function was reported for acute beer intake [56]. Similarly, beneficial acute beer intake effects were reported on arterial function and structure [57,58] in healthy young lean subjects. So far, to our knowledge, there are not data regarding a long-term effect of beer on vascular dysfunction and atherosclerosis related arterial biomarkers, such as flow mediated dilatation (FMD) and augmentation index (AI). Here, assessment of the endothelial function (EndoPAT technique) at baseline and after four-week beer consumption did not induce any change in endothelial vascular reactivity and function. Indeed, the reported beneficial effects of beer on endothelial function after acute beer intake were lost four hours after the intake of the alcoholic beverage [56], suggesting that beer intake may induce beneficial acute short-term changes on the vascular endothelium.

The current study has some limitations that warrant discussion. Although this study is based on a well-characterized cohort of healthy but overweight/obese individuals, it has a small sample size that does not represent a more general population of individuals with metabolic syndrome. Moreover, due to the limited number of women in the study, we cannot exclude that some sex related effects could result from a small but differential response in the peri-menopausal women group (women median [IQR] age: 50 (44–54) years) of our study and might not reflect the effects of beer intake in women in general. However, the longitudinal cross-over design gives strength to the results of the study minimizing inter-individual variability for the effects observed with the traditional and alcohol-free beer. A second aspect is the short duration of the intervention for each type of beer. Although many studies that focus in variables like those analyzed here use these same intervention periods, our results might not reflect the potential risks/benefits of longer-term moderate beer consumption.

5. Conclusions

In summary, moderate intake of beer (traditional and alcohol-free) does not exert vascular detrimental effects nor increases body weight in obese but otherwise healthy individuals during the eight-week intervention study. In contrast, moderate intake of beer was associated with favorable effects on HDL-function increasing its capacity to protect against LDL oxidation and to enhance cholesterol efflux, which may prevent lipid deposition in the vessel wall. The results of the study may merit new studies with longer intervention periods and a larger sample size to further define the long-term balance of benefits/risks of moderate beer intake in cardiovascular health.

Supplementary Materials: The following are available online at http://www.mdpi.com/2072-6643/10/9/1237/s1, Supplementary Table S1: Phenolic composition of the beers used in the study, Supplementary Table S2: Anthropometric and hemodynamic variables, biochemical parameter and hemogram profile before and after four-week dietary intervention with alcohol-free and traditional and beer in men (N = 21), Supplementary Table S3: Anthropometric and hemodynamic variables, biochemical parameter and hemogram profile before and after four-week dietary intervention with alcohol-free and traditional and beer in women (N = 15).

Author Contributions: T.P. designed, conducted, and supervised the research; analyzed data and performed the statistical analysis; and wrote the manuscript. N.M.-G. designed and conducted the research; analyzed data and performed the statistical analysis; and wrote the manuscript. G.V. designed and supervised the research; analyzed data and performed the statistical analysis; and wrote the manuscript. P.C. designed and supervised the research; analyzed data and performed the statistical analysis; and wrote the manuscript. A.D. designed and conducted the research; analyzed data and performed the statistical analysis; and wrote the manuscript. R.M.A. designed the research, supervised the clinical study, and analyzed the data; L.B. designed and supervised the research; analyzed data and performed the statistical analysis; and wrote and revised the manuscript. All authors had primary responsibility for the final content and approved the final version of the manuscript.

Funding: This research was funded by an unrestricted grant of Fundacion Cerveza y Salud, Madrid, Spain and from The European Foundation for Alcohol Research (ERAB) EA1659 (to LB), Rue Washington 40, Brussels. Additional support came from the Spanish Ministry of Economy and Competitiveness of Science [PNS2016-76819-R to L.B and PNS 2015-71653-R to GV.]; Institute of Health Carlos III, ISCIII [FIS PI16/01915 to T.P]; FEDER "Una Manera de Hacer Europa". NMG is recipient of a pre-doctoral grant from the Cardiovascular Program ICCC, AD of a "Beca Manuel de Oya" from Fundacion Cerveza y Salud, and PC was a "bolsista do CNPq-Brasil, Universidade Federal de Santa Maria". We thank FIC-Fundacion Jesús Serra, Barcelona, Spain, for their continuous support.

Acknowledgments: The technical assistance of Montse-Gomez Pardo and the Technical personal of the CIM is gratefully acknowledged.

Conflicts of Interest: The authors declare no conflict of interest.

References

1. Costanzo, S.; Di Castelnuovo, A.; Donati, M.B.; Iacoviello, L.; de Gaetano, G. Alcohol Consumption and Mortality in Patients With Cardiovascular Disease. A Meta-Analysis. *J. Am. Coll. Cardiol.* **2010**, *55*, 1339–1347. [CrossRef] [PubMed]

2. O'Keefe, J.H.; Bybee, K.A.; Lavie, C.J. Alcohol and Cardiovascular Health. The Razor-Sharp Double-Edged Sword. *J. Am. Coll. Cardiol.* **2007**, *50*, 1009–1014. [CrossRef] [PubMed]

3. Goel, S.; Sharma, A.; Garg, A. Effect of Alcohol Consumption on Cardiovascular Health. *Curr. Cardiol. Rep.* **2018**, *20*, 19. [CrossRef] [PubMed]

4. Volcik, K.A.; Ballantyne, C.M.; Fuchs, F.D.; Sharrett, A.R.; Boerwinkle, E. Relationship of Alcohol Consumption and Type of Alcoholic Beverage Consumed With Plasma Lipid Levels: Differences Between Whites and African Americans of the ARIC Study. *Ann. Epidemiol.* **2008**, *18*, 101–107. [CrossRef] [PubMed]

5. Chiva-Blanch, G.; Magraner, E.; Condines, X.; Valderas-Martínez, P.; Roth, I.; Arranz, S.; Casas, R.; Navarro, M.; Hervas, A.; Sisó, A.; et al. Effects of alcohol and polyphenols from beer on atherosclerotic biomarkers in high cardiovascular risk men: A randomized feeding trial. *Nutr. Metab. Cardiovasc. Dis.* **2015**, *25*, 36–45. [CrossRef] [PubMed]

6. Huang, S.; Li, J.; Shearer, G.C.; Lichtenstein, A.H.; Zheng, X.; Wu, Y.; Jin, C.; Wu, S.; Gao, X. Longitudinal study of alcohol consumption and HDL concentrations: A community-based study. *Am. J. Clin. Nutr.* **2017**, *105*, 905–912. [CrossRef] [PubMed]

7. Mukamal, K.J.; Conigrave, K.M.; Mittleman, M.A.; Camargo, C.A.; Stampfer, M.J.; Willett, W.C.; Rimm, E.B. Roles of drinking pattern and type of alchohol consumed in coronary heart disease in men. *N. Engl. J. Med.* **2003**, *348*, 109–118. [CrossRef] [PubMed]

8. Leong, D.P.; Smyth, A.; Teo, K.K.; McKee, M.; Rangarajan, S.; Pais, P.; Liu, L.; Anand, S.S.; Yusuf, S. Patterns of alcohol consumption and myocardial infarction risk: Observations from 52 countries in the INTERHEART case-control study. *Circulation* **2014**, *130*, 390–398. [CrossRef] [PubMed]

9. Stockwell, T.; Zhao, J.; Panwar, S.; Roemer, A.; Naimi, T.; Chikritzhs, T. Do "Moderate" Drinkers Have Reduced Mortality Risk? A Systematic Review and Meta-Analysis of Alcohol Consumption and All-Cause Mortality. *J. Stud. Alcohol Drugs* **2016**, *77*, 185–198. [CrossRef] [PubMed]

10. Naimi, T.S.; Brown, D.W.; Brewer, R.D.; Giles, W.H.; Mensah, G.; Serdula, M.K.; Mokdad, A.H.; Hungerford, D.W.; Lando, J.; Naimi, S.; et al. Cardiovascular risk factors and confounders among nondrinking and moderate-drinking U.S. adults. *Am. J. Prev. Med.* **2005**, *28*, 369–373. [CrossRef] [PubMed]

11. Naimi, T.S.; Xuan, Z.; Brown, D.W.; Saitz, R. Confounding and studies of "moderate" alcohol consumption: The case of drinking frequency and implications for low-risk drinking guidelines. *Addiction* **2013**, *108*, 1534–1543. [CrossRef] [PubMed]

12. Hansel, B.; Thomas, F.; Pannier, B.; Bean, K.; Kontush, A.; Chapman, M.J.; Guize, L.; Bruckert, E. Relationship between alcohol intake, health and social status and cardiovascular risk factors in the urban Paris-Ile-De-France Cohort: Is the cardioprotective action of alcohol a myth. *Eur. J. Clin. Nutr.* **2010**, *64*, 561–568. [CrossRef] [PubMed]

13. Gronbaek, M.; Becker, U.; Johansen, D.; Gottschau, A.; Schnohr, P.; Hein, H.O.; Jensen, G.; Sorensen, T.I.A. Type of alcohol consumed and mortality from all causes, coronary heart disease, and cancer. *Ann. Intern. Med.* **2000**, *133*, 411–419. [CrossRef] [PubMed]

14. Di Castelnuovo, A.; Rotondo, S.; Iacoviello, L.; Donati, M.B.; De Gaetano, G. Meta-analysis of wine and beer consumption in relation to vascular risk. *Circulation* **2002**, *105*, 2836–2844. [CrossRef] [PubMed]

15. Costanzo, S.; Di Castelnuovo, A.; Donati, M.B.; Iacoviello, L.; De Gaetano, G. Wine, beer or spirit drinking in relation to fatal and non-fatal cardiovascular events: A meta-analysis. *Eur. J. Epidemiol.* **2011**, *26*, 833–850. [CrossRef] [PubMed]

16. Arranz, S.; Chiva-Blanch, G.; Valderas-Martínez, P.; Medina-Remón, A.; Lamuela-Raventós, R.M.; Estruch, R. Wine, beer, alcohol and polyphenols on cardiovascular disease and cancer. *Nutrients* **2012**, *4*, 759–781. [CrossRef] [PubMed]

17. De Gaetano, G.; Costanzo, S.; Di Castelnuovo, A.; Badimon, L.; Bejko, D.; Alkerwi, A.; Chiva-Blanch, G.; Estruch, R.; La Vecchia, C.; Panico, S.; et al. Effects of moderate beer consumption on health and disease: A consensus document. *Nutr. Metab. Cardiovasc. Dis.* **2016**, *26*, 443–467. [CrossRef] [PubMed]

18. World Health Organisation. Global Status Report on Alcohol and Health 2014. Available online: http://www.who.int/substance_abuse/publications/global_alcohol_report/en/ (accessed on 2 April 2018).

19. Pi-Sunyer, F.; Becker, D.; Bouchard, C.; Carletom, R.; Colditz, G.; Dietz, W.; Foreyt, J.; Garrison, R.; Grundy, R.; Hansen, B.; et al. Clinical Guidelines on the Identification, Evaluation, and Treatment of Overweight and Obesity in Adults: Executive Summary. *Am. J. Clin. Nutr.* **1998**, *68*, 899–917.

20. Levey, A.S.; Stevens, L.A.; Schmid, C.H.; Zhang, Y.L.; Castro, A.F.; Feldman, H.I.; Kusek, J.W.; Eggers, P.; Van Lente, F.; Greene, T.; et al. A new equation to estimate glomerular filtration rate. *Ann. Intern. Med.* **2009**, *150*, 604–612. [CrossRef] [PubMed]

21. Havel, R.J.; Eder, H.A.; Bradgon, J.H. The distribution and chemical composition of ultracentrifugally separated lipoproteins in human serum. *J. Clin. Investig.* **1955**, *34*, 1345–1353. [CrossRef] [PubMed]

22. De Juan-Franco, E.; Pérez, A.; Ribas, V.; Sánchez-Hernández, J.A.; Blanco-Vaca, F.; Ordóñez-Llanos, J.; Sánchez-Quesada, J.L. Standardization of a method to evaluate the antioxidant capacity of high-density lipoproteins. *Int. J. Biomed. Sci.* **2009**, *5*, 402–410. [PubMed]

23. Esterbauer, H.; Striegl, G. Continuous Monitoring of in Vitro Oxidation of Human Low Density Lipoprotein. *Free Radic. Biol. Med.* **1989**, *6*, 67–75.

24. Valkonen, M.; Kuusi, T. Spectrophotometric assay for total peroxyl radical-trapping antioxidant potential in human serum. *J. Lipid Res.* **1997**, *38*, 823–833. [PubMed]

25. Aldini, G.; Yeum, K.J.; Russell, R.M.; Krinsky, N.I. A method to measure the oxidizability of both the aqueous and lipid compartments of plasma. *Free Radic. Biol. Med.* **2001**, *31*, 1043–1050. [CrossRef]

26. Escolà-Gil, J.C.; Lee-Rueckert, M.; Santos, D.; Cedó, L.; Blanco-Vaca, F.; Julve, J. Quantification of in vitro macrophage cholesterol efflux and in vivo macrophage-specific reverse cholesterol transport. In *Methods in Molecular Biology*; Springer Science + Business Media: New York, NY, USA, 2015; Volume 1339, pp. 211–233, ISBN 978-1-4939-2928-3.

27. Padró, T.; Cubedo, J.; Camino, S.; Béjar, M.T.; Ben-Aicha, S.; Mendieta, G.; Escolà-Gil, J.C.; Escate, R.; Gutiérrez, M.; Casani, L.; et al. Detrimental Effect of Hypercholesterolemia on High-Density Lipoprotein Particle Remodeling in Pigs. *J. Am. Coll. Cardiol.* **2017**, *70*, 165–178. [CrossRef] [PubMed]

28. Riso, P.; Klimis-Zacas, D.; Del Bo', C.; Martini, D.; Campolo, J.; Vendrame, S.; Møller, P.; Loft, S.; De Maria, R.; Porrini, M. Effect of a wild blueberry (*Vaccinium angustifolium*) drink intervention on markers of oxidative stress, inflammation and endothelial function in humans with cardiovascular risk factors. *Eur. J. Nutr.* **2013**, *52*, 949–961. [CrossRef] [PubMed]

29. Hard Coronary Heart Disease (10-Year Risk). Available online: https://www.framinghamheartstudy.org/fhs-risk-functions/hard-coronary-heart-disease-10-year-risk/ (accessed on 30 July 2018).

30. Ronksley, P.E.; Brien, S.E.; Turner, B.J.; Mukamal, K.J.; Ghali, W.A. Association of alcohol consumption with selected cardiovascular disease outcomes: A systematic review and meta-analysis. *BMJ* **2011**, *342*, 479. [CrossRef] [PubMed]

31. Badimon, L.; Vilahur, G.; Padro, T. Nutraceuticals and atherosclerosis: Human trials. *Cardiovasc. Ther.* **2010**, *28*, 202–215. [CrossRef] [PubMed]

32. Vilahur, G.; Casani, L.; Guerra, J.M.; Badimon, L. Intake of fermented beverages protect against acute myocardial injury: Target organ cardiac effects and vasculoprotective effects. *Basic Res. Cardiol.* **2012**, *107*. [CrossRef] [PubMed]

33. Bell, S.; Daskalopoulou, M.; Rapsomaniki, E.; George, J.; Britton, A.; Bobak, M.; Casas, J.P.; Dale, C.E.; Denaxas, S.; Shah, A.D.; et al. Association between clinically recorded alcohol consumption and initial presentation of 12 cardiovascular diseases: Population based cohort study using linked health records. *BMJ* **2017**, *356*. [CrossRef] [PubMed]

34. Wood, A.M.; Kaptoge, S.; Butterworth, A.S.; Willeit, P.; Warnakula, S.; Bolton, T.; Paige, E.; Paul, D.S.; Sweeting, M.; Burgess, S.; et al. Risk thresholds for alcohol consumption: Combined analysis of individual-participant data for 599 912 current drinkers in 83 prospective studies. *Lancet* **2018**, *391*, 1513–1523. [CrossRef]

35. Anastasius, M.; Kockx, M.; Jessup, W.; Sullivan, D.; Rye, K.A.; Kritharides, L. Cholesterol efflux capacity: An introduction for clinicians. *Am. Heart J.* **2016**, *180*, 1–10. [CrossRef] [PubMed]

36. Romeo, J.; González-Gross, M.; Wärnberg, J.; Díaz, L.E.; Marcos, A. Effects of moderate beer consumption on blood lipid profile in healthy Spanish adults. *Nutr. Metab. Cardiovasc. Dis.* **2008**, *18*, 365–372. [CrossRef] [PubMed]

37. Balkau, B.; Deanfield, J.E.; Després, J.-P.; Bassand, J.-P.; Fox, K.A.A.; Smith, S.C.; Barter, P.; Tan, C.-E.; Van Gaal, L.; Wittchen, H.-U.; et al. International Day for the Evaluation of Abdominal Obesity (IDEA): A study of waist circumference, cardiovascular disease, and diabetes mellitus in 168,000 primary care patients in 63 countries. *Circulation* **2007**, *116*, 1942–1951. [CrossRef] [PubMed]

38. Yu, J.-H.; Yim, S.H.; Yu, S.H.; Lee, J.Y.; Kim, J.D.; Seo, M.H.; Jeon, W.S.; Park, S.-E.; Park, C.-Y.; Lee, W.-Y.; et al. The relationship of body composition and coronary artery calcification in apparently healthy Korean adults. *Endocrinol. Metab.* **2013**, *28*, 33–40. [CrossRef] [PubMed]

39. Flegal, K.M.; Kit, B.K.; Orpana, H.; Graubard, B.I. Association of all-cause mortality with overweight and obesity using standard body mass index categories: A systematic review and meta-analysis. *JAMA* **2013**, *309*, 71–82. [CrossRef] [PubMed]

40. Pischon, T.; Boeing, H.; Hoffmann, K.; Bergmann, M.; Schulze, M.B.; Overvad, K.; van der Schouw, Y.T.; Spencer, E.; Moons, K.G.M.; Tjønneland, A.; et al. General and Abdominal Adiposity and Risk of Death in Europe. *N. Engl. J. Med.* **2008**, *359*, 2105–2120. [CrossRef] [PubMed]

41. O'Keefe, J.H.; Bhatti, S.K.; Bajwa, A.; DiNicolantonio, J.J.; Lavie, C.J. Alcohol and cardiovascular health: The dose makes the poison or the remedy. *Mayo Clin. Proc.* **2014**, *89*, 382–393. [CrossRef] [PubMed]

42. Baliunas, D.O.; Taylor, B.J.; Irving, H.; Roerecke, M.; Patra, J.; Mohapatra, S.; Rehm, J. Alcohol as a risk factor for type 2 diabetes: A systematic review and meta-analysis. *Diabetes Care* **2009**, *32*, 2123–2132. [CrossRef] [PubMed]

43. Kim, J.Y.; Lee, D.Y.; Lee, Y.J.; Park, K.J.; Kim, K.H.; Kim, J.W.; Kim, W.-H. Chronic alcohol consumption potentiates the development of diabetes through pancreatic β-cell dysfunction. *World J. Biol. Chem.* **2015**, *6*, 1–15. [CrossRef] [PubMed]

44. Cederbaum, A.I.; Lu, Y.; Wu, D. Role of oxidative stress in alcohol-induced liver injury. *Arch. Toxicol.* **2009**, *83*, 519–548. [CrossRef] [PubMed]

45. Pochareddy, S.; Edenberg, H.J. Chronic Alcohol Exposure Alters Gene Expression in HepG2 Cells. *Alcohol. Clin. Exp. Res.* **2012**, *36*, 1021–1033. [CrossRef] [PubMed]

46. Rader, D.J.; Alexander, E.T.; Weibel, G.L.; Billheimer, J.; Rothblat, G.H. The role of reverse cholesterol transport in animals and humans and relationship to atherosclerosis. *J. Lipid Res.* **2009**, *50*, S189–S194. [CrossRef] [PubMed]

47. Van der Velde, A.E. Reverse cholesterol transport: From classical view to new insights. *World J. Gastroenterol.* **2010**, *16*, 5908–5915. [PubMed]

48. Beulens, J.W.J.; Sierksma, A.; van Tol, A.; Fournier, N.; van Gent, T.; Paul, J.-L.; Hendriks, H.F.J. Moderate alcohol consumption increases cholesterol efflux mediated by ABCA1. *J. Lipid Res.* **2004**, *45*, 1716–1723. [CrossRef] [PubMed]

49. Davidson, W.S.; Heink, A.; Sexmith, H.; Melchior, J.T.; Gordon, S.M.; Kuklenyik, Z.; Woollett, L.; Barr, J.R.; Jones, J.I.; Toth, C.A.; et al. The effects of apolipoprotein B depletion on HDL subspecies composition and function. *J. Lipid Res.* **2016**, *57*, 674–686. [CrossRef] [PubMed]

50. Stockley, C.S. The relationships between alcohol, wine and cardiovascular diseases—A review. *Nutr. Aging* **2016**, *3*, 55–88. [CrossRef]

51. Vilahur, G.; Casani, L.; Mendieta, G.; Lamuela-Raventos, R.M.; Estruch, R.; Badimon, L. Beer elicits vasculoprotective effects through Akt/eNOS activation. *Eur. J. Clin. Investig.* **2014**, *44*, 1177–1188. [CrossRef] [PubMed]

52. Hines, L.M. Moderate alcohol consumption and coronary heart disease: A review. *Postgrad. Med. J.* **2001**, *77*, 747–752. [CrossRef] [PubMed]

53. Estruch, R.; Lamuela-Raventós, R.M. Wine, alcohol, polyphenols and cardiovascular disease. *Nutr. Aging* **2014**, *2*, 101–109.

54. Shaw, J.; Anderson, T. Coronary endothelial dysfunction in non-obstructive coronary artery disease: Risk, pathogenesis, diagnosis and therapy. *Vasc. Med.* **2016**, *21*, 146–155. [CrossRef] [PubMed]

55. Veerasamy, M.; Bagnall, A.; Neely, D.; Allen, J.; Sinclair, H.; Kunadian, V. Endothelial dysfunction and coronary artery disease: A state of the art review. *Cardiol. Rev.* **2015**, *23*, 119–129. [CrossRef] [PubMed]

56. Tousoulis, D.; Ntarladimas, I.; Antoniades, C.; Vasiliadou, C.; Tentolouris, C.; Papageorgiou, N.; Latsios, G.; Stefanadis, C. Acute effects of different alcoholic beverages on vascular endothelium, inflammatory markers and thrombosis fibrinolysis system. *Clin. Nutr.* **2008**, *27*, 594–600. [CrossRef] [PubMed]

57. Karatzi, K.; Rontoyanni, V.G.; Protogerou, A.D.; Georgoulia, A.; Xenos, K.; Chrysou, J.; Sfikakis, P.P.; Sidossis, L.S. Acute effects of beer on endothelial function and hemodynamics: Asingle-blind, crossover study in healthy volunteers. *Nutrition* **2013**, *29*, 1122–1126. [CrossRef] [PubMed]

58. Nishiwaki, M.; Kora, N.; Matsumoto, N. Ingesting a small amount of beer reduces arterial stiffness in healthy humans. *Physiol. Rep.* **2017**, *5*. [CrossRef] [PubMed]

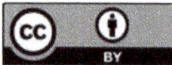

nutrients

MDPI

Article

Dietary Cows' Milk Protein A1 Beta-Casein Increases the Incidence of T1D in NOD Mice

Joanne S. J. Chia [1,†], Jennifer L. McRae [1,†], Ashwantha Kumar Enjapoori [2,†],
Christophe M. Lefèvre [3,4,5], Sonja Kukuljan [6] and Karen M. Dwyer [1,2,7,*]

[1] Immunology Research Centre, St. Vincent's Hospital, Fitzroy, Victoria 3065, Australia;
    joannesj.chia@gmail.com (J.S.J.C.); jennifer.mcrae@svha.org.au (J.L.M.)
[2] Metabolic Research Unit, School of Medicine, Deakin University, Geelong, Victoria 3216, Australia;
    ashwantha.enjapoori@deakin.edu.au
[3] Division of Bioinformatics, The Walter and Eliza Hall Institute of Medical Research,
    Parkville, Victoria 3000, Australia; lefevre.c@wehi.edu.au
[4] Department of Pharmacology and Therapeutics, The University of Melbourne,
    Melbourne, Victoria 3010, Australia
[5] Peter MacCallum Cancer Centre, Melbourne, Victoria 3010, Australia
[6] Freedom Foods Group Ltd., Sydney, New South Wales 2229, Australia; skukuljan@ffgl.com.au
[7] Department of Nephrology, St. Vincent's Health, Melbourne, Victoria 3065, Australia
* Correspondence: Karen.dwyer@deakin.edu.au; Tel.: +61-3-522-714-21
† These authors contributed equally to this work.

Received: 3 August 2018; Accepted: 8 September 2018; Published: 12 September 2018

Abstract: The contribution of cows' milk containing beta-casein protein A1 variant to the development of type 1 diabetes (T1D) has been controversial for decades. Despite epidemiological data demonstrating a relationship between A1 beta-casein consumption and T1D incidence, direct evidence is limited. We demonstrate that early life exposure to A1 beta-casein through the diet can modify progression to diabetes in non-obese diabetic (NOD) mice, with the effect apparent in later generations. Adult NOD mice from the F0 generation and all subsequent generations (F1 to F4) were fed either A1 or A2 beta-casein supplemented diets. Diabetes incidence in F0–F2 generations was similar in both cohorts of mice. However, diabetes incidence doubled in the F3 generation NOD mice fed an A1 beta-casein supplemented diet. In F4 NOD mice, subclinical insulitis and altered glucose handling was evident as early as 10 weeks of age in A1 fed mice only. A significant decrease in the proportion of non-conventional regulatory T cell subset defined as CD4$^+$CD25$^-$FoxP3$^+$ was evident in the F4 generation of A1 fed mice. This feeding intervention study demonstrates that dietary A1 beta-casein may affect glucose homeostasis and T1D progression, although this effect takes generations to manifest.

Keywords: type 1 diabetes; beta-casein; cows' milk; epigenetics; NOD mice

---

1. Introduction

Type 1 diabetes (T1D) results from the autoimmune destruction of insulin-producing beta cells in the pancreatic islets of Langerhans [1–3], culminating in the loss of blood-glucose homeostasis. T1D poses a serious health problem: the inability to regulate blood glucose levels necessitates exogenous insulin for survival; however, suboptimal glycemic control may lead to long-term complications resulting in substantial disability and reduced lifespan [4]. The International Diabetes Federation estimated that there were 437,500 children that have diabetes worldwide in 2007. Of all individuals with T1D, 70,000 young children under the age of 14 years, developing per year and the incidence will rise by 3% globally [5,6]. The data was significant as it comes from a large childhood

T1D registry of 44 centres representing most countries in Europe [6]. T1D is a global disease, although there is geographical variation with respect to incidence and prevalence [7]. The cause of geographical variation could be due to differences in genetic and environmental risk factors [8].

Genetic predisposition, immunological and environmental factors such as dietary factors [9–11], infections [12], viruses [13] and gut microbiota [14,15] are all involved in the initiation, development and progression of T1D [5,7,16]. Studies of T1D genetics have revealed that individuals with specific human leukocyte antigen (HLA) genotypes, HLA DR and HLA DQ genotypes have an increased risk of developing the disease [17,18]. However, not everyone who has this genetic predisposition develops T1D, suggesting that environmental factors are needed to trigger and drive the disease [5,19]. Cows' milk, one of the first foods introduced early to infants, is one such putative environmental factor [20]. Indeed, the identification of T1D-associated autoantibodies as biomarkers of pre-symptomatic disease in the birth cohort study, Diabetes Autoimmunity Study in the Young (DAISY), found that children who have the low to moderate HLA-DR genotype paired with a greater dietary intake of cows' milk protein may be at an increased risk of developing islet autoimmunity and progression to T1D [21]. More recently, results of a randomized trial to reduce insulin dependent diabetes in the genetically at risk (TRIGR type 1 diabetes primary prevention pilot study) reported that cows' milk consumption was associated with increased risk of beta-cell autoimmunity and T1D in children with genetic susceptibility [22].

The World Health Organization (WHO) recommends that infants be exclusively breast fed for six months and breastfeeding should continue beyond the second year to ensure healthy growth and development [23,24]. Beyond weaning, cows' milk is introduced into the diets of infants [25]. Cows' milk itself is introduced into the diet of infants as they age. Beta-casein is one of the major proteins contained in cows' milk and constitutes up to 35% of the total protein in cows' milk [26]. Currently, thirteen beta-casein genetic variants have been identified [27]. The most common are the A1 and A2 genetic variants, the former differing from the latter in one amino acid substitution (Pro_{67} to His_{67}) [28]. The amino acid substitution is associated with physiochemical properties of A1 beta-casein digestion at position 67. During *in-vivo* and *in vitro* digestion, only the A1 variant produces a seven amino acid peptide called beta-casomorphin 7 (BCM-7) [29–31]. The impact of BCM-7 on human disease, in particular T1D, is the subject of intense debate [32–35].

Most compelling is the data analysis by Laugesen and Elliott, which demonstrated a positive correlation ($r = 0.92$) between cows' milk A1 beta-casein supply per-capita and T1D in 19 developed countries [36]. The 19 countries included in the analysis were the USA, Canada, Venezuela, Oceania (Australia and New Zealand), East Asia (Japan) and Middle East (Israel). A higher incidence rate was observed in Finland and Sweden (highest A1 β-casein consumption/per capita) and very low rates have been found in Venezuela and Japan (lowest A1 β-casein consumption/per capita) [36].

The association between beta-casein consumption and T1D has been investigated in rodent models although mechanisms have been difficult to define. Two publications highlighted the relationship between cows' milk consumption and T1D. Firstly, in 1997, Elliot et al. reported that NOD mice fed a 2% casein supplemented diet at weaning developed T1D at a greater rate than NOD mice fed base (Pregestimil powder) diet (14.6% versus 1% at 250 days) [37]. Later, in 1997, Elliot et al. reported that a 28% of female NOD mice fed whole A1 beta-casein developed T1D at 250 days compared with 2% on the Pregestimil diet [38]. Given the controversy surrounding the purported association between A1 beta-casein consumption and T1D, we sought to test whether a diet supplemented with A1 or A2 beta-casein would increase the incidence of T1D in genetically susceptible female NOD mice over generations.

2. Materials and Methods

2.1. Animal Experiments

Newly weaned 3–4 week old male and female NOD/ShiLtJArc mice were obtained from the Animal Recourses Centre, Canning Vale, Western Australia, Australia. Mice were housed in a pathogen-free environment in the Experimental Medical Surgery Unit, St Vincent's Hospital, Melbourne. These mice (designated F0) were immediately separated into two cohorts and fed a nutritionally balanced milk-based diet containing either the A1 or A2 beta-casein component. The diets were prepared by Specialty Feeds (Glen Forrest, Western Australia, 6071) (Table 1), in accordance with strict manufacturing protocols. Feeds were produced every three months and stored under strict temperature controlled environments, in order to ensure that the quality and freshness of the diets was maintained.

Mice were fed ad libitum and had free access to drinking water. Non-fasting blood glucose levels (BGLs) were monitored weekly throughout the 30-week study.

All animal experiments in this study were approved by the St. Vincent's Hospital Animal Ethics Committee (Melbourne, Australia).

Table 1. The nutrient composition of the experimental A1 and A2 beta-casein supplemented diets for mice.

Ingredients (g/100 g)	A1A1 Skim Milk Diet	A2A2 Skim Milk Diet
Sucrose	25.753	25.753
Skim milk powder (as supplement)	60.528	60.529
Instruction	Standard mixing	
COPHA hydrogenated vegetable oil	1.366	1.366
Palm oil	3.709	3.709
Safflower oil (High Linoleic)	0.787	0.787
Flax oil	0.462	0.462
Instructions	Standard mixing	
Cellulose	5.000	5.000
Instructions	Standard mixing	
dl Methionine	0.904	0.904
A1N_93_Trace minerals	0.140	0.140
Salt (Fine sodium chloride)	0.100	0.100
AIN_93_Vitamins	1.000	1.000
Choline chloride 75% w/w	0.250	0.250
Red food colour	0.001	-
Instructions	Standard mixing	
Total	100.000	100.000

2.2. Breeding Program

For breeding further generations, 6–8 week old mice were mated. Brother/sister breeding pairs from the A1- and A2-fed F0 cohort were mated to generate F1 offspring. Similarly, breeding pairs from the F1 generation were mated to produce the F2 generation. Two further generations (i.e., F3 and F4) were produced. This resulted in all offspring from F1 to F4 being exposed to either A1 or A2 beta-casein only from conception.

2.3. Blood Glucose Monitoring and Diabetes Incidence

Weekly BGLs were monitored from 6 to 30 weeks of age. Mice were deemed diabetic if they had a reading of more than 20 mM. Diabetes incidence at any week in time was determined by the formula:

$$\text{Diabetes incidence} = \frac{Number\ of\ mice\ fed\ a\ particular\ beta - casein\ diet\ with\ BGL\ > \ 20\ mM}{Total\ number\ of\ mice\ fed\ a\ particular\ beta - casein\ diet}. \quad (1)$$

2.4. Intraperitoneal Glucose Tolerance Test

Female NOD mice at 10- to 12-weeks old from the F4 generation were made to fast overnight (12–16 h). The mice were injected intraperitoneally with glucose (2 g/kg body weight). BGLs were measured from blood samples collected from the tail at 0, 15, 30, 45, 60, 90, and 120 min.

2.5. Insulin Tolerance Test

Insulin (0.75 IU/kg body weight) was administered intraperitoneally into 10-week old female mice from the F4 generation after a 12-h overnight fast. BGLs were determined from blood samples obtained from the tail at 0, 15, 30, 45, 60, 90, and 120 min after the injection.

2.6. Immune Profiling

Leukocytes were obtained from peripheral lymphoid organs (spleen, thymus, pancreatic and mesenteric lymph nodes) and blood. Red blood cells were cleared using 0.9% ammonium chloride solution. The leukocytes were then washed and spun down and were stained with antibodies for various leukocyte populations. The antibodies used were as follows: Fc block (anti-mouse FcRγIII/II mAb, 2.4G2, BD Biosciences, Franklin Lakes, NJ, USA), CD3-FITC (Clone: 17A2, BD Biosciences), CD4-PeCy5 (Clone: H129.19, BD Biosciences), CD8-APC-Cy7 (Clone: 53-6.7, BD Biosciences), CD19-PeCy7 (Clone: 1D3, BD Biosciences), CD25-APC-Cy7 (Clone: PC61, BD Biosciences), CD45 Pacific Blue (Clone: 30-F11, Biolegend, San Diego, CA, USA), and F4/80-APC (Clone: BM8, Invitrogen, Carlsbad, CA, USA). For intracellular FoxP3 staining, cells were incubated with FcRγIII/II, surface stained for CD4 and CD25, fixed and permeabilised as per manufacturer's instructions (eBioscience, Waltham, MA, USA), and stained for FoxP3 (Clone: FJK-16S, eBioscience). Cells were then analysed using a FACSCanto flow cytometer (BD Biosciences) and Diva software (BD Biosciences). A total of 1×10^6 cells were analysed.

2.7. Treg Suppression Assays

Mouse CD4$^+$CD25$^+$ Treg and CD4$^+$CD25$^-$ Tresp populations were purified using the CD4$^+$CD25$^+$ Regulatory T cell isolation kit (Catalog number: 130-091-041) and AUTOMACS (Miltenyi Biotec Australia, Macquarie Park, NSW, Australia) as per manufacturer's instructions. Tresp were stained with CFSE using the CellTrace™ CFSE Cell Proliferation Kit (Molecular Probes™, Thermo Scientific, Melbourne, VIC, Australia). Accessory cells were irradiated CD4-depleted splenocytes. In each well, a total of 1×10^5 Tresp cells and 1×10^5 accessory cells were incubated with 1 µg/mL anti-CD3 antibody (WEHI) in complete medium (RPMI-1640 containing Glutamax, 1 mM Pen-Strep, 1 mM Na-Pyruvate (Gibco™, Thermo Scientific, Melbourne, VIC, Australia), 10% mouse sera and 50 µM 2-mercaptoethanol (Sigma-Aldrich, Castle Hill, NSW, Australia)). To assess suppressive activity, Treg were co-cultured at Treg: Tresp ratios of 1:1 to 1:16 for 3 days. Following culture, wells were washed and cells were incubated with anti-mouse CD4-APC Ab (Clone: RM4-5, eBiosciences) at room temperature. 7AAD (BD Biosciences) was added to exclude dead cells prior to FACS analysis. CD4$^+$ cells were gated and Tresp proliferation assessed using FlowJo v7.6 Proliferation Platform (Tree Star, Ashland, OR, USA), on a FACSCanto (BD Biosciences).

2.8. Peptide Extraction from Whole Blood, Lymph Tissues and Mass Spectrometry

Whole blood samples from female NOD mice fed on A1 diet (each generation F0–F4; $n = 10$) were collected in vials containing dipeptidyl peptidase -IV inhibitor, immediately aliquoted and stored at $-80\ ^\circ$C until the time of analysis. The peptides were extracted from whole blood using a previously described procedure [39]. Peptide analysis was carried out on a QExactive plus Orbitrap mass spectrometer (Thermo Scientific).

Female NOD mice from F0 generation ($n = 12$) mesenteric and pancreatic lymph nodes were collected in vials and immediately stored at $-80\ ^\circ$C until the time of analysis. In brief, the tissues samples were finely diced using a scalpel and then homogenised on ice in 600 μL of ice-cold lysis buffer (10 mM Tris, pH 7.5; 25 mM KCl; 250 mM sucrose; 1 mM EDTA; 150 mM NaCl; 1 mM PMSF). The samples were left for 30 min and then spun at 12,000× *g* for 15 min at 4 °C to pellet any insoluble material. For peptide recovery, 500 μL of tissue supernatant were mixed with 1 mL of acidic acetonitrile and acetone, containing individual labelled internal standard for each targeted beta-casomorphin peptide (BCM-5, BCM-7, and BCM-9). The mixtures were spun at 12,000× *g* for 15 min at 4 °C and 1200 μL of supernatant from each extract was recovered to a new Lo-bind tube, evaporated to dryness, and reconstituted for HLB Prime solid phase extraction (SPE) clean-up. Peptides recovered from the SPE clean-up were again evaporated to dryness and reconstituted for the final analysis by LC-MS/MS (Sciex 6500 TripleQuad). LC separation was performed on a Water XSelect® HSS T3 2.5 μm column (2.1 × 50 mm). The mass spectrometer was operated in SRM mode, alternating between detection of BCM-5, BCM-7, and BCM-9 transition ions.

2.9. Bacterial DNA Preparation

Faecal samples were collected from F0 generation female NOD mice (A1 diet *n* = 6; A2 diet *n* = 6) and stored at −80 °C immediately after collection until further use. Genomic DNA from faeces was extracted using a QIAamp DNA stool mini kit (Qiagen, Germantown, MD, USA) according to the manufacturer's instructions, with some modifications. Briefly, an aliquot (~100 mg) of each fecal sample was suspended in 1 mL of inhibit EX buffer. Microbial cells were then lysed by mechanical disruption with a TissueLyser II (Qiagen) for 3 min at 30 Hz. After centrifugation, the supernatant was digested with proteinase K and DNA was precipitated with ethanol. DNA was further washed and purified by a QIAamp spin column. DNA was eluted in 0.2 mL of elution buffer ATE. The quality and quantity of the genomic DNA was measured using the NanoDrop assay. DNA concentrations were adjusted to 100 ng/μL for subsequent Metagenome shotgun pyrosequencing.

2.10. High-Throughput Sequence Analysis

Sequencing was performed by Macrogen (Seoul, Korea) using paired-end sequencing with read length 101 nucleotides using TruSeq Nano DNA kit sample library preparation protocol (Part #15041110 Rev. A) on a HiSeq 25000 System (Part #15011190 Rev. V HCS 2.2.70). For each of the six samples from mice fed the A1 and A2 diets, 8 to 12 million reads were obtained. The data was annotated using the Centrifuge software and a mapping threshold of 80 nucleotides minimum match length was apply to filter poor confidence matches [40]. Results were analysed with the R packages Phyloseq [41] and DESeq2 version 1.2.10 [42,43].

2.11. Histological Staining

Intestinal sections from the jejunum, proximal ileum and distal ileum and pancreatic tissues of F4 generation NOD mice were collected. These tissues were fixed in 10% phosphate-buffered formalin overnight at room temperature and embedded in paraffin. Sections (intestinal: 1–2 μm, pancreatic: 4 μm) were stained with hematoxylin and eosin (H&E; Merck, Darmstadt, Germany) using standard techniques. H&E-stained tissue sections were visualized and evaluated under a standard light microscopy using an AxioImager Z1 microscope (Carl Zeiss MicroI-maging, Jena, Germany).

2.12. Statistical Analysis

Results are reported as mean ± standard error of the mean (SEM). Statistical analysis was performed by one-way ANOVA and Student's *t*-test. *p* < 0.05 was considered a statistical significance between groups.

3. Results

3.1. Effect of A1 Beta-Casein Supplemented Diet on Incidence of T1D in NOD Mice

To investigate the potential effects of the A1 and A2 beta-casein on the development of T1D, NOD mice were fed with either diet separately for five generations and monitored for 30 weeks. No difference in diabetes incidence was observed between the two cohorts from F0 to F2 generations (F1: A1 18.4% vs. A2 21.6%; F2: A1 18.2% vs. A2 13.2%). In the F3 generation, at 30 weeks, the diabetes incidence was doubled in the cohort fed A1 beta-casein compared to the A2 cohort (A1: 40% vs. A2: 20.7%) (Figure 1).

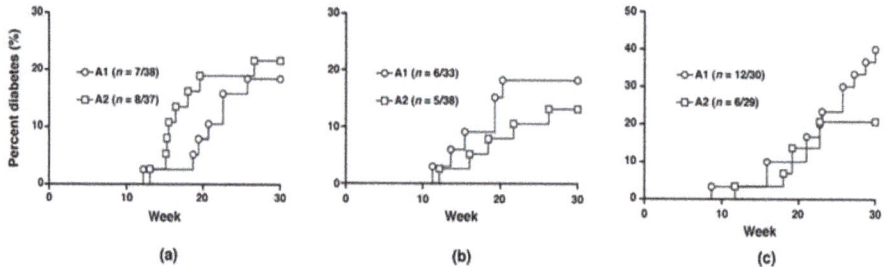

Figure 1. Diabetes incidence in female mice. Diabetes incidence of mice in the (**a**) F1 generation; (**b**) F2 generation; (**c**) F3 generation.

In the F4 generation, the glucose handling capacity was assessed prior to the onset of T1D at 10 weeks of age. Fasting BGLs was significantly higher in NOD mice fed the A1 beta-casein supplemented diet compared with mice fed the A2 beta-casein supplemented diet (A1: 7.0 ± 0.4 mM vs. A2: 5.5 ± 0.5 mM, $p < 0.05$) (Figure 2a). This was associated with lower body weights in the cohort fed an A1 beta-casein supplemented diet (A1: 21.5 ± 0.6 g vs. A2: 23.6 ± 0.3 g, $p < 0.05$) (Figure 2b). NOD mice fed A1 beta-casein had higher 2-h BGLs compared to A2 beta-casein fed mice (A1: 7.9 ± 0.4 mM vs. A2: 5.5 ± 0.4 mM, $p < 0.05$) (Figure 2c). In both cohorts, glycemic response to insulin tolerance testing was preserved (Figure 2d) indicating normal insulin sensitivity. Insulitis was evident in 80% of islets graded in the A1 beta-casein fed mice and among those, 55% were graded as severe with a grade 3 or 4, whereas the majority of islets (~70%) from the A2 beta-casein cohort were free from insulitis (Figure 2e). Together, these data suggest that an A1 beta-casein diet alters glucose handling capacity by promoting islet inflammation.

While human studies report no change in peripheral blood Treg numbers, suppressive capacities are reduced [44–48]. We evaluated splenic CD4$^+$CD25$^+$FoxP3$^+$Treg, CD4$^+$CD25$^-$FoxP3$^+$ Treg, macrophage, CD4$^+$, CD8$^+$ and B cell numbers from NOD mice fed with A1 and A2 beta-casein supplemented diet across the generations. We observed no change in number (Figure 3a) and function (Supplementary Figure S1) of conventional CD4$^+$CD25$^+$FoxP3$^+$Tregs in the F4 generation NOD mice fed with A1 and A2 diets. However, there was a significant decrease in the Treg subset defined by CD4$^+$CD25$^-$FoxP3$^+$ in the A1-fed mice compared to the A2-fed cohort (Figure 3b). The numbers of CD4$^+$, CD8$^+$, B cells and macrophages were unaltered (Figure 3c–f).

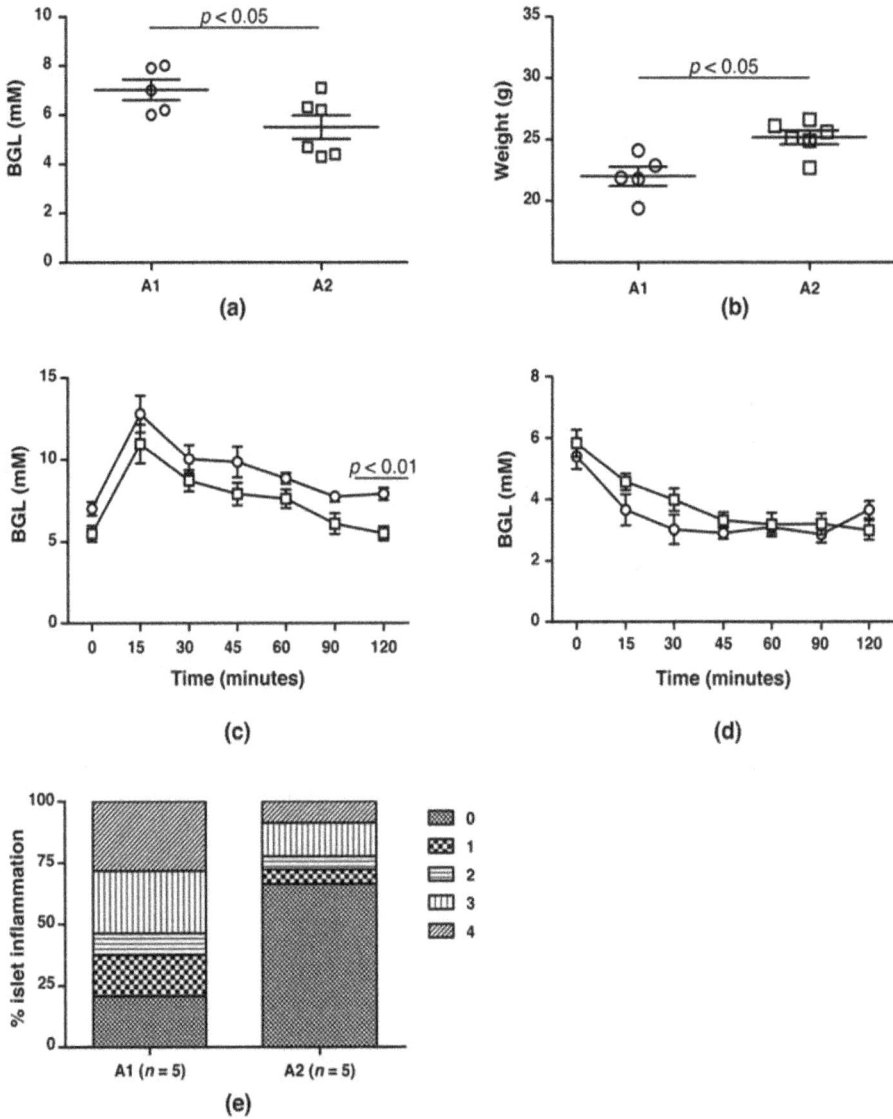

Figure 2. Glucose handling capacity in F4 generation female NOD mice. (**a**) fasting blood glucose levels and (**b**) body weights of 10- to 12-week old A1 (–O–) and A2 (–□–) beta-casein fed female mice. BGLs of female mice assessed in (**c**) glucose and (**d**) insulin tolerance tests. (**e**) distribution of insulitis in islets represented as a percentage of islet infiltration in 10-week old female mice fed either A1 or A2 beta-casein supplemented diets. Islets were scored blindly from individual mice. Islet inflammation was calculated on a scale from 0 to 4. 0—islets devoid of mononuclear cells; 1—minimal (<10%) focal islet infiltrate; 2—peri-islet infiltrate in <25% of islet circumference; 3—peri-islet infiltrate in >25% but <50% intra-islet and 4—>50% intra-islet infiltration.

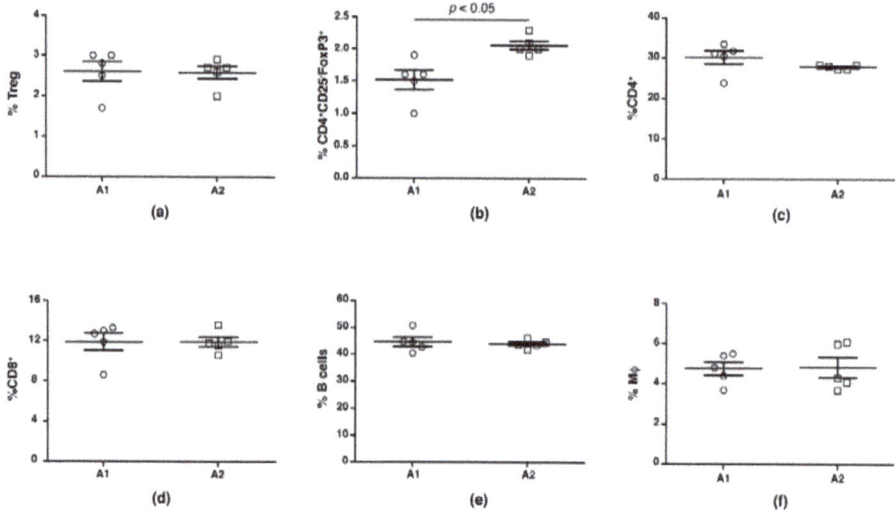

Figure 3. Immune profile in F4 generation mice fed A1 and A2 beta-casein supplemented diets. Splenic leukocytes were obtained and stained with various antibodies. The percentages of the different immune subsets in the spleen were then assessed via flow cytometry. (**a**) conventional Tregs (CD4$^+$CD25$^+$FoxP3$^+$); (**b**) non-conventional Tregs (CD4$^+$CD25$^-$Foxp3$^+$); (**c**) CD4$^+$; (**d**) CD8$^+$; (**e**) B cells; and (**f**) macrophages.

3.2. Isolation and Analysis of Peptides from Whole Blood and Lymph Tissues by Mass Spectrometry

To test for the presence of BCM-7 peptide in the whole blood and lymph tissues of NOD mice, peptides were isolated and analysed by LC-MS/MS and triple-quadrupole mass spectrometry, respectively. No BCM-7 peptide was detected in either sample type (data not shown).

3.3. The Effect of A1 Beta-Casein Supplemented Diet on Intestinal Microbial Communities of Female NOD Mice in the F0 Generation

To test whether A1 beta-casein supplemented diet altered the gut microbiota in mice, we performed metagenome shotgun sequencing on the faecal samples obtained from the F0 generation of female NOD mice fed A1 and A2 supplemented diets for six weeks. There were small differences in bacterial diversity (Supplementary Figure S2), but no significant differences in microbial abundances at the phylum level between the A1 and A2 diet groups. We did find some operational taxonomic units (OTUs) that exhibited a trend towards differential expression. Compared to A2 beta-casein fed NOD mice, A1 beta-casein supplementation increased the level of several bacterial species, some of which have been shown to produce effects on diabetes, including *Streptococcus pyogenes* [49] and *Streptococcus suis.* [50]. In contrast, *Enterobacter cloacae*, *Enterobacter hormaechei* and *Klebsiella oxytoca* at the species level were reduced by A1 beta-casein supplemented diet.

3.4. A1 Beta-Casein Diet Consumption Did Not Alter the Gastrointestinal Integrity in Female NOD Mice in the F4 Generation

In mice, a leaky gut with increased gut permeability, disturbed microbial balance and impaired intestinal mucosal immunity are associated with T1D [51]. The impact of A1 and A2 supplemented diets on the cellularity and architecture of the small intestine in the NOD F4 mice was assessed histologically. Neither an A1 nor A2 supplemented diet impacted the gastrointestinal integrity of the mice (data not shown).

4. Discussion

Despite a number of reports demonstrating a positive correlation between dairy consumption and risk of T1D [36,52,53], conclusive evidence of causation is lacking. This feeding intervention study demonstrates that the consumption of A1 beta-casein in genetically susceptible mice increases the incidence of T1D, which only becomes evident in later generations. We chose to study female NOD mice as these mice have a heightened susceptibility to T1D [54–56] and monitored mice for a number of generations. Later generations showed an increased incidence of T1D, altered glucose handling and associated weight loss and a reduction in a non-conventional Treg cell subset.

The main finding in this study was the doubling of T1D incidence in the F3 generation and presence of subclinical insulitis in 10-week old F4 female NOD mice, suggesting the onset of T1D is influenced by an epigenetic phenomenon [57,58]. It has been reported that diet alone [59] and diet and microbiota mediated epigenetic programming can affect the expression of insulin resistance and insulin signalling genes [60]. In addition to genetic and environmental factors, epigenetic modifications may contribute to the etio-pathogenesis of T1D, necessitating studies with long follow-up durations to capture incidence and enable identification of dietary associations. Indeed, inconsistent findings from some animal studies of A1 beta-casein diet supplementation and T1D associations might be a consequence of the very long latency for T1D development.

We found a reduction in the CD4$^+$CD25$^-$Foxp3$^+$ T cell subset. Although not currently described in the T1D setting, changes in this population have been described in autoimmune systemic lupus erythematosus during active disease [61,62]. Questions as to their role remain, however these 'atypical' Tregs share similar expression profiles with CD4$^+$CD25$^+$FoxP3$^+$ Tregs and display some suppressive capacity [61]. Plasticity in Treg populations subsets has been well described [63] and may contribute to the differences in proportions of CD4$^+$CD25$^+$FoxP3$^+$ and CD4$^+$CD25$^-$FoxP3$^+$ in this study. One study described CD4$^+$CD25$^-$FoxP3$^+$ as a "replenishment pool" that can be recruited and regain their CD25 expression to help combat autoreactive immune cells following disease onset [64]. Thus, the CD4$^+$CD25$^-$FoxP3$^+$ increase observed in the A2-fed NOD mice may represent an effort to regulate autoreactive immune cells. Further investigations are warranted to elucidate the nature of this T cell subset and their role in T1D.

Following A1 beta-casein milk or supplemented diet intake, the BCM-7 peptide has been detected in animal and human biofluids [31,65–67]. BCM-7 was not detected in peripheral blood and mesenteric lymph nodes of NOD mice fed an A1 supplemented diet by mass spectrometry. This may be due to lower than limit-of-detection levels of BCM-7 in the samples, timing of lymph node retrieval or the complex blood peptide samples. We are currently investigating whether BCM-7 has a direct effect on islet development.

Although others have shown changes in gastrointestinal architecture and inflammation after short periods of exposure to A1 beta-casein [68], we did not see such changes, even in the fifth generation of mice. The different rodent strains may account for these disparate findings—where the other studies were performed with male Swiss albino mice [69] and Wistar rats [70], our study utilised NOD mice.

Recently, it was reported that casein supplemented diets modulate the composition of rat gut bacteria [71,72]. The rats fed with casein had a higher abundance of Bacteroidetes at phylum level [72]. At the family level, the composition of bacteria had lowest abundance of *Lactobacillaceae* and highest of *Lachnospiraceae* [72]. The *Lactobacillaceae* members have been proposed to play a key role in host metabolic homeostasis by protecting the gut integrity against pathogens disruption and can reduce inflammation [72]. Intestinal inflammation is a recognised trigger of T1D [51]. We did not observe a significant change in gastrointestinal microbiome composition in F0 generation of mice, and due to funding limitations we did not collect faecal samples in the generations in which increased diabetes incidence was observed. Faecal samples from the later generations in which diabetes incidence was increased would provide greater insight into the potential role of the microbiome in the onset of T1D.

A positive association between food allergy and *Helicobacter pylori* infection has been reported [73], and children with *H. pylori* infection have been shown to exhibit elevated IgE responses to cow's milk [74]. It is therefore possible that *H. pylori* infection at least partly explains the observed relationship between A1 beta-casein consumption and the increased incidence of T1D [36]. *H. pylori* infection reportedly increases epithelial permeability and permits the non-selective passage of allergens to cross the intestinal barrier [73]; a similar cascade of events could permit the passage A1 beta-casein derived BCM-7 to cross the epithelial barrier. If so, the previously reported immunological cross reactivity or molecular mimicry between an epitope on the pancreatic beta-cell-specific glucose-transporter GLUT-2 and the BCM-7 peptide may explain some of the interplay between T1D and A1 beta-casein [75]. Here, exposure to A1 beta-casein may promote the development of autoantibodies that ultimately contribute to the cascade of events leading to type 1 diabetes development. Autoantibodies to GLUT-2 have been detected in patients with recent onset T1D [76] and reactivity of beta-casein T-cell lines to human insulinoma extracts and GLUT-2 have been reported [77]. However, the full implications of these findings are open to speculation because beta-cell autoantibodies may not necessarily be pathogenic: rather, they may represent reproducible biomarkers of the pathogenesis.

This study had a number of limitations that should be considered. The cumulative incidence of diabetes in our NOD colony was low, impacted by in-house microbiota colonisation [54]. We only investigated changes in the microbiome from the F0 generation between A1 and A2 fed mice and data on BCM-7 detection is limited to lymph nodes and blood. The major strength of this study is that experimental conditions were stringently controlled throughout and diabetes incidence across multiple generations were analysed, which to our knowledge has not previously been done.

Despite the limitations described above, we propose that A1 beta-casein influences T1D incidence through a number of potential mechanisms mediated via BCM-7. We hypothesise that BCM-7 released from A1 beta-casein may influence the immune response [38], gut architecture and microbiota [71,72,78] and/or impart direct islet toxicity. Together, these effects may induce epigenetic alterations predisposing pancreatic beta-cells to an autoimmune response (Figure 4) [60,79].

The specific contribution of these mechanisms to the development of T1D, as well as their ability to compensate for each other, is unknown. Furthermore, in milk, caseins form complex aggregates with calcium phosphate called casein micelles [80]. Casein micelles are the source of calcium phosphate and proteins to the young for the growth of bone and teeth [81]. A recent study revealed that cows' milk A1 beta-casein forms a larger micelle compared to A2 beta-casein, which may influence their function [82]. Whether casein micelles were operational in this model was not investigated.

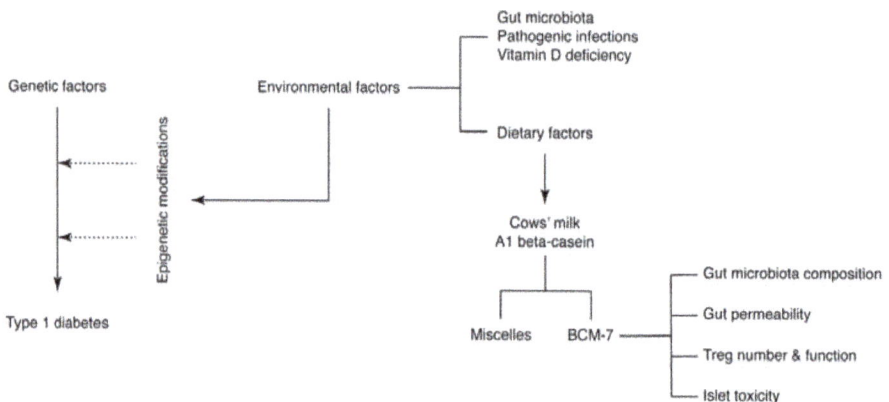

Figure 4. A1 beta-casein supplemented diet associated mechanisms in T1D development in NOD mice.

5. Conclusions

The data presented in this study are provocative and suggest an interaction between dietary protein consumption and the incidence of T1D that differs across generations in NOD mice. This study, alongside others [36–38,83–86], raises questions regarding widespread consumption and timing of introduction of A1 beta-casein in early childhood. Many other environmental factors, such as infections, air pollution, vaccines, location of residence, family environment and stress [87], have been postulated as potential environmental triggers [11]. It is feasible that a combination of environmental triggers in the genetically susceptible host is required. Because cows' milk is the only alternative source of nutrition after breast milk for neonatal feeding in the general population, definitive testing of the hypothesis is clearly warranted.

Supplementary Materials: The following are available online at http://www.mdpi.com/2072-6643/10/9/1291/s1, Figure S1: Treg-mediated suppression in the F4 generation NOD mice, and Figure S2: The diversity of gut bacteria in faecal contents level of A1 and A2 beta-casein fed F0 NOD mice according to several diversity indices.

Author Contributions: Conceptualization, S.K. and K.M.D.; Methodology, J.S.J.C., J.L.M., A.K.E. and C.M.L.; Formal Analysis, J.S.J.C., J.L.M., A.K.E., C.M.L., S.K. and K.M.D.; Investigation, J.S.J.C., J.L.M., A.K.E. and C.M.L.; Resources, J.S.J.C. and J.L.M.; Data Curation, J.S.J.C., J.L.M., A.K.E. and C.M.L.; Writing—Original Draft Preparation, A.K.E. and K.M.D.; Writing—Review and Editing, J.S.J.C., J.L.M., A.K.E., C.M.L., S.K. and K.M.D.; Supervision, S.K. and K.M.D.; Project Administration, S.K. and K.M.D.; Funding Acquisition, S.K. and K.M.D.

Funding: This work was supported through an Innovation Connections Grant (ICG number: RC54051) of the Department of Industry, Innovation and Science, Australia and funding from a2 Infant Nutrition Australia Private Limited, Sydney, NSW, Australia.

Conflicts of Interest: Sonja Kukuljan was a previous salaried employee of a2 Infant Nutrition Australia Private Limited. The remaining authors declare no conflict of interest.

References

1. Jeker, L.T.; Bour-Jordan, H.; Bluestone, J.A. Breakdown in peripheral tolerance in type 1 diabetes in mice and humans. *Cold Spring Harb. Perspect. Med.* **2012**, *2*, a007807. [CrossRef] [PubMed]

2. Mathis, D.; Vence, L.; Benoist, C. beta-Cell death during progression to diabetes. *Nature* **2001**, *414*, 792–798. [CrossRef] [PubMed]

3. Atkinson, M.A.; Eisenbarth, G.S.; Michels, A.W. Type 1 diabetes. *Lancet* **2014**, *383*, 69–82. [CrossRef]

4. Polychronakos, C.; Li, Q. Understanding type 1 diabetes through genetics: Advances and prospects. *Nat. Rev. Genet.* **2011**, *12*, 781–792. [CrossRef] [PubMed]

5. Burn, P. Type 1 diabetes. *Nat. Rev. Drug Discov.* **2010**, *9*, 187–188. [CrossRef] [PubMed]

6. Patterson, C.C.; Dahlquist, G.G.; Gyurus, E.; Green, A.; Soltesz, G. Incidence trends for childhood type 1 diabetes in Europe during 1989–2003 and predicted new cases 2005-20: A multicentre prospective registration study. *Lancet* **2009**, *373*, 2027–2033. [CrossRef]

7. Katsarou, A.; Gudbjornsdottir, S.; Rawshani, A.; Dabelea, D.; Bonifacio, E.; Anderson, B.J.; Jacobsen, L.M.; Schatz, D.A.; Lernmark, A. Type 1 diabetes mellitus. *Nat. Rev. Dis. Primers* **2017**, *3*, 17016. [CrossRef] [PubMed]

8. Delli, A.J.; Lernmark, Å. Chapter 39–Type 1 (Insulin-Dependent) Diabetes Mellitus: Etiology, Pathogenesis, Prediction, and Prevention. In *Endocrinology: Adult and Pediatric*, 7 ed.; Jameson, J.L., De Groot, L.J., de Kretser, D.M., Giudice, L.C., Grossman, A.B., Melmed, S., Potts, J.T., Weir, G.C., Eds.; W.B. Saunders: Philadelphia, PA, USA, 2016; pp. 672–690. [CrossRef]

9. Bluestone, J.A.; Herold, K.; Eisenbarth, G. Genetics, pathogenesis and clinical interventions in type 1 diabetes. *Nature* **2010**, *464*, 1293–1300. [CrossRef] [PubMed]

10. Nielsen, D.S.; Krych, L.; Buschard, K.; Hansen, C.H.; Hansen, A.K. Beyond genetics. Influence of dietary factors and gut microbiota on type 1 diabetes. *FEBS Lett.* **2014**, *588*, 4234–4243. [CrossRef] [PubMed]

11. Rewers, M.; Ludvigsson, J. Environmental risk factors for type 1 diabetes. *Lancet* **2016**, *387*, 2340–2348. [CrossRef]

12. Mustonen, N.; Siljander, H.; Peet, A.; Tillmann, V.; Harkonen, T.; Ilonen, J.; Hyoty, H.; Knip, M. Early childhood infections precede development of beta-cell autoimmunity and type 1 diabetes in children with HLA-conferred disease risk. *Pediatr. Diabetes* 2017. [CrossRef] [PubMed]

13. Zhao, G.; Vatanen, T.; Droit, L.; Park, A.; Kostic, A.D.; Poon, T.W.; Vlamakis, H.; Siljander, H.; Harkonen, T.; Hamalainen, A.M.; et al. Intestinal virome changes precede autoimmunity in type I diabetes-susceptible children. *Proc. Natl. Acad. Sci. USA* **2017**, *114*, E6166–E6175. [CrossRef] [PubMed]

14. Kostic, A.D.; Gevers, D.; Siljander, H.; Vatanen, T.; Hyotylainen, T.; Hamalainen, A.M.; Peet, A.; Tillmann, V.; Poho, P.; Mattila, I.; et al. The dynamics of the human infant gut microbiome in development and in progression toward type 1 diabetes. *Cell Host Microbe* **2015**, *17*, 260–273. [CrossRef] [PubMed]

15. Wen, L.; Ley, R.E.; Volchkov, P.Y.; Stranges, P.B.; Avanesyan, L.; Stonebraker, A.C.; Hu, C.; Wong, F.S.; Szot, G.L.; Bluestone, J.A.; et al. Innate immunity and intestinal microbiota in the development of Type 1 diabetes. *Nature* **2008**, *455*, 1109–1113. [CrossRef] [PubMed]

16. Herold, K.C.; Vignali, D.A.A.; Cooke, A.; Bluestone, J.A. Type I Diabetes: Translating Mechanistic Observations into Effective Clinical Outcomes. *Nat. Rev. Immunol.* **2013**, *13*, 243–256. [CrossRef] [PubMed]

17. Ziegler, A.G.; Rewers, M.; Simell, O.; Simell, T.; Lempainen, J.; Steck, A.; Winkler, C.; Ilonen, J.; Veijola, R.; Knip, M.; et al. Seroconversion to multiple islet autoantibodies and risk of progression to diabetes in children. *JAMA* **2013**, *309*, 2473–2479. [CrossRef] [PubMed]

18. Krischer, J.P.; Lynch, K.F.; Schatz, D.A.; Ilonen, J.; Lernmark, A.; Hagopian, W.A.; Rewers, M.J.; She, J.X.; Simell, O.G.; Toppari, J.; et al. The 6 year incidence of diabetes-associated autoantibodies in genetically at-risk children: The TEDDY study. *Diabetologia* **2015**, *58*, 980–987. [CrossRef] [PubMed]

19. Knip, M.; Simell, O. Environmental Triggers of Type 1 Diabetes. *Cold Spring Harb. Perspect. Med.* **2012**, *2*, a007690. [CrossRef] [PubMed]

20. Chia, J.S.J.; McRae, J.L.; Kukuljan, S.; Woodford, K.; Elliott, R.B.; Swinburn, B.; Dwyer, K.M. A1 beta-casein milk protein and other environmental pre-disposing factors for type 1 diabetes. *Nutr. Diabetes* **2017**, *7*, e274. [CrossRef] [PubMed]

21. Lamb, M.M.; Miller, M.; Seifert, J.A.; Frederiksen, B.; Kroehl, M.; Rewers, M.; Norris, J.M. The effect of childhood cow's milk intake and HLA-DR genotype on risk of islet autoimmunity and type 1 diabetes: The Diabetes Autoimmunity Study in the Young. *Pediatr. Diabetes* **2015**, *16*, 31–38. [CrossRef] [PubMed]

22. Knip, M.; Virtanen, S.M.; Seppa, K.; Ilonen, J.; Savilahti, E.; Vaarala, O.; Reunanen, A.; Teramo, K.; Hamalainen, A.M.; Paronen, J.; et al. Dietary intervention in infancy and later signs of beta-cell autoimmunity. *N. Engl. J. Med.* **2010**, *363*, 1900–1908. [CrossRef] [PubMed]

23. Kramer, M.S.; Kakuma, R. The optimal duration of exclusive breastfeeding: A systematic review. *Adv. Exp. Med. Biol.* **2004**, *554*, 63–77. [PubMed]

24. Chowdhury, R.; Sinha, B.; Sankar, M.J.; Taneja, S.; Bhandari, N.; Rollins, N.; Bahl, R.; Martines, J. Breastfeeding and maternal health outcomes: A systematic review and meta-analysis. *Acta Paediatr.* **2015**, *104*, 96–113. [CrossRef] [PubMed]

25. Haug, A.; Hostmark, A.T.; Harstad, O.M. Bovine milk in human nutrition—A review. *Lipids Health Dis.* **2007**, *6*, 25. [CrossRef] [PubMed]

26. Huppertz, T.; Fox, P.F.; Kelly, A.L. 3–The caseins: Structure, stability, and functionality A2–Yada, Rickey Y. In *Proteins in Food Processing*, 7th ed.; Woodhead Publishing: Cambridge, UK, 2018; pp. 49–92.

27. Kaminski, S.; Cieslinska, A.; Kostyra, E. Polymorphism of bovine beta-casein and its potential effect on human health. *J. Appl. Genet.* **2007**, *48*, 189–198. [CrossRef] [PubMed]

28. De Noni, R.J.; FitzGerald, H.J.T.; Korhonen, Y.; Le Roux, C.T.; Livesey, I.; Thorsdottir, D.; Tomé, R.W. Scientific Report of EFSA prepared by a DATEX Working Group on the potential health impact of β-casomorphins and related peptides. *Eur. Food Saf. Auth.* **2009**, *231*, 1–107.

29. Brantl, V.; Teschemacher, H.; Henschen, A.; Lottspeich, F. Novel opioid peptides derived from casein (beta-casomorphins). I. Isolation from bovine casein peptone. *Hoppe-Seyler Z. Physiol. Chem.* **1979**, *360*, 1211–1216. [CrossRef] [PubMed]

30. Henschen, A.; Lottspeich, F.; Brantl, V.; Teschemacher, H. Novel opioid peptides derived from casein (beta-casomorphins). II. Structure of active components from bovine casein peptone. *Hoppe-Seyler Z. Physiol. Chem.* **1979**, *360*, 1217–1224. [PubMed]

31. Boutrou, R.; Gaudichon, C.; Dupont, D.; Jardin, J.; Airinei, G.; Marsset-Baglieri, A.; Benamouzig, R.; Tome, D.; Leonil, J. Sequential release of milk protein-derived bioactive peptides in the jejunum in healthy humans. *Am. J. Clin. Nutr.* **2013**, *97*, 1314–1323. [CrossRef] [PubMed]

32. Clemens, R.A. Milk A1 and A2 peptides and diabetes. *Nestle Nutr. Workshop Ser. Paediatr. Prog.* **2011**, *67*, 187–195. [CrossRef]

33. Elliott, R.B.; Harris, D.P.; Hill, J.P.; Bibby, N.J.; Wasmuth, H.E. Type I (insulin-dependent) diabetes mellitus and cow milk: Casein variant consumption. *Diabetologia* **1999**, *42*, 292–296. [CrossRef] [PubMed]

34. Knip, M. Environmental triggers and determinants of beta-cell autoimmunity and type 1 diabetes. *Rev. Endocr. Metab. Disord.* **2003**, *4*, 213–223. [CrossRef] [PubMed]

35. Harrison, L.C.; Honeyman, M.C. Cow's milk and type 1 diabetes: The real debate is about mucosal immune function. *Diabetes* **1999**, *48*, 1501–1507. [CrossRef] [PubMed]

36. Laugesen, M.; Elliott, R. Ischaemic heart disease, Type 1 diabetes, and cow milk A1 beta-casein. *N. Zeal. Med. J.* **2003**, *116*, U295.

37. Elliott, R.B.; Reddy, S.N.; Bibby, N.J.; Kida, K. Dietary prevention of diabetes in the non-obese diabetic mouse. *Diabetologia* **1988**, *31*, 62–64. [PubMed]

38. Elliott, R.B.; Wasmuth, W.H.; Bibby, N.J.; Hill, J.P. The role of β-casein variants in the induction of insulin-dependent diabetes in the non-obese diabetic mouse and humans. In *Milk Protein Polymorphism*; IDF Special Issue No. 9702; Food and Agriculture Organization: Brussels, Belgium, 1997; pp. 445–453.

39. Johnsen, E.; Leknes, S.; Wilson, S.R.; Lundanes, E. Liquid chromatography-mass spectrometry platform for both small neurotransmitters and neuropeptides in blood, with automatic and robust solid phase extraction. *Sci. Rep.* **2015**, *5*, 9308. [CrossRef] [PubMed]

40. Kim, D.; Song, L.; Breitwieser, F.P.; Salzberg, S.L. Centrifuge: Rapid and sensitive classification of metagenomic sequences. *Genome Res.* **2016**, *26*, 1721–1729. [CrossRef] [PubMed]

41. McMurdie, P.J.; Holmes, S. Phyloseq: An R package for reproducible interactive analysis and graphics of microbiome census data. *PLoS ONE* **2013**, *8*, e61217. [CrossRef] [PubMed]

42. Love, M.; Anders, S.; Huber, W. Differential Analysis of Count Data–The deseq2 Package. *Genome Biol.* **2014**, *15*, 10–1186.

43. Love, M.I.; Huber, W.; Anders, S. Moderated estimation of fold change and dispersion for RNA-seq data with DESeq2. *Genome Biol.* **2014**, *15*, 550. [CrossRef] [PubMed]

44. Brusko, T.; Wasserfall, C.; McGrail, K.; Schatz, R.; Viener, H.L.; Schatz, D.; Haller, M.; Rockell, J.; Gottlieb, P.; Clare-Salzler, M.; et al. No alterations in the frequency of FOXP3+ regulatory T-cells in type 1 diabetes. *Diabetes* **2007**, *56*, 604–612. [CrossRef] [PubMed]

45. Brusko, T.M.; Wasserfall, C.H.; Clare-Salzler, M.J.; Schatz, D.A.; Atkinson, M.A. Functional defects and the influence of age on the frequency of CD4$^+$CD25$^+$ T-cells in type 1 diabetes. *Diabetes* **2005**, *54*, 1407–1414. [CrossRef] [PubMed]

46. Lindley, S.; Dayan, C.M.; Bishop, A.; Roep, B.O.; Peakman, M.; Tree, T.I. Defective suppressor function in CD4$^+$CD25$^+$ T-cells from patients with type 1 diabetes. *Diabetes* **2005**, *54*, 92–99. [CrossRef] [PubMed]

47. Ryba-Stanislawowska, M.; Rybarczyk-Kapturska, K.; Mysliwiec, M.; Mysliwska, J. Elevated levels of serum IL-12 and IL-18 are associated with lower frequencies of CD4$^+$CD25^{high}FOXP3$^+$ regulatory t cells in young patients with type 1 diabetes. *Inflammation* **2014**, *37*, 1513–1520. [CrossRef] [PubMed]

48. Haseda, F.; Imagawa, A.; Murase-Mishiba, Y.; Terasaki, J.; Hanafusa, T. CD4$^+$CD45RA$^-$FoxP3^{high} activated regulatory T cells are functionally impaired and related to residual insulin-secreting capacity in patients with type 1 diabetes. *Clin. Exp. Immunol.* **2013**, *173*, 207–216. [CrossRef] [PubMed]

49. Davies, H.D.; McGeer, A.; Schwartz, B.; Green, K.; Cann, D.; Simor, A.E.; Low, D.E. Invasive Group A Streptococcal Infections in Ontario, Canada. *N. Engl. J. Med.* **1996**, *335*, 547–554. [CrossRef] [PubMed]

50. Hughes, J.M.; Wilson, M.E.; Wertheim, H.F.L.; Nghia, H.D.T.; Taylor, W.; Schultsz, C. *Streptococcus suis*: An Emerging Human Pathogen. *Clin. Infect. Dis.* **2009**, *48*, 617–625. [CrossRef]

51. Vaarala, O.; Atkinson, M.A.; Neu, J. The "perfect storm" for type 1 diabetes: The complex interplay between intestinal microbiota, gut permeability, and mucosal immunity. *Diabetes* **2008**, *57*, 2555–2562. [CrossRef] [PubMed]

52. Scott, F.W. Cow milk and insulin-dependent diabetes mellitus: Is there a relationship? *Am. J. Clin. Nutr.* **1990**, *51*, 489–491. [CrossRef] [PubMed]

53. Dahl-Jorgensen, K.; Joner, G.; Hanssen, K.F. Relationship between cows' milk consumption and incidence of IDDM in childhood. *Diabetes Care* **1991**, *14*, 1081–1083. [CrossRef] [PubMed]

54. Pozzilli, P.; Signore, A.; Williams, A.J.; Beales, P.E. NOD mouse colonies around the world–recent facts and figures. *Immunol. Today* **1993**, *14*, 193–196. [CrossRef]

55. Markle, J.G.; Frank, D.N.; Mortin-Toth, S.; Robertson, C.E.; Feazel, L.M.; Rolle-Kampczyk, U.; von Bergen, M.; McCoy, K.D.; Macpherson, A.J.; Danska, J.S. Sex differences in the gut microbiome drive hormone-dependent regulation of autoimmunity. *Science* **2013**, *339*, 1084–1088. [CrossRef] [PubMed]

56. Pearson, J.A.; Wong, F.S.; Wen, L. The importance of the Non Obese Diabetic (NOD) mouse model in autoimmune diabetes. *J. Autoimmun.* **2016**, *66*, 76–88. [CrossRef] [PubMed]

57. Jerram, S.T.; Dang, M.N.; Leslie, R.D. The Role of Epigenetics in Type 1 Diabetes. *Curr. Diabetes Rep.* **2017**, *17*, 89. [CrossRef] [PubMed]

58. Dang, M.N.; Buzzetti, R.; Pozzilli, P. Epigenetics in autoimmune diseases with focus on type 1 diabetes. *Diabetes/Metab. Res. Rev.* **2013**, *29*, 8–18. [CrossRef] [PubMed]

59. Huypens, P.; Sass, S.; Wu, M.; Dyckhoff, D.; Tschop, M.; Theis, F.; Marschall, S.; de Angelis, M.H.; Beckers, J. Epigenetic germline inheritance of diet-induced obesity and insulin resistance. *Nat. Genet.* **2016**, *48*, 497–499. [CrossRef] [PubMed]

60. Krautkramer, K.A.; Kreznar, J.H.; Romano, K.A.; Vivas, E.I.; Barrett-Wilt, G.A.; Rabaglia, M.E.; Keller, M.P.; Attie, A.D.; Rey, F.E.; Denu, J.M. Diet-Microbiota Interactions Mediate Global Epigenetic Programming in Multiple Host Tissues. *Mol. Cell* **2016**, *64*, 982–992. [CrossRef] [PubMed]

61. Bonelli, M.; Savitskaya, A.; Steiner, C.W.; Rath, E.; Smolen, J.S.; Scheinecker, C. Phenotypic and functional analysis of CD4$^+$CD25$^-$Foxp3$^+$ T cells in patients with systemic lupus erythematosus. *J. Immunol.* **2009**, *182*, 1689–1695. [CrossRef] [PubMed]

62. Yang, H.X.; Zhang, W.; Zhao, L.D.; Li, Y.; Zhang, F.C.; Tang, F.L.; He, W.; Zhang, X. Are CD4$^+$CD25$^-$Foxp3$^+$ cells in untreated new-onset lupus patients regulatory T cells? *Arthritis Res. Ther.* **2009**, *11*, R153. [CrossRef] [PubMed]

63. DuPage, M.; Bluestone, J.A. Harnessing the plasticity of CD4$^+$ T cells to treat immune-mediated disease. *Nat. Rev. Immunol.* **2016**, *16*, 149–163. [CrossRef] [PubMed]

64. Zelenay, S.; Lopes-Carvalho, T.; Caramalho, I.; Moraes-Fontes, M.F.; Rebelo, M.; Demengeot, J. Foxp3$^+$ CD25$^-$CD4 T cells constitute a reservoir of committed regulatory cells that regain CD25 expression upon homeostatic expansion. *Proc. Natl. Acad. Sci. USA* **2005**, *102*, 4091–4096. [CrossRef] [PubMed]

65. Svedberg, J.; de Haas, J.; Leimenstoll, G.; Paul, F.; Teschemacher, H. Demonstration of beta-casomorphin immunoreactive materials in in vitro digests of bovine milk and in small intestine contents after bovine milk ingestion in adult humans. *Peptides* **1985**, *6*, 825–830. [CrossRef]

66. Umbach, M.; Teschemacher, H.; Praetorius, K.; Hirschhauser, R.; Bostedt, H. Demonstration of a beta-casomorphin immunoreactive material in the plasma of newborn calves after milk intake. *Regul. Pept.* **1985**, *12*, 223–230. [CrossRef]

67. Barbé, F.; Le Feunteun, S.; Rémond, D.; Ménard, O.; Jardin, J.; Henry, G.; Laroche, B.; Dupont, D. Tracking the in vivo release of bioactive peptides in the gut during digestion: Mass spectrometry peptidomic characterization of effluents collected in the gut of dairy matrix fed mini-pigs. *Food Res. Int.* **2014**, *63*, 147–156. [CrossRef]

68. Brooke-Taylor, S.; Dwyer, K.; Woodford, K.; Kost, N. Systematic Review of the Gastrointestinal Effects of A1 Compared with A2 beta-Casein. *Adv. Nutr.* **2017**, *8*, 739–748. [CrossRef] [PubMed]

69. Ul Haq, M.R.; Kapila, R.; Sharma, R.; Saliganti, V.; Kapila, S. Comparative evaluation of cow beta-casein variants (A1/A2) consumption on Th2-mediated inflammatory response in mouse gut. *Eur. J. Nutr.* **2014**, *53*, 1039–1049. [CrossRef] [PubMed]

70. Barnett, M.P.; McNabb, W.C.; Roy, N.C.; Woodford, K.B.; Clarke, A.J. Dietary A1 beta-casein affects gastrointestinal transit time, dipeptidyl peptidase-4 activity, and inflammatory status relative to A2 beta-casein in Wistar rats. *Int. J. Food Sci. Nutr.* **2014**, *65*, 720–727. [CrossRef] [PubMed]

71. Zhu, Y.; Lin, X.; Zhao, F.; Shi, X.; Li, H.; Li, Y.; Zhu, W.; Xu, X.; Li, C.; Zhou, G. Meat, dairy and plant proteins alter bacterial composition of rat gut bacteria. *Sci. Rep.* **2015**, *5*, 15220. [CrossRef] [PubMed]

72. Zhu, Y.; Lin, X.; Li, H.; Li, Y.; Shi, X.; Zhao, F.; Xu, X.; Li, C.; Zhou, G. Intake of Meat Proteins Substantially Increased the Relative Abundance of Genus Lactobacillus in Rat Feces. *PLoS ONE* **2016**, *11*, e0152678. [CrossRef] [PubMed]

73. Ma, Z.F.; Majid, N.A.; Yamaoka, Y.; Lee, Y.Y. Food Allergy and Helicobacter pylori Infection: A Systematic Review. *Front. Microbiol.* **2016**, *7*, 368. [CrossRef] [PubMed]

74. Kolho, K.L.; Haapaniemi, A.; Haahtela, T.; Rautelin, H. Helicobacter pylori and specific immunoglobulin E antibodies to food allergens in children. *J. Pediatr. Gastroenterol. Nutr.* **2005**, *40*, 180–183. [CrossRef] [PubMed]

75. Pozzilli, P. Beta-casein in cow's milk: A major antigenic determinant for type 1 diabetes? *J. Endocrinol. Invest.* **1999**, *22*, 562–567. [CrossRef]

76. Inman, L.R.; McAllister, C.T.; Chen, L.; Hughes, S.; Newgard, C.B.; Kettman, J.R.; Unger, R.H.; Johnson, J.H. Autoantibodies to the GLUT-2 glucose transporter of beta cells in insulin-dependent diabetes mellitus of recent onset. *Proc. Natl. Acad. Sci. USA* **1993**, *90*, 1281–1284. [CrossRef] [PubMed]

77. Monetini, L.; Barone, F.; Stefanini, L.; Petrone, A.; Walk, T.; Jung, G.; Thorpe, R.; Pozzilli, P.; Cavallo, M.G. Establishment of T cell lines to bovine beta-casein and beta-casein-derived epitopes in patients with type 1 diabetes. *J. Endocrinol.* **2003**, *176*, 143–150. [CrossRef] [PubMed]

78. Kar, S.K.; Jansman, A.J.M.; Benis, N.; Ramiro-Garcia, J.; Schokker, D.; Kruijt, L.; Stolte, E.H.; Taverne-Thiele, J.J.; Smits, M.A.; Wells, J.M. Dietary protein sources differentially affect microbiota, mTOR activity and transcription of mTOR signaling pathways in the small intestine. *PLoS ONE* **2017**, *12*, e0188282. [CrossRef] [PubMed]

79. Wu, H.; Deng, Y.; Feng, Y.; Long, D.; Ma, K.; Wang, X.; Zhao, M.; Lu, L.; Lu, Q. Epigenetic regulation in B-cell maturation and its dysregulation in autoimmunity. *Cell. Mol. Immunol.* **2018**. [CrossRef] [PubMed]

80. Dalgleish, D.G.; Corredig, M. The structure of the casein micelle of milk and its changes during processing. *Annu. Rev. Food Sci. Technol.* **2012**, *3*, 449–467. [CrossRef] [PubMed]

81. De Kruif, C.G.; Huppertz, T. Casein micelles: Size distribution in milks from individual cows. *J. Agric. Food Chem.* **2012**, *60*, 4649–4655. [CrossRef] [PubMed]

82. Raynes, J.K.; Day, L.; Augustin, M.A.; Carver, J.A. Structural differences between bovine A(1) and A(2) beta-casein alter micelle self-assembly and influence molecular chaperone activity. *J. Dairy Sci.* **2015**, *98*, 2172–2182. [CrossRef] [PubMed]

83. Gerstein, H.C.; VanderMeulen, J. The relationship between cow's milk exposure and type 1 diabetes. *Diabet. Med.* **1996**, *13*, 23–29. [CrossRef]

84. Virtanen, S.M.; Hypponen, E.; Laara, E.; Vahasalo, P.; Kulmala, P.; Savola, K.; Rasanen, L.; Aro, A.; Knip, M.; Akerblom, H.K. Cow's milk consumption, disease-associated autoantibodies and type 1 diabetes mellitus: A follow-up study in siblings of diabetic children. Childhood Diabetes in Finland Study Group. *Diabet. Med.* **1998**, *15*, 730–738. [CrossRef]

85. Birgisdottir, B.E.; Hill, J.P.; Harris, D.P.; Thorsdottir, I. Variation in consumption of cow milk proteins and lower incidence of Type 1 diabetes in Iceland vs the other 4 Nordic countries. *Diabetes Nutr. Metab.* **2002**, *15*, 240–245. [PubMed]

86. Beales, P.E.; Elliott, R.B.; Flohe, S.; Hill, J.P.; Kolb, H.; Pozzilli, P.; Wang, G.S.; Wasmuth, H.; Scott, F.W. A multi-centre, blinded international trial of the effect of A(1) and A(2) beta-casein variants on diabetes incidence in two rodent models of spontaneous Type I diabetes. *Diabetologia* **2002**, *45*, 1240–1246. [CrossRef] [PubMed]

87. Butalia, S.; Kaplan, G.G.; Khokhar, B.; Rabi, D.M. Environmental Risk Factors and Type 1 Diabetes: Past, Present, and Future. *Can. J. Diabetes* **2016**, *40*, 586–593. [CrossRef] [PubMed]

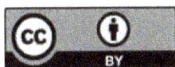

nutrients

MDPI

Article

Gastric Emptying and Dynamic In Vitro Digestion of Drinkable Yogurts: Effect of Viscosity and Composition

Olivia Ménard [1], Marie-Hélène Famelart [1], Amélie Deglaire [1], Yann Le Gouar [1], Sylvie Guérin [2], Charles-Henri Malbert [3] and Didier Dupont [1,*]

[1] Institut National de la Recherche Agronomique (INRA)-Agrocampus Ouest, Science et Technologie du Lait et de l'œuf (STLO), 65 rue de Saint-Brieuc, 35042 Rennes CEDEX, France; olivia.menard@inra.fr (O.M.); marie-helene.famelart@inra.fr (M.-H.F.); amelie.deglaire@agrocampus-ouest.fr (A.D.); yann.le-gouar@inra.fr (Y.L.G.)
[2] Institut Nutrition-Métabolisme-Cancer, INRA, Institut National de la Santé et de la Recherche Médicale (INSERM), Université Rennes 1, Domaine de la prise, 35590 Saint-Gilles, France; sylvie.guerin@inra.fr
[3] INRA, ANI-SCAN Unit, Domaine de la Prise, 35590 Saint-Gilles, France; charles-henri.malbert@inra.fr
* Correspondence: didier.dupont@inra.fr; Tel.: +33-223-48-5335

Received: 9 August 2018; Accepted: 11 September 2018; Published: 14 September 2018

Abstract: Gastric emptying of food is mainly driven by the caloric concentration, the rheological properties of the chyme, and the physical state (liquid/solid) of food once in the stomach. The present work investigated: (1) The effect of the composition and the viscosity of drinkable yogurts on gastric emptying in pigs, and (2) the behavior of yogurts during dynamic in vitro digestion. Three isocaloric liquid yogurts were manufactured: Two enriched in protein and fiber showing either a low (LV) or high (HV) viscosity, one control enriched in sugar and starch (CT). They were labelled with ^{99m}Tc-sulfur colloid and given to pigs (n = 11) to determine gastric emptying pattern by gamma scintigraphy. Then dynamic in vitro digestion of the yogurts was done using the parameters of gastric emptying determined in vivo. Gastric emptying half-times were significantly longer for LV than CT, whereas HV exhibited an intermediate behavior. In vitro gastric digestion showed a quick hydrolysis of caseins, whereas whey proteins were more resistant in the stomach particularly for LV and HV. During the intestinal phase, both whey proteins and caseins were almost fully hydrolyzed. Viscosity was shown to affect the behavior of yogurt in the small intestine.

Keywords: gastric emptying; gamma-scintigraphy; yogurt; in vitro digestion; casein; whey protein; satiety

1. Introduction

Until recently, it was considered that the structure of the food matrix had a limited impact on food digestion and food could be described only according to its composition in proteins, lipids, and carbohydrates. During the last years, new evidences have clearly demonstrated that the food matrix structure plays a key role on the kinetics of transit and hydrolysis of the macronutrients [1–4]. Several parameters have been shown to affect food intake, transit, and digestion. Even before food arrives in the gastrointestinal tract, cognitive and sensory signals generated by the sight and smell of food and by the oro-sensory experience of food in the oral cavity influence the amount of food ingested for that eating episode, but also for an extended period of time during which no ingestion takes place. Aside the sensory component, the composition of food could also play a key role and the effect of the type of macronutrients on food intake has been further investigated in many studies. For example, dietary protein has been observed to increase satiety and suppress short-term food intake beyond what would be expected by an iso-energetic amount from carbohydrates and fats [5,6]. The development of protein-supplemented foods has been used as a strategy for either modulating appetite in healthy adults [7] or increasing the protein intake of elderly people suffering from malnutrition [8,9]. However, the extent to which the source of the protein matters is uncertain. Whey and casein, two milk derived protein sources, have more commonly been studied with regard to their effects on satiety and food intake. Whey proteins account for 20% of the total milk protein and are rich in essential amino acids, whereas casein is the major protein of milk accounting for ~80% of the total protein [10]. Whey protein and casein are both heterogeneous groups of proteins containing all amino acids and are especially rich in the essential ones, although in different proportions. Whey protein is reported as more satiating than casein [11,12], although this statement is still controversial. Indeed, a recent review indicates that whey is more satiating in the short term, whereas casein is more satiating in the long term [13] because of different mechanisms of action. Whey tends to stimulate the secretion of the incretin hormones glucagon-like peptide-1 (GLP-1) and glucose-dependent insulinotropic polypeptide, whereas casein is more active on the satiety (cholecystokinin, peptide YY) and hunger-stimulating (ghrelin) hormones.

Another food ingredient that can have beneficial effects on food intake is dietary fiber [14]. Fiber is thought to affect satiety in many ways, depending on the fiber type, and relating to its ability to bulk foods, increase viscosity, gel in the stomach, and ferment in the distal part of the gut [15]. When reviewing the literature available on the effect of fiber on satiety, it has been shown that fibers characterized as being more viscous (e.g., pectins, β-glucans and guar gum) reduced appetite more often than the less viscous fibers. However, overall, effects on energy intake and body weight were relatively small [16].

Post-ingestive signals encoding for nutrient content [17,18] and volume [19] arising from the stomach and intestine also affect satiety. Gastric signals are only of physical nature and are transmitted locally and centrally after the selective involvement of stretch receptors. These intramural receptors are sensitive to the amount of food present within the stomach and therefore are detecting the level of distension and the rate of emptying. Indirectly, via a chemical mediated duodenal detection of the amount of nutrient, and more specifically, the energy contents of the duodenal juice, where the satiation signals are transmitted centrally. Furthermore, part of the duodenal signal is transmitted to the enteric nervous system to alter locally gastric motility and emptying [20]. The increase in satiety through gastric distension has been demonstrated through alteration of the gastric emptying rate using isovolumetric and isocaloric liquid and semisolid meals [21–23].

Viscosity has been shown to have an effect on satiation and satiety in multiple studies [24–27] and it has been hypothesized that this effect of viscosity was due to its action on gastric emptying. Indeed, most of the published studies have shown that increasing the viscosity delayed the gastric emptying rate [23,27,28]. However, increasing the viscosity of the meal to slow down gastric emptying appears to be less effective than increasing its caloric content [29].

In this context, two fiber and protein-enriched yogurts (similar composition but different viscosity) and a control yogurt were formulated. All three yogurts had similar caloric content. The aim of the present study was to investigate whether protein and fiber enrichment could affect gastric emptying and, consequently, the kinetics of protein digestion. Yogurt digestion was studied using a dynamic in vitro model that had been previously validated against in vivo data [30]. In order to define the parameters of the model, gastric emptying half-time, and the shape of the emptying curve were determined by gamma-scintigraphy using the pig as a model. Gamma-scintigraphy, like Magnetic Resonance Imaging, is a direct method for assessing gastric emptying that has been shown to be more relevant than indirect methods such as ^{13}C breath tests that can be biased by the food matrix as recently described [31]. Then, an in vitro dynamic digestion was conducted on the three yogurts using the parameters determined in vivo. The gastric and intestinal behavior of the three matrices were compared and the proteolysis kinetics were monitored.

2. Materials and Methods

Three isocaloric yogurts with different compositions and structure kindly provided by Senoble (Jouy, France) were submitted to in vivo and in vitro assays. The three yogurts, for which the composition is given in Table 1, had a control yogurt (CT) and two yogurts enriched in protein and fibers both with different textures, i.e., Low Viscosity (LV) or High Viscosity (HV).

Table 1. Composition and texture of the three yogurts.

	Control	Low Viscosity	High Viscosity
Protein (g/100 g)	3.1	8.1	8.1
Lipid (g/100 g)	0.1	0.2	0.2
Sugar (g/100 g)	17.3	11.6	11.6
Fiber (g/100 g)	0	2.5	2.5
Starch (%)	0.53	0.18	0.18
Energy (kcal/100 g)	82	85	85
Texture	standard	liquid	thick liquid

2.1. Viscosity Analysis

Yogurt viscosity was measured using a cone-plan (6 cm diameter, 4 degree angle) geometry on an AR 2000 rheometer (TA Instruments, Leatherhead, UK). Yogurt was carefully sampled from the center of the cup, deposited on the plate at 4 °C and the cone was slowly lowered into the sample. A logarithm shear rate increase ranging from 0.2 to 100 s^{-1} at 4 °C was applied ($n = 2$) on 2 independent batches of the 3 yogurts. Since the study of gastric emptying on pigs and the in vitro digestion experiments occurred up to 15 days after manufacture, viscosity- of yogurts was assessed 4 days (D + 4) and -5 days (D + 15) after manufacture to check for a possible evolution of the viscosity during storage. Typical flow behaviors following the model of Herschel-Bulkley [32] were observed for yogurts. The apparent viscosities (Viscosity$_{app}$) at 100 s^{-1} were deduced. They were significantly different for the 3 yogurts, but not between the days (Table 2).

Table 2. Apparent viscosity of the three yogurts measured 4 days (D + 4) and 15 days (D + 15) after manufacture.

Viscosity$_{app}$ (Pa·s)	CT	LV	HV
D + 4	1.26 ± 0.12	0.32 ± 0.04	2.20 ± 0.11
D + 15	1.30 ± 0.05	0.37 ± 0.04	2.07 ± 0.20

Note: Viscosity$_{app}$, apparent viscosities; CT, control yogurt; LV: low viscosity; HV: high viscosity.

2.2. Gastric Emptying Assessment by Gamma-Scintigraphy on Pigs

All procedures were in accordance with the European Community guidelines for the use of laboratory animals (L358-86/609/EEC). The study received prior approval by the local animal ethic committee (agreement number: R-2013-CHM-01). The facilities have the authorization to use animals (agreement number: A35-622) and radioisotopes (agreement number: T35-0282).

The animals used were 11 young Large White sows of about 3 months old and 30–35 kg body weight. During the week before the experiment, the animals were trained to consume the food while in quadrupedal position within a Pavlov stand. Furthermore, they were trained to eat 529 g (450 kcal) of yogurt within 5 min and then stay still for two hours in front of the gamma camera. On the day of experiment, conscious pigs were installed in a Pavlov stand and fed with 529 g of one of the three yogurt radiolabeled with 20 MBq, ^{99m}Tc-colloid sulfur CK1 (CISBio International, Saclay, France), as described in previous studies [33]. The gamma camera was calibrated for energy and uniformity weekly. Data acquisition was performed using high-resolution low energy collimator and with a 64 × 64 pixel matrix. Gastric emptying was followed by gamma scintigraphy during 2 h after meal ingestion using sequential images taken every minute for 15 s each. During the 2 h of the experiment, animals had no access to water. Each animal received the 3 yogurts on separate days and each animal was therefore its own control.

The dynamic image series were analyzed with the OSIRIX MD software (Pixmeo SARL, Bernex, Switzerland) and with dedicated software. This software allowed to re-aligns the images to compensate the movements of the animal relative to the camera head during acquisition. Gastric emptying half-time ($T_{1/2}$, time needed for 50% of the radioactivity to be transferred from the stomach into the small intestine) and the shape of the gastric emptying curve (β) that describes the length of the initial phase and the shape of the curve after the lag phase [34] were determined. The adequacy of the power exponential fit was evaluated using modified-stretch exponential (MSE).

2.3. Yogurt Dynamic In Vitro Digestion

A dynamic in vitro gastro-intestinal digestion system (DIDGI®, Institut national de la recherche agronomique (INRA), Rennes CEDEX, France) was used to simulate the digestion of the three yogurts and investigate the kinetics of milk protein hydrolysis during digestion. The gastric emptying half-time and the shape of the gastric emptying curve determined in vivo by gamma-scintigraphy on the three different matrices were entered in the simulator software to simulate the gastric emptying using the Elashoff equation [34]. Each matrix was digested in duplicate. In the gastric phase, aliquots were sampled at G0 (undigested yogurts) and after 120 min digestion (G120). In the intestinal phase, samples were taken after 180 min (I180) for the three yogurts and 240 min (I240) digestion for only the low and high viscosity yogurts (milk protein digestion in the control yogurt was already completed after 180 min). Except the gastric emptying parameters that were deduced from the in vivo experiment, the other parameters used in the digestion experiments were set up to simulate the adult gastro-intestinal, as proposed in Egger et al. [35]. They are summarized in Table 3.

Table 3. Gastro-intestinal parameters for in vitro dynamic digestions.

Gastric Conditions (37 °C)			
Simulated Gastric Fluid (SGF)	Na+		100 mmol/L
(stock solution adjusted at pH 6.5)	Ca^{2+}		1 mmol/L
Fasted state/initial conditions	SGF		24 mL
	pH		1.8
Yogurt	Ingested amount		150 g
Gastric pH (acidification curve)	pH = 1.68 + 3.82($-t/42$) (with t: time after ingestion in min)		
	Pepsin		2000 U/mL of gastric content
SGF + pepsin (porcine)	Flow rate		1 mL/min from 0 to 5 min
	Flow rate		0.5 mL/min from 5 to 180 min
	CT	$T_{1/2}$ *	58 min
		β	1.1
Gastric emptying (Elashoff fitting)	LV	$T_{1/2}$	73 min
		β	1.0
	HV	$T_{1/2}$	65 min
		β	1.1
Intestinal Conditions (37 °C)			
Simulated Intestinal Fluid (SIF)	Na$^+$		100 mmol/L
(stock solution adjusted at pH 6.2)	Ca^{2+}		1 mmol/L
Intestinal pH	pH		6.6
	Bile		4% from 0 to 30 min
SIF + bile (bovine)	Bile		2% from 30 min to the end
	Flow rate		0.5 mL/min from 0 to the end
SIF + pancreatin (porcine)	Pancreatin		7%
	Flow rate		0.25 mL/min from 0 to the end
Intestinal emptying (Elashoff fitting)	$T_{1/2}$		160 min
	β		1.6

* $T_{1/2}$ = gastric emptying half-time.

2.4. SDS-PAGE

Milk protein extent of hydrolysis was assessed during the gastric and the intestinal phase by Sodium dodecyl sulfate polyacrylamide gel electrophoresis (SDS-PAGE) analysis. Briefly, the electrophoretic analyses were performed using 4–12% polyacrylamide NuPAGE® Novex® Bis-Tris 15 well precast gels (Invitrogen, Carlsbad, CA, USA) in accordance with the manufacturer's instructions. All samples were diluted with NuPAGE® LDS sample buffer and then treated with 0.5 M DL-dithiothreitol and distilled water. Mark 12 Unstained Standard (Invitrogen) was used as a molecular weight (MW) marker—as a reference of the position of the bands. Gels were fixed in 30% (*v/v*) ethanol, 10% (*v/v*) acetic acid, and 60% (*v/v*) deionized water. They were rinsed in deionized water before staining with Bio-Safe Coomassie stain (Bio-Rad Laboratories, Marnes-la-Coquette, France). Discoloration of gels were performed with water Image analysis of SDS-PAGE gels was carried out using Image Scanner III (General Electric (GE) Healthcare Europe GbmH, Velizy-Villacoublay, France). After digitization of gels, the bands were selected and their gray intensity determined by densitometry using the software Image Quant TL™ (GE Healthcare Europe GbmH, Velizy-Villacoublay, France). Densitometry analyses of the SDS-PAGE gels were used for the semi-quantification of protein levels. The percentage of each intact protein remaining in the gastric and intestinal compartment was estimated in comparison with the undigested yogurt sample.

2.5. Statistics

The difference of proteolysis kinetics between yogurts was examined by a two-way Analysis of variance (ANOVA) with yogurt and time as factors and with time as a repeated measure using the SAS software 9.3 (SAS, Cary, NC, USA). Post-hoc comparison was performed using a Tukey test. The value of $p < 0.05$ was considered statistically significant.

3. Results

3.1. Gastric Emptying

The results are summarized in Table 4 and an example of a video recorded is available as Supplementary Material. The $T_{1/2}$ obtained for the LV yogurt was significantly different from the CT yogurt ($p < 0.05$) with 72.7 ± 5.1 and 57.7 ± 3.9 min (mean ± standard deviation (SD)), respectively. In contrast, although the $T_{1/2}$ for the HV yogurt was higher than that of the CT yogurt, it was not statistically different ($p = 0.12$). There was no significant difference between the β factor calculated from the gastric emptying curve of the three yogurts.

Table 4. Gastric emptying half-time ($T_{1/2}$) and shape of the emptying curve (β) observed on the 3 yogurts.

	$T_{1/2}$ (min)	β
Control	57.7 ± 3.9	1.1 ± 0.05
Low viscosity	72.7 ± 5.1 *	1.0 ± 0.04
High viscosity	65.3 ± 3.5	1.1 ± 0.03

* indicates a statistically significant difference ($p < 0.05$) between the control and the low viscosity yogurt.

The modelling of the mean gastric empting curves is presented in Figure 1.

A difference of filling of the proximal part of the small intestine according to the type of yogurt was observed. The control yogurt did not stay in the duodenum but was spread all over the first segments of the small intestine. In contrast, the high viscosity yogurt accumulated in the proximal part of the small intestine, whereas the low viscosity yogurt had a similar behavior to that of the control, as shown in Figure 2. This was only an observation made for eight out of 11 pigs; quantifying this phenomenon would require a specific experiment.

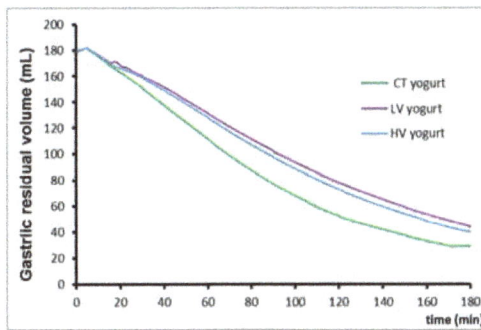

Figure 1. Gastric residual volume for the three yogurts. CT, LV, HV stand for control, low viscosity and high viscosity yogurts, respectively. $T_{1/2}$ means gastric emptying half-time.

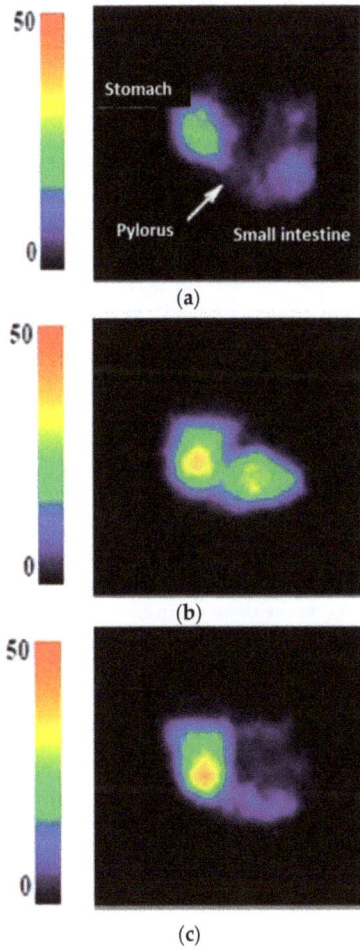

Figure 2. Images of the gastrointestinal region taken 60 min after meal ingestion for the control yogurt (**a**) the low viscosity yogurt; (**b**) and the high viscosity yogurt; and (**c**) The output of the radio-isotopic counter was expressed through a scale ranging from 0 to 50.

3.2. Dynamic In Vitro Digestion

Figure 3 shows the evolution of the three main milk proteins during gastrointestinal digestion. The decrease in the band intensity is due to the concomitant dilution by the secretions and proteolysis occurring during the digestion process. Caseins, shown in Figure 4a, were extensively degraded during gastric digestion and almost totally disappeared in all the samples after 120 min of gastric digestion. The percentage of residual caseins at the end of the gastric phase, compared to the amount of caseins in the undigested product, represented 4%, 4.9%, and 2.2% for the control, the low viscosity and the high viscosity yogurt, respectively. Casein digestion was finalized in the intestinal compartment resulting in the total disappearance of the caseins bands after 180 min of gastrointestinal digestion.

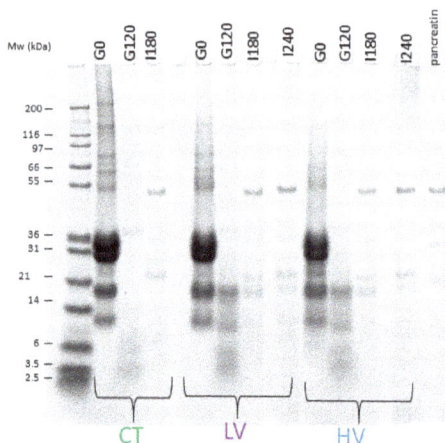

Figure 3. SDS-PAGE of the undigested 3 yogurts, i.e., control (CT), low (LV), and high (HV) viscosity before digestion (G0), after 120 min gastric digestion (G120) and 180 and/or 240 intestinal digestion (I180, I240).

The situation was different for β-lactoglobulin, where whey was the major protein (Figure 4b). In comparison, β-lactoglobulin was extensively hydrolyzed in the control yogurt with only 3.1% remaining after 120 min of gastric digestion, this protein was more resistant to digestion for the low viscosity and high viscosity with 49.8% and 39.1% remaining at 120 min of the gastric phase, respectively. After 180 min (CT) and 240 min (LV and HV) of intestinal digestion, β-lactoglobulin was shown to be extensively hydrolyzed in the three yogurts with 2.3%, 4.8%, and 3.2% remaining for the control, the low viscosity, and the high viscosity yogurt, respectively.

Finally, α-lactalbumin was sensitive to gastric digestion in the control yogurt with 6.4% being intact after 120 min digestion (Figure 4c). It was shown to be more resistant during gastric digestion in the low viscosity yogurt (73.9%), whereas it was partly digested in the high viscosity yogurt (36.2%). After 180 min (CT) and 240 min (LV and HV) of intestinal digestion, α-lactalbumin was also shown, like β-lactoglobulin, to be highly degraded in the three different yogurts with 6%, 6%, and 6.5% remaining for the control, the low viscosity, and the high viscosity yogurt, respectively.

(a)

(b)

(c)

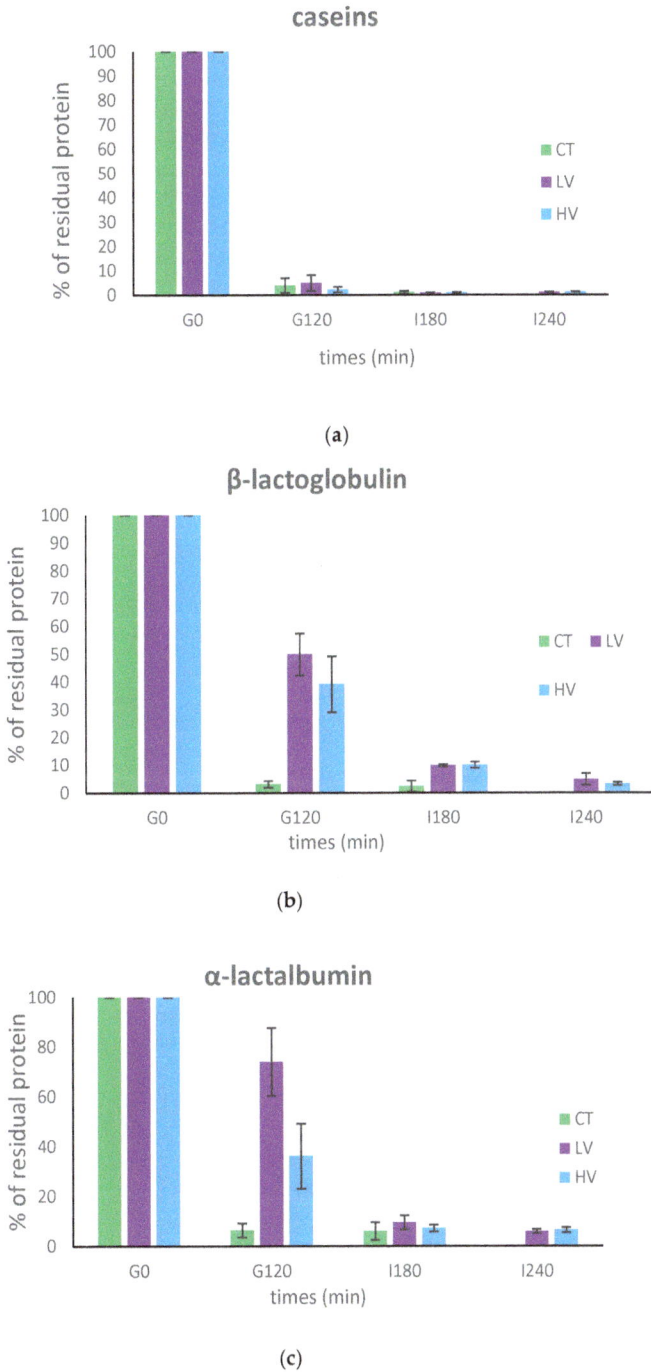

Figure 4. Residual % of casein (**a**), α-lactoglobulin (**b**), and α-lactalbumin (**c**) before digestion (G0), after 120 gastric digestion (G120) and after 180 (I180) and 240 (I240) min of intestinal digestion in the control (green), low viscosity (violet), and high viscosity (blue) yogurts.

4. Discussion

The present study indicated that enriching a yogurt with protein and fiber slows down gastric emptying. Indeed, the control yogurt, that has an identical caloric content as the low viscosity yogurt but a 2.5-fold reduction in protein content and no fiber, exhibited a 20% lower gastric emptying half-time (57.7 min vs. 72.7 min). This confirms the role that enrichment with milk proteins and fiber plays on the transit of the food in the gastrointestinal tract. Gastric emptying half-time of the control yogurt was lower than that of the high viscosity yogurt, but the difference was not statistically significant. Low and high viscosity yogurts did not show statistical differences in gastric emptying indicating that viscosity of the undigested yogurt was not a crucial parameter impacting gastric emptying in the present study. Finally, no significant differences were observed between the β factors calculated from the gastric emptying curve of the three yogurts. The β factor reflects the shape of the emptying curve and can be highly impacted by the physical state of the food (e.g., liquid vs. solid). In the present case, the three test foods were all gels and exhibited emptying curves of exponential power nature, typical for this kind of material. It should also be noted that a high inter-individual variability was observed in this in vivo assay, probably limiting the significance of the differences observed between the three yogurts. Therefore, a new experiment with a higher number of pigs would be required to emphasize the differences of behavior of the three yogurts in the gastrointestinal tract and see whether the high viscosity one is different than that of the control. In the hierarchy of satiating effects, proteins have been shown to be more effective than carbohydrates and fat [36]. The possible physiological mechanisms underlying this effect include diet induced thermogenesis [37] and gastrointestinal hormonal signaling [38], although more recent studies have suggested that the sensory experience of ingesting protein is also important [26,39].

The limit of the present study was that low and high viscosity yogurts differed from the control not only by their protein content but also by the presence of fibers. Hence, it is impossible to conclude which of these two components had the most important effect on gastric emptying. The effect of fibers on gastric emptying highly depends on the nature and the characteristics of the molecule and the interaction it can have with the other food constituents. A review systematically investigated the available literature on the relationship between dietary fiber types, appetite, acute and long-term energy intake, and body weight [16]. It was observed that more viscous fibers presumably affect subjective appetite and acute energy intake, whereas no evident association between physicochemical properties and long-term energy intake or body weight was found. A recent systematic review on the effect of fiber on satiety showed that most of the acute fiber treatment (78%) did not reduce food intake [14]. A recent study on the combined effect of high protein content (casein or pea) and dietary fiber (pectin) on food intake was carried out on obese rats [40]. It showed that dietary pectin, but not high protein, decreased food intake and decreased body weight. However, the protein content was two times lower and the fiber content and four times higher than in the present study. Therefore, further research on decoupling the two parameters is mandatory to generate a definite conclusion.

Interestingly, the low and high viscosity yogurts had different behaviors when entering in the small intestine, even though they exhibited similar gastric emptying half-times. The high viscosity yogurt accumulated in the proximal part of the small intestine, whereas the low viscosity yogurt did not stay in the duodenum but spread along the first segments of the small intestine. This could result in different intestinal transit time of the two yogurts. Unfortunately, although this phenomenon was visible for eight out of the 11 pigs used in the study, in the absence of a reference anatomical imaging co-registered with gamma-scintigraphy, we were not able to quantitatively assess the intestinal time of transit of the different yogurts and could not be simulated in the in vitro dynamic digestions. Nevertheless, our data strongly suggest that the effect of yogurt viscosity is not on the time of residence of the yogurt in the stomach, but further in the small intestine. To our knowledge, such a result has never been published.

Dynamic in vitro digestion using the $T_{1/2}$ and β parameters, determined in vivo, allowed for the following of the evolution of the three main milk proteins i.e., casein, β-lactoglobulin, and α-lactalbumin in the gastrointestinal tract. Caseins were shown to be extensively hydrolyzed in the stomach, compared to whey proteins as previously described [35,41]. Caseins have a flexible and loose structure that makes them highly sensitive to digestive enzymes [42]. In contrast, the globular structure of whey proteins make them partly resistant to digestion by pepsin [43,44]. In the present case, the heat treatment applied to milk during yogurt manufacture made these proteins less resistant to digestion than the native form, due to conformational changes as previously shown [45–47]. In vitro digestion also showed some differences in the hydrolysis of whey proteins between the control yogurt and the low or high viscosity yogurt. Indeed β-lactoglobulin was less affected by pepsin in the gastric phase for the low and high viscosity yogurts than for the control yogurt where the protein was extensively hydrolyzed. This difference might be explained by the differences of enzyme/substrate ratio that were present between the control yogurt and the low or high viscosity yogurts. The control yogurt had 2.5 times less proteins than the two other yogurts, and for the three yogurts, the amount of pepsin provided during digestion was the same. Interestingly, whey proteins appeared to be more sensitive to pepsin hydrolysis when present in the high viscosity versus the low viscosity yogurt. This might be explained by the different behaviors of the two yogurts observed by gamma scintigraphy when entering the small intestine. Thus, it is possible that gastric conditions affect the microstructure of the two gels, leading to differences in the accessibility of whey proteins in the chyme.

Finally, dynamic in vitro digestion also demonstrated that, even though the amounts of milk proteins were 2.5 higher in the low or high viscosity yogurt than in the control one, the milk protein enriched yogurts are still well digested. This confirms that dairy proteins, even at high concentration, are highly digestible, as has been shown previously [48]. Indeed, most of the available studies indicated digestibility of milk proteins to be around 95% [49] (which means from 5% of undigested proteins at the extremity of the small intestine), which is coherent with the values we have found in the present study. Together with excellent profiles in essential amino acids, it emphasizes that milk proteins are very high in nutritional properties.

In the present study, we have not investigated the hormonal profile after the ingestion of the experimental diets. It could be highly interesting to repeat the experiment to identify the alteration in GLP-1, Cholecystokinin (CCK), ghrelin, etc., and other peptides in relation to emptying. This could clarify the mechanisms of action of the milk protein enriched yogurts in generating satiety.

Supplementary Materials: The following are available online at http://www.mdpi.com/2072-6643/10/9/1308/s1, Video S1: Yogurt gastric emptying followed by gamma-scintigraphy.

Author Contributions: Conceptualization, D.D.; Investigation, M.-H.F., A.D., Y.L.G., S.G. and C.-H.M.; Writing—original draft, O.M.

Funding: This research was performed the Satiarome project which was supported by Vitagora pole, DGCIS and local authorities with the financial support of Bpifrance and FEDER.

Acknowledgments: The authors wish to thank the PRISM platform for having performed the experiments of gamma scintigraphy on pigs.

Conflicts of Interest: The authors declare no conflict of interest.

References

1. Turgeon, S.L.; Rioux, L.E. Food matrix impact on macronutrients nutritional properties. *Food Hydrocoll.* **2011**, *25*, 1915–1924. [CrossRef]

2. Mao, L.K.; Miao, S. Structuring food emulsions to improve nutrient delivery during digestion. *Food Eng. Rev.* **2015**, *7*, 439–451. [CrossRef]

3. Guo, Q.; Ye, A.Q.; Bellissimo, N.; Singh, H.; Rousseau, D. Modulating fat digestion through food structure design. *Prog. Lipid Res.* **2017**, *68*, 109–118. [CrossRef] [PubMed]

4. Dupont, D.; Le Feunteun, S.; Marze, S.; Souchon, I. Structuring food to control its disintegration in the gastrointestinal tract and optimize nutrient bioavailability. *Innov. Food Sci. Emerg. Technol.* **2018**, *46*, 83–90. [CrossRef]

5. Bensaid, A.; Tome, D.; Gietzen, D.; Even, P.; Morens, C.; Gausseres, N.; Fromentin, G. Protein is more potent than carbohydrate for reducing appetite in rats. *Physiol. Behav.* **2002**, *75*, 577–582. [CrossRef]

6. Anderson, G.H.; Moore, S.E. Dietary proteins in the regulation of food intake and body weight in humans. *J. Nutr.* **2004**, *134*, 974S–979S. [CrossRef] [PubMed]

7. Dougkas, A.; Ostman, E. Protein-enriched liquid preloads varying in macronutrient content modulate appetite and appetite-regulating hormones in healthy adults. *J. Nutr.* **2016**, *146*, 637–645. [CrossRef] [PubMed]

8. Giezenaar, C.; Trahair, L.G.; Luscombe-Marsh, N.D.; Hausken, T.; Standfield, S.; Jones, K.L.; Lange, K.; Horowitz, M.; Chapman, I.; Soenen, S. Effects of randomized whey-protein loads on energy intake, appetite, gastric emptying, and plasma gut-hormone concentrations in older men and women. *Am. J. Clin. Nutr.* **2017**, *106*, 865–877. [CrossRef] [PubMed]

9. Giezenaar, C.; van der Burgh, Y.; Lange, K.; Hatzinikolas, S.; Hausken, T.; Jones, K.L.; Horowitz, M.; Chapman, I.; Soenen, S. Effects of substitution, and adding of carbohydrate and fat to whey-protein on energy intake, appetite, gastric emptying, glucose, insulin, ghrelin, cck and glp-1 in healthy older men—A randomized controlled trial. *Nutrients* **2018**, *10*, 113. [CrossRef] [PubMed]

10. Aimutis, W.R. Bioactive properties of milk proteins with particular focus on anticariogenesis. *J. Nutr.* **2004**, *134*, 989S–995S. [CrossRef] [PubMed]

11. Hall, W.L.; Millward, D.J.; Long, S.J.; Morgan, L.M. Casein and whey exert different effects on plasma amino acid profiles, gastrointestinal hormone secretion and appetite. *Br. J. Nutr.* **2003**, *89*, 239–248. [CrossRef] [PubMed]

12. Veldhorst, M.A.B.; Nieuwenhuizen, A.G.; Hochstenbach-Waelen, A.; Van Vught, A.J.A.H.; Westerterp, K.R.; Engelen, M.P.K.J.; Brummer, R.J.M.; Deutz, N.E.P.; Westerterp-Plantenga, M.S. Dose-dependent satiating effect of whey relative to casein or soy. *Physiol. Behav.* **2009**, *96*, 675–682. [CrossRef] [PubMed]

13. Bendtsen, L.Q.; Lorenzen, J.K.; Bendsen, N.T.; Rasmussen, C.; Astrup, A. Effect of dairy proteins on appetite, energy expenditure, body weight, and composition: A review of the evidence from controlled clinical trials. *Adv. Nutr.* **2013**, *4*, 418–438. [CrossRef] [PubMed]

14. Clark, M.J.; Slavin, J.L. The effect of fiber on satiety and food intake: A systematic review. *J. Am. Coll. Nutr.* **2013**, *32*, 200–211. [CrossRef] [PubMed]

15. Slavin, J.; Green, H. Dietary fibre and satiety. *Nutr. Bull.* **2007**, *32*, 32–42. [CrossRef]

16. Wanders, A.J.; van den Borne, J.; de Graaf, C.; Hulshof, T.; Jonathan, M.C.; Kristensen, M.; Mars, M.; Schols, H.A.; Feskens, E.J.M. Effects of dietary fibre on subjective appetite, energy intake and body weight: A systematic review of randomized controlled trials. *Obes. Rev.* **2011**, *12*, 724–739. [CrossRef] [PubMed]

17. Clegg, M.E.; Ranawana, V.; Shafat, A.; Henry, C.J. Soups increase satiety through delayed gastric emptying yet increased glycaemic response. *Eur. J. Clin. Nutr.* **2013**, *67*, 8–11. [CrossRef] [PubMed]

18. Ritter, R.C. Gastrointestinal mechanisms of satiation for food. *Physiol. Behav.* **2004**, *81*, 249–273. [CrossRef] [PubMed]

19. Bell, E.A.; Roe, L.S.; Rolls, B.J. Sensory-specific satiety is affected more by volume than by energy content of a liquid food. *Physiol. Behav.* **2003**, *78*, 593–600. [CrossRef]

20. Andrews, J.M.; Doran, S.M.; Hebbard, G.S.; Malbert, C.H.; Horowitz, M.; Dent, J. Nutrient-induced spatial patterning of human duodenal motor function. *Am. J. Physiol. Gastrointest. Liver Physiol.* **2001**, *280*, G501–G509. [CrossRef] [PubMed]

21. Rolls, B.J.; Castellanos, V.H.; Halford, J.C.; Kilara, A.; Panyam, D.; Pelkman, C.L.; Smith, G.P.; Thorwart, M.L. Volume of food consumed affects satiety in men. *Am. J. Clin. Nutr.* **1998**, *67*, 1170–1177. [CrossRef] [PubMed]

22. Wang, G.J.; Tomasi, D.; Backus, W.; Wang, R.; Telang, F.; Geliebter, A.; Korner, J.; Bauman, A.; Fowler, J.S.; Thanos, P.K.; et al. Gastric distention activates satiety circuitry in the human brain. *Neuroimage* **2008**, *39*, 1824–1831. [CrossRef] [PubMed]

23. Mackie, A.R.; Rafiee, H.; Malcolm, P.; Salt, L.; van Aken, G. Specific food structures supress appetite through reduced gastric emptying rate. *Am. J. Physiol Gastrointest. Liver Physiol.* **2013**, *304*, G1038–G1043. [CrossRef] [PubMed]

24. Zijlstra, N.; Mars, M.; de Wijk, R.A.; Westerterp-Plantenga, M.S.; de Graaf, C. The effect of viscosity on ad libitum food intake. *Int. J. Obes. (Lond.)* **2008**, *32*, 676–683. [CrossRef] [PubMed]

25. Wanders, A.J.; Jonathan, M.C.; van den Borne, J.; Mars, M.; Schols, H.A.; Feskens, E.J.M.; de Graaf, C. The effects of bulking, viscous and gel-forming dietary fibres on satiation. *Br. J. Nutr.* **2013**, *109*, 1330–1337. [CrossRef] [PubMed]

26. Bertenshaw, E.J.; Lluch, A.; Yeomans, M.R. Perceived thickness and creaminess modulates the short-term satiating effects of high-protein drinks. *Br. J. Nutr.* **2013**, *110*, 578–586. [CrossRef] [PubMed]

27. Zhu, Y.; Hsu, W.H.; Hollis, J.H. The impact of food viscosity on eating rate, subjective appetite, glycemic response and gastric emptying rate. *PLoS ONE* **2013**, *8*, e67482. [CrossRef] [PubMed]

28. Clegg, M.E.; Shafat, A. The effect of agar jelly on energy expenditure, appetite, gastric emptying and glycaemic response. *Eur. J. Nutr.* **2014**, *53*, 533–539. [CrossRef] [PubMed]

29. Camps, G.; Mars, M.; de Graaf, C.; Smeets, P.A.M. Empty calories and phantom fullness: A randomized trial studying the relative effects of energy density and viscosity on gastric emptying determined by MRI and satiety. *Am. J. Clin. Nutr.* **2016**, *104*, 73–80. [CrossRef] [PubMed]

30. Ménard, O.; Cattenoz, T.; Guillemin, H.; Souchon, I.; Deglaire, A.; Dupont, D.; Picque, D. Validation of a new in vitro dynamic system to simulate infant digestion. *Food Chem.* **2014**, *145*, 1039–1045. [CrossRef] [PubMed]

31. Camps, G.; Mars, M.; Witteman, B.J.M.; de Graaf, C.; Smeets, P.A.M. Indirect vs direct assessment of gastric emptying: A randomized crossover trial comparing c-isotope breath analysis and MRI. *Neurogastroenterol. Motil.* **2018**, *30*, e13317. [CrossRef] [PubMed]

32. Herschel, W.H.; Bulkley, R. Konsistenzmessungen von gummi-benzollosungen. *Colloid Polym. Sci.* **1926**, *39*, 291–300. [CrossRef]

33. Val-Laillet, D.; Guerin, S.; Malbert, C.H. Slower eating rate is independent to gastric emptying in obese minipigs. *Physiol. Behav.* **2010**, *101*, 462–468. [CrossRef] [PubMed]

34. Elashoff, J.D.; Reedy, T.J.; Meyer, J.H. Analysis of gastric-emptying data. *Gastroenterology* **1982**, *83*, 1306–1312. [PubMed]

35. Egger, L.; Ménard, O.; Baumann, C.; Duerr, D.; Schlegel, P.; Stoll, P.; Vergères, G.; Dupont, D.; Portmann, R. Digestion of milk proteins: Comparing static and dynamic in vitro digestion systems with in vivo data. *Food Res. Int.* **2017**, in press. [CrossRef]

36. Blundell, J.E.; Macdiarmid, J.I. Fat as a risk factor for overconsumption: Satiation, satiety, and patterns of eating. *J. Am. Diet. Assoc.* **1997**, *97*, S63–S69. [CrossRef]

37. Halton, T.L.; Hu, F.B. The effects of high protein diets on thermogenesis, satiety and weight loss: A critical review. *J. Am. Coll. Nutr.* **2004**, *23*, 373–385. [CrossRef] [PubMed]

38. Veldhorst, M.; Smeets, A.; Soenen, S.; Hochstenbach-Waelen, A.; Hursel, R.; Diepvens, K.; Lejeune, M.; Luscombe-Marsh, N.; Westerterp-Plantenga, M. Protein-induced satiety: Effects and mechanisms of different proteins. *Physiol. Behav.* **2008**, *94*, 300–307. [CrossRef] [PubMed]

39. Masic, U.; Yeomans, M.R. Does monosodium glutamate interact with macronutrient composition to influence subsequent appetite? *Physiol. Behav.* **2013**, *116*, 23–29. [CrossRef] [PubMed]

40. Adam, C.L.; Gratz, S.W.; Peinado, D.I.; Thomson, L.M.; Garden, K.E.; Williams, P.A.; Richardson, A.J.; Ross, A.W. Effects of dietary fibre (pectin) and/or increased protein (casein or pea) on satiety, body weight, adiposity and caecal fermentation in high fat diet-induced obese rats. *PLoS ONE* **2016**, *11*, e0155871. [CrossRef] [PubMed]

41. Barbe, F.; Menard, O.; Le Gouar, Y.; Buffiere, C.; Famelart, M.H.; Laroche, B.; Le Feunteun, S.; Dupont, D.; Remond, D. The heat treatment and the gelation are strong determinants of the kinetics of milk proteins digestion and of the peripheral availability of amino acids. *Food Chem.* **2013**, *136*, 1203–1212. [CrossRef] [PubMed]

42. Dupont, D.; Mandalari, G.; Molle, D.; Jardin, J.; Rolet-Repecaud, O.; Duboz, G.; Leonil, J.; Mills, E.N.C.; Mackie, A.R. Food processing increases casein resistance to simulated infant digestion. *Mol. Nutr. Food Res.* **2010**, *54*, 1677–1689. [CrossRef] [PubMed]

43. Macierzanka, A.; Sancho, A.I.; Mills, E.N.C.; Rigby, N.M.; Mackie, A.R. Emulsification alters simulated gastrointestinal proteolysis of beta-casein and beta-lactoglobulin. *Soft Matter* **2009**, *5*, 538–550. [CrossRef]

44. Mandalari, G.; Adel-Patient, K.; Barkholt, V.; Baro, C.; Bennett, L.; Bublin, M.; Gaier, S.; Graser, G.; Ladics, G.; Mierzejewska, D.; et al. In vitro digestibility of beta-casein and beta-lactoglobulin under simulated human gastric and duodenal conditions: A multi-laboratory evaluation. *Regul. Toxicol. Pharmacol.* **2009**, *55*, 372–381. [CrossRef] [PubMed]

45. Rahaman, T.; Vasiljevic, T.; Ramchandran, L. Digestibility and antigenicity of beta-lactoglobulin as affected by heat, pH and applied shear. *Food Chem.* **2017**, *217*, 517–523. [CrossRef] [PubMed]
46. Sanchez-Rivera, L.; Menard, O.; Recio, I.; Dupont, D. Peptide mapping during dynamic gastric digestion of heated and unheated skimmed milk powder. *Food Res. Int.* **2015**, *77*, 132–139. [CrossRef]
47. Singh, T.K.; Oiseth, S.K.; Lundin, L.; Day, L. Influence of heat and shear induced protein aggregation on the in vitro digestion rate of whey proteins. *Food Funct.* **2014**, *5*, 2686–2698. [CrossRef] [PubMed]
48. Mathai, J.K.; Liu, Y.H.; Stein, H.H. Values for digestible indispensable amino acid scores (diaas) for some dairy and plant proteins may better describe protein quality than values calculated using the concept for protein digestibility-corrected amino acid scores (pdcaas). *Br. J. Nutr.* **2017**, *117*, 490–499. [CrossRef] [PubMed]
49. Bos, C.; Mahé, S.; Gaudichon, C.; Benamouzig, R.; Gausserès, N.; Luengo, C.; Ferrière, F.; Rautureau, J.; Tomé, D. Assessment of net postprandial protein utilization of 15N-labelled milk nitrogen in human subjects. *Br. J. Nutr.* **1999**, *81*, 221–226. [PubMed]

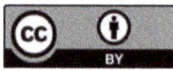

MDPI

St. Alban-Anlage 66

4052 Basel

Switzerland

Tel. +41 61 683 77 34

Fax +41 61 302 89 18

www.mdpi.com

Nutrients Editorial Office

E-mail: nutrients@mdpi.com

www.mdpi.com/journal/nutrients

www.ingramcontent.com/pod-product-compliance
Lightning Source LLC
Chambersburg PA
CBHW051903210326

41597CB00033B/6006